AAPC CPC

Study Guide

Medical Coding Certification Exam Prep with 700+ Practice Questions and Answer Explanations

Nedrial TestPrep

AAPC CPC Study Guide: Medical Coding Certification Exam Prep with 650+ Practice Questions and Answer Explanations

Disclaimer: This study guide is designed to help candidates prepare for the AAPC CPC certification examination. The content is based on publicly available information and the author's expertise in medical coding. This guide is not affiliated with, endorsed by, or sponsored by the American Academy of Professional Coders (AAPC). CPC® and Certified Professional Coder® are registered trademarks of the AAPC, which does not endorse this product.

The information in this guide is accurate as of the publication date. Medical coding guidelines and exam content may change. Candidates should always verify current requirements with official AAPC resources.

Published by Nedrial TestPrep

First Edition: 2025

Printed in the United States of America

TABLE OF CONTENTS

FOREWORD

Congratulations on taking the first step toward earning your Certified Professional Coder (CPC) credential. This journey represents more than just passing an exam—you're entering a stable, growing healthcare field where your skills will directly impact patient care and healthcare operations.

Medical coding has evolved into one of healthcare's most essential functions. Every patient encounter, procedure, and diagnosis must be accurately translated into standardized codes that facilitate billing, research, and quality improvement. As healthcare becomes increasingly complex, the demand for skilled medical coders continues to grow, making CPC certification your gateway to a rewarding career.

This study guide was created with one goal in mind: helping you pass the CPC exam on your first attempt. We've analyzed thousands of exam questions, studied successful test-taking strategies, and distilled the most critical information into a format that works with your busy schedule.

You have what it takes to succeed. The path ahead requires dedication and consistent effort, but every successful CPC before you has walked this same journey. Trust the process, follow the study plan, and remember that each practice question brings you closer to your goal.

Your future in medical coding starts now.

The Nedrial TestPrep Team

ABOUT THIS GUIDE

The healthcare industry employs over 350,000 medical coders, with job growth projected at 13% through 2032—much faster than average for all occupations. Your decision to pursue CPC certification positions you at the forefront of this expanding field.

This study guide serves as your comprehensive companion through CPC exam preparation. Unlike generic study materials, every chapter is specifically designed around the actual CPC exam content outline, ensuring you focus your valuable study time on what matters most.

What Makes This Guide Different:

Exam-Focused Content: Every topic covered appears on the actual CPC exam. We've eliminated unnecessary information that might distract from your core preparation goals.

Practical Application: Rather than just memorizing facts, you'll learn to apply coding principles through realistic scenarios that mirror actual exam questions.

Proven Study Methods: The strategies in this guide are based on learning science research and feedback from thousands of successful CPC candidates.

Current and Accurate: All content reflects the latest 2025-2026 coding guidelines and exam requirements.

This guide contains:

- Comprehensive coverage of all CPC exam content areas
- 650+ practice questions with detailed answer explanations
- Three full-length practice exams
- Strategic study plans for different timelines
- Test-taking techniques specific to the CPC format
- Current coding updates and guidelines

Who Should Use This Guide:

This study guide is designed for anyone preparing for the CPC examination, whether you're new to medical coding or have years of healthcare experience. The content assumes no prior coding knowledge while providing the depth needed for exam success.

Success on the CPC exam requires understanding both coding fundamentals and practical application. This guide bridges that gap, taking you from basic concepts to complex coding scenarios with confidence.

Your investment in this guide represents an investment in your future. Medical coding offers stability, growth potential, and the satisfaction of contributing to quality healthcare. Let's begin this journey together.

HOW TO USE THIS STUDY GUIDE EFFECTIVELY

Success on the CPC exam isn't about spending countless hours studying—it's about studying smart. This section will help you maximize your preparation time and increase your chances of passing on the first attempt.

Before You Begin: Assess Your Starting Point

Take a few minutes to honestly evaluate your current knowledge level:

Medical Terminology: Can you break down medical terms into prefixes, suffixes, and root words? Do you understand basic anatomy and physiology?

Coding Experience: Have you worked with medical codes before, or will this be your first exposure to CPT®, ICD-10-CM, and HCPCS Level II?

Available Study Time: How many hours per week can you realistically dedicate to studying? Be honest—overestimating leads to unrealistic schedules that create stress.

Learning Style: Do you learn better through reading, practice questions, visual aids, or hands-on application?

Understanding your starting point helps you choose the right study approach and timeline.

Creating Your Study Schedule

Successful CPC candidates typically study for 2-4 months, depending on their background and available time. Here are three proven approaches:

Intensive 8-Week Plan (15-20 hours per week):

- Weeks 1-2: Chapters 1-5 (Foundation and Medical Terminology)
- Weeks 3-4: Chapters 6-8 (ICD-10-CM Diagnosis Coding)
- Weeks 5-6: Chapters 9-15 (CPT® Procedure Coding)
- Weeks 7-8: Practice exams and weak area review

Balanced 12-Week Plan (10-12 hours per week):

- Weeks 1-3: Chapters 1-5 (Foundation building)
- Weeks 4-6: Chapters 6-8 (Diagnosis coding mastery)
- Weeks 7-9: Chapters 9-15 (Procedure coding mastery)
- Weeks 10-12: Practice exams and final preparation

Extended 16-Week Plan (6-8 hours per week):

- Weeks 1-4: Chapters 1-5 (Thorough foundation)
- Weeks 5-8: Chapters 6-8 (Diagnosis coding with practice)
- Weeks 9-12: Chapters 9-15 (Procedure coding with practice)
- Weeks 13-16: Extensive practice and review

Choose the plan that fits your schedule and stick to it. Consistency beats intensity every time.

How to Study Each Chapter

Step 1: Preview (5 minutes)

- Read the chapter objectives
- Scan headings and subheadings
- Review any charts or tables
- Read the chapter summary

Step 2: Active Reading (20-30 minutes)

- Read one section at a time
- Take notes on key concepts
- Write questions about unclear topics
- Complete any embedded exercises

Step 3: Practice Questions (10-15 minutes)

- Answer all chapter practice questions
- Review explanations for both correct and incorrect answers
- Identify patterns in questions you miss

Step 4: Review and Reinforce (10 minutes)

- Summarize key points in your own words
- Create flashcards for important terms or concepts
- Schedule review time for this material

Maximizing Practice Questions

The 650+ practice questions in this guide are your most valuable preparation tool. Here's how to use them effectively:

Don't Rush: Take time to read each question carefully. CPC exam questions often include extra information designed to test your ability to identify relevant details.

Think Before Looking: Try to answer each question before looking at the options. This builds confidence and prevents you from talking yourself out of correct answers.

Learn from Mistakes: Wrong answers are learning opportunities. Read every explanation, not just for questions you missed, but for questions where you guessed correctly.

Track Your Progress: Keep a log of your practice test scores. Seeing improvement motivates continued effort and helps identify when you're ready for the real exam.

Simulate Exam Conditions: Take at least one practice exam under timed conditions to build stamina and test your pacing strategies.

Managing Test Anxiety

Even well-prepared candidates can struggle with exam anxiety. These techniques help maintain calm confidence:

Preparation Confidence: Nothing reduces anxiety like thorough preparation. Trust your study plan and the time you've invested.

Practice Relaxation: Learn simple breathing techniques you can use during the exam. Practice them during study sessions so they become automatic.

Positive Visualization: Spend a few minutes each day imagining yourself succeeding on the exam. Mental rehearsal improves actual performance.

Day-Before Strategy: The day before your exam, do light review only. Trust your preparation and focus on rest and relaxation.

Final Recommendations

Join Study Groups: Connect with other CPC candidates online or in your area. Explaining concepts to others reinforces your own understanding.

Use Multiple Resources: While this guide provides comprehensive preparation, supplement with AAPC's official resources and practice exams when possible.

Stay Current: Medical coding changes frequently. Follow AAPC updates and coding news to ensure your knowledge remains current.

Think Long-Term: The CPC exam is just the beginning. The habits you develop during preparation will serve you throughout your coding career.

Remember, thousands of people pass the CPC exam every year. You have the same opportunity they had. The difference between success and failure often comes down to preparation, persistence, and believing in yourself.

You're ready to begin. Let's start with understanding exactly what the CPC exam will ask of you.

PART I: EXAM OVERVIEW & PREPARATION STRATEGIES

Chapter 1: Understanding the CPC Exam

"Success is where preparation and opportunity meet." - Bobby Unser

The CPC exam represents your opportunity to demonstrate mastery of medical coding principles and join the ranks of healthcare's most essential professionals. Understanding exactly what this exam entails—its structure, content, and requirements—forms the foundation of your preparation strategy.

This chapter will demystify the CPC examination, giving you a clear picture of what to expect and how to approach each component strategically. By the end of this chapter, you'll understand not just what's on the exam, but how to tackle it with confidence.

What is the CPC Certification?

The Certified Professional Coder (CPC) credential, administered by the American Academy of Professional Coders (AAPC), represents the gold standard in outpatient medical coding. Established in 1988, AAPC has certified over 200,000 medical coding professionals, making CPC the most widely recognized coding credential in healthcare.

Why Pursue CPC Certification?

Career Stability: Healthcare continues to grow, and accurate coding is essential for every patient encounter. The Bureau of Labor Statistics projects 13% job growth for medical records specialists through 2032.

Income Potential: CPC-certified coders earn significantly more than non-certified peers. According to AAPC's 2024 salary survey, certified coders earn an average of $59,428 annually, with experienced coders earning $70,000 or more.

Professional Recognition: CPC certification demonstrates your commitment to accuracy, ethics, and continuous learning. Employers prefer certified coders because they understand the direct impact on revenue and compliance.

Career Flexibility: CPC certification opens doors in physician offices, hospitals, insurance companies, consulting firms, and remote work opportunities.

The CPC Role in Healthcare

As a Certified Professional Coder, you serve as the crucial link between clinical care and healthcare administration. Your daily responsibilities include:

- Reviewing medical documentation to identify diagnoses and procedures
- Assigning appropriate ICD-10-CM, CPT®, and HCPCS Level II codes
- Ensuring compliance with coding guidelines and regulations
- Supporting accurate billing and reimbursement processes
- Maintaining patient privacy and data security

Accuracy is paramount. A single coding error can result in claim denials, compliance violations, or patient care issues. The CPC exam tests your ability to code accurately under time pressure—a skill essential to professional success.

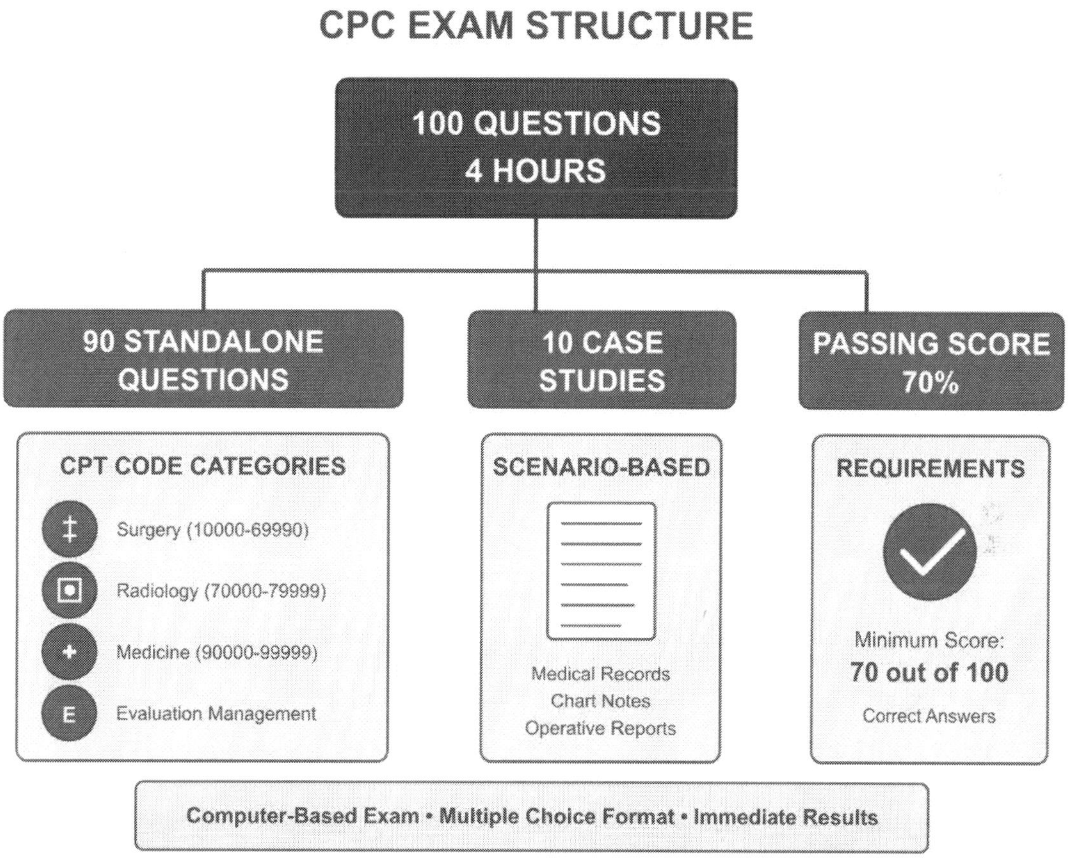

Exam Structure and Format

The CPC exam is a computer-based test administered at Pearson VUE testing centers nationwide. Understanding the exam's structure helps you allocate study time and develop test-taking strategies.

Basic Exam Facts:

- **Questions:** 100 multiple-choice questions
- **Time Limit:** 4 hours
- **Format:** Computer-based (some locations offer paper-based)
- **Passing Score:** 70% (70 questions correct)
- **Reference Materials:** You may bring your own coding books (CPT®, ICD-10-CM, HCPCS Level II)

Question Types:

The exam includes two distinct question formats:

Standalone Questions (90 questions): These test specific coding knowledge, guidelines, anatomy, or medical terminology. Examples:

- "What is the correct ICD-10-CM code for Type 2 diabetes with diabetic nephropathy?"
- "Which CPT® modifier indicates a bilateral procedure?"

Case Studies (10 questions): These present clinical scenarios requiring you to identify relevant information and assign appropriate codes. Case studies typically include:

- Patient demographics and medical history
- Chief complaint and symptoms
- Physical examination findings
- Procedures performed or planned
- Physician's assessment and plan

Time Management Reality

Four hours might seem generous, but successful candidates report time pressure as a significant challenge. Here's the math:

- 100 questions ÷ 240 minutes = 2.4 minutes per question
- Account for reviewing answers: approximately 2 minutes per question
- Case studies require more time than standalone questions

Effective preparation includes building speed and accuracy simultaneously.

Knowledge Areas Breakdown and Weightings

The CPC exam tests 17 distinct knowledge areas. Understanding the weight of each area helps you prioritize study time effectively.

High-Weight Areas (Focus Your Energy Here):

1. 10000 Series CPT® - Integumentary System (6 questions)

- Skin lesion removal and repair
- Wound care and debridement
- Breast procedures

2. 20000 Series CPT® - Musculoskeletal System (6 questions)

- Fracture repair and casting
- Arthroscopy procedures
- Joint replacements

3. 30000 Series CPT® - Respiratory System (6 questions)

- Endoscopy procedures
- Lung and bronchus surgery
- Sinus procedures

4. 40000 Series CPT® - Digestive System (6 questions)

- Endoscopy procedures
- Hernia repairs
- Gallbladder and appendix surgery

5. 50000 Series CPT® - Urinary System (6 questions)

- Kidney and bladder procedures
- Prostate surgery
- Dialysis services

Medium-Weight Areas (Solid Understanding Required):

6. 60000 Series CPT® - Endocrine System (4 questions)

7. 70000 Series CPT® - Radiology (6 questions)

8. 80000 Series CPT® - Pathology and Laboratory (6 questions)

9. 90000 Series CPT® - Medicine (6 questions)

10. Evaluation and Management (12 questions)

11. Anesthesia (4 questions)

12. ICD-10-CM (12 questions)

13. HCPCS Level II (4 questions)

Lower-Weight Areas (Basic Understanding Sufficient):

14. Medical Terminology (4 questions)

15. Anatomy (4 questions)

16. Compliance and Regulatory (4 questions)

17. Cases (10 questions - mixed content)

Strategic Study Approach:

Spend 60% of your time on high-weight areas, 30% on medium-weight areas, and 10% on lower-weight areas. This allocation maximizes your score potential while ensuring comprehensive coverage.

Scoring and Pass/Fail Requirements

Passing Score: 70% (70 out of 100 questions correct)

The CPC exam uses scaled scoring, meaning your raw score (number correct) is converted to a scaled score between 300-900. A scaled score of 700 represents passing.

Why Scaled Scoring?

Different exam versions may have slight difficulty variations. Scaled scoring ensures fairness by adjusting for these differences. Your goal remains the same: answer at least 70 questions correctly.

Score Reporting:

You'll receive preliminary results immediately after completing the exam. Official results arrive within 7-10 business days and include:

- Your scaled score
- Pass/fail status
- Performance by knowledge area
- Retake eligibility information

What if You Don't Pass?

Approximately 70% of first-time test-takers pass the CPC exam. If you don't pass on your first attempt:

- You can retake the exam after a 10-day waiting period
- There's no limit on retake attempts
- Each retake requires a new exam fee
- Your score report identifies weak areas for focused study

The mindset difference between passers and non-passers: Successful candidates treat practice questions like the real exam and the real exam like another practice question.

Registration Process and Requirements

Before You Can Test:

1. AAPC Membership Required

- Student membership: $125/year
- Regular membership: $190/year
- Membership includes study resources and networking opportunities

2. Education Requirements You must demonstrate coding competency through:

- AAPC-approved training program completion, OR
- Equivalent work experience in medical coding, OR
- Relevant degree in health information management

3. Exam Registration

- Log into your AAPC account
- Select "Register for Certification Exam"
- Choose exam date and location
- Pay exam fee

Exam Fees (as of 2025):

- Single attempt: $349
- Dual attempt: $449 (second attempt included)
- Student discount: Available with valid student membership

Scheduling Your Exam:

Best Times to Test:

- Tuesday through Thursday (fewer distractions)
- Morning appointments (when you're mentally fresh)
- Avoid Mondays and Fridays (testing center disruptions)

Book Early: Popular testing dates fill quickly, especially in major metropolitan areas.

Rescheduling Policy: You can reschedule up to 24 hours before your appointment for a $35 fee.

Test Day Logistics and What to Expect

What to Bring:

Required:

- Two forms of identification (one photo ID)
- Your coding books (CPT®, ICD-10-CM, HCPCS Level II)

Allowed:

- Highlighters and pens (for marking books only)
- Calculator (basic four-function; provided by testing center)

Prohibited:

- Cell phones or electronic devices
- Food and beverages

- Reference materials other than coding books
- Notes or study materials

Book Preparation:

Your coding books are your lifeline during the exam. Proper preparation makes the difference between passing and failing:

Tabbing Strategy:

- Use small, labeled tabs for major sections
- Color-code by book (e.g., green for ICD-10-CM, blue for CPT®)
- Mark important guidelines and tables
- Practice using tabs during study sessions

Testing Center Experience:

Arrival: Arrive 30 minutes early for check-in procedures **Storage:** Personal items go in a locked locker **Testing Room:** Individual computer stations with minimal distractions **Breaks:** Unscheduled breaks are allowed but count against your time **Environment:** Temperature-controlled, quiet environment with minimal interruptions

During the Exam:

Technical Issues: Notify the proctor immediately if you experience any computer problems **Questions:** You cannot ask content questions, but can ask about technical issues **Bathroom Breaks:** Allowed but count against your exam time

After the Exam:

Preliminary Results: Displayed immediately upon completion **Official Results:** Emailed within 7-10 business days **Next Steps:** If you pass, you'll receive information about maintaining your certification

Building Your Confidence

The CPC exam is challenging but passable. Every year, thousands of candidates with backgrounds similar to yours earn their certification. The key differentiators among candidates are:

Preparation Quality: Systematic study following a proven plan **Practice Volume:** Exposure to hundreds of realistic practice questions **Test-Taking Skills:** Strategies for managing time and handling difficult questions **Mindset:** Confidence built through thorough preparation

You now understand what the CPC exam entails. The next chapter will teach you how to prepare effectively, transforming this knowledge into a passing score.

Chapter 1 Summary

The CPC exam consists of 100 multiple-choice questions administered over four hours at computer-based testing centers. The exam tests 17 knowledge areas with varying weights, requiring a 70% passing score. Registration requires AAPC membership and demonstration of coding competency through education or experience.

Understanding the exam structure allows you to:

- Allocate study time proportionally to question weights
- Develop time management strategies
- Prepare your reference materials effectively
- Set realistic expectations for exam day

Success Formula: Thorough preparation + strategic approach + confident execution = CPC certification

Your journey to CPC certification continues with learning how to study effectively and efficiently.

Chapter 1 Practice Questions

Test your understanding of the CPC exam basics with these practice questions:

1. How many questions are on the CPC exam? a) 75 b) 100 c) 125 d) 150

Answer: B) 100 *Explanation: The CPC exam consists of exactly 100 multiple-choice questions that must be completed within 4 hours.*

2. What is the passing score for the CPC exam? a) 65% b) 70% c) 75% d) 80%

Answer: B) 70% *Explanation: Candidates must answer at least 70 out of 100 questions correctly to pass the CPC exam.*

3. Which knowledge area has the most questions on the CPC exam? a) ICD-10-CM b) Medical Terminology c) Evaluation and Management d) Cases

Answer: C) Evaluation and Management *Explanation: Evaluation and Management coding accounts for 12 questions, making it the highest-weighted single knowledge area.*

4. What reference materials are you allowed to bring to the CPC exam? a) Any medical reference books b) CPT®, ICD-10-CM, and HCPCS Level II code books only c) Notes and study guides d) Electronic devices with medical apps

Answer: B) CPT®, ICD-10-CM, and HCPCS Level II code books only *Explanation: Only official coding books are permitted as reference materials during the CPC exam.*

5. How long do you have to complete the CPC exam? a) 3 hours b) 3.5 hours c) 4 hours d) 5 hours

Answer: C) 4 hours *Explanation: The CPC exam allows 4 hours (240 minutes) for completion, including any breaks you choose to take.*

Chapter 2: Proven Study Strategies for CPC Success

"The will to win, the desire to succeed, the urge to reach your full potential... these are the keys that will unlock the door to personal excellence." - Confucius

Passing the CPC exam isn't about how many hours you study—it's about how effectively you study. This chapter reveals the strategies used by successful CPC candidates, based on learning science research and analysis of thousands of exam results.

You'll discover how to create a personalized study plan, manage your time efficiently, and develop the test-taking skills that separate passing candidates from those who struggle. These aren't generic study tips, but specific techniques proven to work for medical coding exams.

Creating Your Personalized Study Plan

The Foundation: Honest Self-Assessment

Before creating your study plan, you need a clear picture of your starting point. Complete this assessment honestly—overestimating your knowledge leads to inadequate preparation, while underestimating creates unnecessary stress.

Medical Terminology Assessment:

- Can you break down "cardiomyopathy" into its component parts?
- Do you know the difference between "anterior" and "posterior"?
- Can you identify basic anatomical structures for each body system?

Coding Experience Assessment:

- Have you worked with medical codes in any capacity?
- Are you familiar with the structure of CPT®, ICD-10-CM, and HCPCS codes?
- Do you understand basic coding principles and guidelines?

Available Time Assessment:

- How many hours per week can you realistically study?
- What time of day are you most alert and focused?
- How many weeks do you have until your exam date?

Learning Style Assessment:

- Do you learn better through reading, practice questions, or hands-on application?

- Do you prefer structured schedules or flexible approaches?
- How do you typically prepare for important tests?

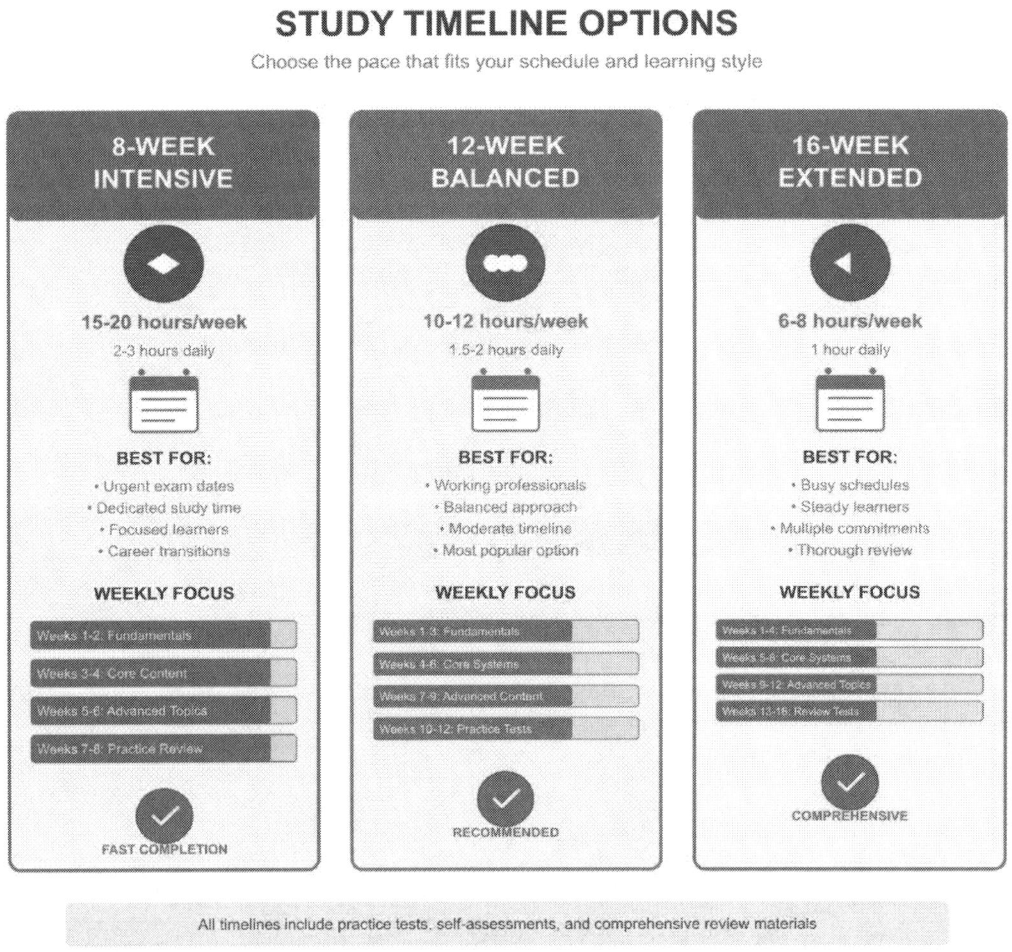

Creating Your Timeline

Based on your assessment, choose one of these proven study approaches:

Intensive 8-Week Plan (15-20 hours/week)

Best for: Candidates with medical background or full-time study availability

Week 1: Foundation Building

- Chapter 1-3: Exam overview and resources
- Chapter 4: Medical terminology mastery
- Begin coding book familiarization
- Target: Complete 50 practice questions

Week 2: Anatomy and ICD-10-CM Basics

- Chapter 5: Anatomy and physiology review
- Chapter 6: ICD-10-CM fundamentals
- Practice: Anatomy identification exercises

- Target: Complete 75 practice questions

Week 3-4: ICD-10-CM Mastery

- Chapter 7-8: ICD-10-CM by body system and complex scenarios
- Daily practice: 25-30 ICD-10-CM coding exercises
- Target: Complete 150 practice questions

Week 5-6: CPT® Coding Mastery

- Chapters 9-15: Complete CPT® review
- Focus on high-weight areas first (10000-50000 series)
- Target: Complete 200 practice questions

Week 7: Integration and Practice Exams

- Chapter 16: HCPCS Level II
- Chapters 17-18: Compliance and reimbursement
- Take Practice Exam 1
- Review weak areas identified

Week 8: Final Preparation

- Take Practice Exams 2 and 3
- Final review of missed question topics
- Light review day before exam

Balanced 12-Week Plan (10-12 hours/week)

Best for: Working professionals with consistent study time

Weeks 1-2: Foundation and Medical Terminology

- Thorough completion of Chapters 1-5
- Build strong terminology base
- Begin book marking and tabbing
- Target: 100 practice questions

Weeks 3-4: ICD-10-CM Fundamentals

- Chapters 6-7: Structure through body systems
- Practice coding 10-15 diagnoses daily
- Master guideline usage
- Target: 100 practice questions

Weeks 5-6: Advanced ICD-10-CM and CPT® Basics

- Chapter 8: Complex ICD-10-CM scenarios
- Chapters 9-10: CPT® fundamentals and E/M
- Target: 125 practice questions

Weeks 7-8: CPT® Surgery Coding

- Chapter 11: All surgical specialties
- Focus extra time on highest-weight areas
- Target: 125 practice questions

Weeks 9-10: Remaining CPT® Sections

- Chapters 12-15: Anesthesia, Radiology, Path/Lab, Medicine
- Chapter 16: HCPCS Level II
- Target: 100 practice questions

Week 11: Integration and First Practice Exam

- Chapters 17-18: Compliance and reimbursement
- Take Practice Exam 1
- Identify and address weak areas

Week 12: Final Preparation

- Take Practice Exams 2 and 3
- Focused review of problem areas
- Final confidence-building activities

Extended 16-Week Plan (6-8 hours/week)

Best for: Part-time studiers or those new to healthcare

Weeks 1-3: Thorough Foundation

- Complete understanding of Chapters 1-5
- Build comprehensive medical terminology base
- Extensive anatomy and physiology review
- Target: 75 practice questions

Weeks 4-6: ICD-10-CM Mastery

- Chapters 6-7: Complete diagnostic coding
- Practice with real medical records
- Master all coding conventions
- Target: 100 practice questions

Weeks 7-9: ICD-10-CM Complex Scenarios

- Chapter 8: Advanced diagnostic coding
- Daily practice with challenging cases
- Build speed and accuracy
- Target: 100 practice questions

Weeks 10-12: CPT® Procedure Coding

- Chapters 9-11: Fundamentals through surgery
- Focus on understanding over memorization
- Target: 125 practice questions

Weeks 13-14: Remaining CPT® and HCPCS

- Chapters 12-16: Complete procedure coding
- Integration of all coding types
- Target: 100 practice questions

Week 15: Comprehensive Practice

- Chapters 17-18: Compliance and reimbursement
- Take Practice Exam 1
- Address identified weaknesses

Week 16: Final Preparation

- Practice Exams 2 and 3
- Light review and confidence building
- Exam day preparation

Customizing Your Plan

Regardless of which timeline you choose, customize it based on your assessment:

If you're weak in medical terminology: Add extra time to Chapter 4 and anatomy review **If you have coding experience:** Focus more time on exam-specific strategies and practice questions **If time is limited:** Prioritize high-weight exam areas and increase practice question volume **If you learn slowly:** Allow extra time for each chapter and increase review frequency

Effective Time Management Techniques

The Pomodoro Technique for Medical Coding

Traditional studying often leads to fatigue and decreased retention. The Pomodoro Technique, adapted for medical coding study, maximizes focus and retention:

25-Minute Study Blocks:

- Study one specific topic (e.g., integumentary system coding)
- Eliminate all distractions
- Take notes or complete exercises actively
- Stop at 25 minutes regardless of progress

5-Minute Breaks:

- Step away from study materials
- Do light physical activity or stretching
- Avoid screens and social media
- Return refreshed for next block

After 4 Blocks (2 hours):

- Take a 15-30 minute break
- Review what you learned
- Plan your next study session
- Reward your progress

Weekly Schedule Optimization

High-Energy Times: Schedule difficult topics (surgery coding, complex E/M) during your peak mental energy hours.

Low-Energy Times: Use for review, practice questions, or administrative tasks like book marking.

Daily Minimums: Establish a minimum daily study time (even 15 minutes) to maintain momentum.

Weekly Goals: Set specific weekly objectives (e.g., "Complete respiratory system coding" or "Master E/M guidelines").

The 80/20 Rule for CPC Study

Focus 80% of your time on the 20% of content most likely to appear on your exam:

High-Priority Content (80% of study time):

- Evaluation and Management coding
- Surgery coding (10000-60000 series)
- ICD-10-CM guidelines and conventions
- Medical terminology and anatomy basics

Lower-Priority Content (20% of study time):

- HCPCS Level II details
- Compliance regulations
- Advanced anatomy concepts
- Rare coding scenarios

Book Marking and Reference Strategies

Your coding books are your lifeline during the exam.

Proper preparation is the difference between confident navigation and frantic searching.

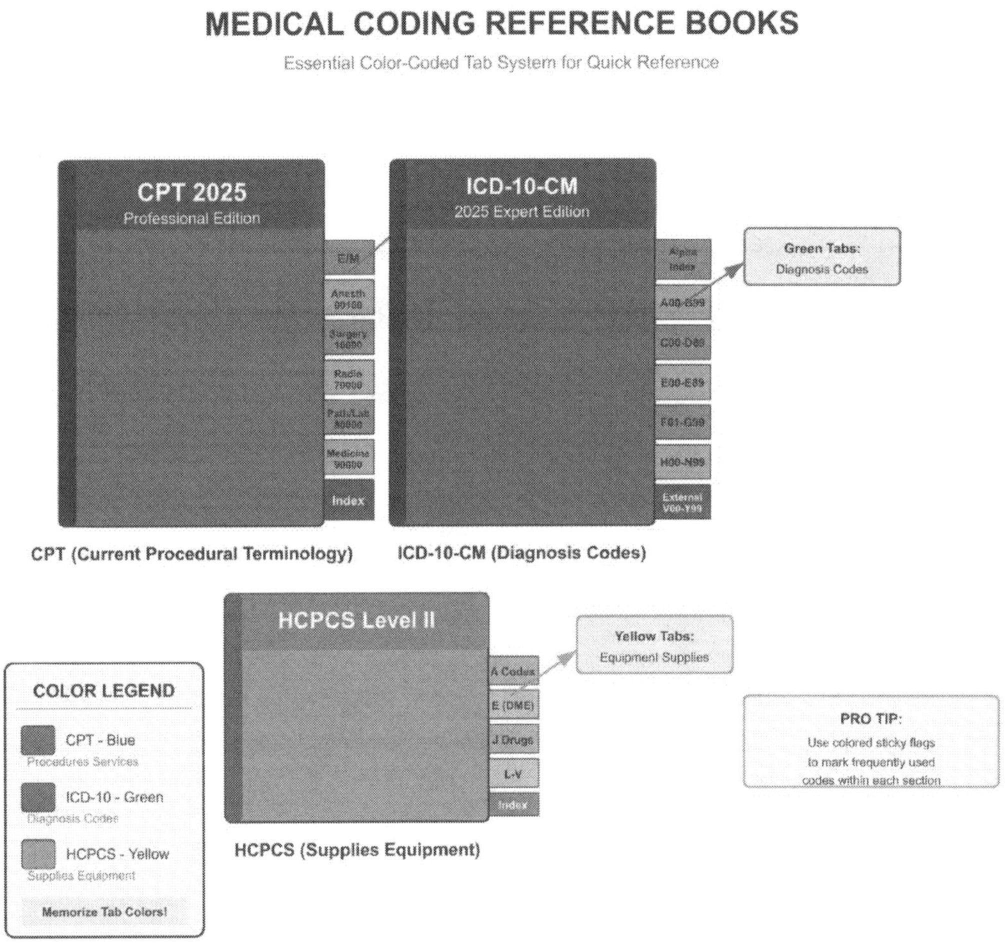

Essential Tabbing Strategy:

CPT® Book Tabs:

- Evaluation and Management (99202-99499)
- Anesthesia (00100-01999)
- Surgery sections by specialty (10000, 20000, 30000, etc.)

- Radiology (70010-79999)
- Pathology/Laboratory (80047-89398)
- Medicine (90281-99607)
- Category II and III codes
- Appendices (especially Appendix A - Modifiers)

ICD-10-CM Book Tabs:

- Official Guidelines for Coding and Reporting
- Alphabetic Index (main sections A-Z)
- Tabular List by chapter (A00-B99, C00-D49, etc.)
- Neoplasm Table
- Table of Drugs and Chemicals
- External Cause Index

HCPCS Level II Book Tabs:

- Transportation Services (A codes)
- Medical and Surgical Supplies (A codes)
- Enteral and Parenteral Therapy (B codes)
- Durable Medical Equipment (E codes)
- Drugs Administered Other than Oral Method (J codes)

Advanced Book Marking Techniques:

Highlighting Strategy: Use different colors systematically:

- **Yellow:** Key guidelines and rules
- **Pink:** Common modifiers and their uses
- **Green:** Important tables and charts
- **Blue:** Exclusion notes and special instructions

Margin Notes: Write brief reminders in margins:

- "Check guidelines" next to complex procedures
- "Multiple codes" for procedures requiring additional codes
- "Modifier required" for procedures needing modifiers

Sticky Notes: Use for frequently referenced pages:

- Modifier tables
- E/M documentation guidelines
- ICD-10-CM coding conventions

Memory Techniques for Medical Terminology

Medical terminology forms the foundation of accurate coding. These proven memory techniques help you master terminology efficiently.

The Building Block Method

Medical terms are built from three basic components:

- **Prefix:** Beginning of the word (modifies meaning)
- **Root:** Main part of the word (core meaning)
- **Suffix:** End of the word (indicates condition, procedure, etc.)

Example Breakdown: Cardiomyopathy

- Cardio- (prefix): relating to the heart
- -myo- (root): relating to muscle
- -pathy (suffix): disease or abnormal condition
- **Translation:** Disease of the heart muscle

Master the Most Common Components:

High-Frequency Prefixes:

- **A-/An-:** Without, not (anemia = without blood)
- **Hyper-:** Above, excessive (hypertension = high blood pressure)
- **Hypo-:** Below, deficient (hypotension = low blood pressure)
- **Inter-:** Between (intercostal = between ribs)
- **Intra-:** Within (intramuscular = within muscle)
- **Pre-:** Before (preoperative = before surgery)
- **Post-:** After (postoperative = after surgery)

Essential Root Words:

- **Cardi/o:** Heart (cardiology = study of the heart)
- **Gastro:** Stomach (gastritis = inflammation of stomach)
- **Nephro:** Kidney (nephrology = study of kidneys)
- **Pneumo:** Lung (pneumonia = lung infection)
- **Osteo:** Bone (osteoporosis = bone loss condition)
- **Derm/dermato:** Skin (dermatitis = skin inflammation)

Common Suffixes:

- **-itis:** Inflammation (appendicitis = appendix inflammation)
- **-ectomy:** Surgical removal (appendectomy = appendix removal)
- **-ology:** Study of (cardiology = study of heart)
- **-osis:** Abnormal condition (cirrhosis = liver scarring)
- **-plasty:** Surgical repair (rhinoplasty = nose surgery)

The Association Method

Create mental links between new terms and familiar concepts:

- **Tachycardia:** "Tachy" sounds like "tacky"—tacky heart beats too fast
- **Bradycardia:** "Brady" like Brady Bunch—slow family, slow heart
- **Rhinoplasty:** "Rhino" like rhinoceros—big nose, nose surgery
- **Nephritis:** "Nephew" has kidney problems—kidney inflammation

The Acronym Method

Create memorable acronyms for related terms:

RICE for injury treatment:

- **R**est
- **I**ce
- **C**ompression
- **E**levation

SAMPLE for patient history:

- **S**igns and symptoms
- **A**llergies
- **M**edications
- **P**ast medical history
- **L**ast meal
- **E**vents leading to illness

Test-Taking Strategies for Multiple Choice Questions

The CPC exam tests not just your coding knowledge, but your ability to apply it under pressure. These strategies help you navigate challenging questions confidently.

The Strategic Reading Method

Step 1: Read the Question Stem Carefully Identify exactly what the question is asking before looking at answer choices. Look for key phrases:

- "Primary diagnosis"
- "Principal procedure"
- "Most appropriate code"
- "According to CPT® guidelines"

Step 2: Predict the Answer Before looking at options, try to answer the question in your own words. This prevents wrong answers from confusing you.

Step 3: Evaluate Each Option Read all options before selecting. Even if option A looks correct, option D might be more specific or accurate.

Step 4: Use Elimination Strategy Cross out obviously wrong answers first, then choose among remaining options.

When You Don't Know the Answer:

Strategy 1: Use Context Clues

- Look for anatomical references
- Identify the type of service or procedure
- Consider patient age, gender, or condition

Strategy 2: Apply Coding Logic

- More specific codes are usually correct over general codes
- Bilateral procedures often require modifiers
- Combination codes take precedence over multiple codes

Strategy 3: Eliminate Impossible Options

- Codes that don't match the described procedure
- Diagnoses that don't fit the patient's condition
- Options that violate basic coding guidelines

Common Question Traps to Avoid:

The "Almost Right" Trap: One option is close but missing a key detail (wrong laterality, incorrect approach, etc.)

The "Too General" Trap: A broad code when a more specific one exists

The "Wrong Category" Trap: Correct procedure but wrong section (surgical vs. medicine codes)

Time Management During Questions:

Easy Questions (30 seconds): Questions you know immediately—answer and move on

Medium Questions (1-2 minutes): Require some thought or reference checking

Hard Questions (3-4 minutes): Complex scenarios requiring careful analysis

If you're spending more than 4 minutes on any question, make your best guess and flag it for review if time permits.

Managing Exam Anxiety and Building Confidence

Exam anxiety can undermine even the best preparation. These evidence-based techniques help you maintain calm confidence throughout your exam.

Pre-Exam Confidence Building

The Power of Positive Visualization: Spend 5-10 minutes daily imagining yourself:

- Walking confidently into the testing center
- Reading questions calmly and clearly
- Finding answers efficiently in your books
- Completing the exam with time to spare
- Receiving your passing score

Success Affirmations: Repeat these daily during study sessions:

- "I am well-prepared for this exam"
- "I trust my knowledge and preparation"
- "I remain calm and focused under pressure"
- "I deserve to pass this exam"

Evidence-Based Preparation: Track your progress with concrete evidence:

- Keep a log of practice test scores
- Note improvement in specific areas
- Document concepts you've mastered
- Celebrate small victories along the way

During-Exam Anxiety Management

The 4-7-8 Breathing Technique: When you feel anxious during the exam:

1. Inhale for 4 counts
2. Hold breath for 7 counts
3. Exhale for 8 counts
4. Repeat 3-4 times

This activates your parasympathetic nervous system, reducing stress hormones.

The Grounding Technique: If you feel overwhelmed:

- Name 5 things you can see (computer screen, desk, etc.)
- Name 4 things you can touch (chair, desk surface, etc.)
- Name 3 things you can hear (air conditioning, typing, etc.)

- Name 2 things you can smell
- Name 1 thing you can taste

This brings your focus back to the present moment.

Progressive Muscle Relaxation: Tense and release muscle groups for 5 seconds each:

- Shoulders (tense, then relax)
- Arms (tense, then relax)
- Face muscles (tense, then relax)
- Legs (tense, then relax)

Building Long-Term Confidence

Competence Leads to Confidence: The most effective way to build confidence is to become genuinely competent. Focus on:

- Understanding concepts rather than memorizing
- Practicing until skills become automatic
- Learning from mistakes rather than avoiding them
- Building on small successes

The Growth Mindset: Adopt beliefs that support learning:

- "I can learn anything with enough practice"
- "Mistakes are learning opportunities"
- "Effort and strategy matter more than natural talent"
- "I'm becoming better at this every day"

Chapter 2 Summary

Effective CPC preparation requires more than just reading—it demands strategic study approaches, efficient time management, and strong test-taking skills. Success comes from:

Personalized Planning: Choose a study timeline that fits your schedule and learning style, then stick to it consistently.

Strategic Time Use: Focus 80% of your effort on high-weight exam areas while ensuring comprehensive coverage.

Book Mastery: Properly marked and tabbed books are your most valuable exam tools.

Terminology Foundation: Strong medical terminology skills accelerate all other learning.

Test-Taking Skills: Strategic approaches to multiple-choice questions can improve your score even when knowledge is incomplete.

Confidence Management: Anxiety management and confidence-building techniques are as important as content knowledge.

Remember: thousands of people pass the CPC exam every year with the same resources available to you. The difference between success and struggle lies in preparation quality, not quantity.

Your next step is mastering the essential resources you'll use throughout your preparation and on exam day.

Chapter 2 Practice Questions

Test your understanding of effective study strategies:

Question 1: What percentage of study time should you spend on high-weight CPC exam areas?

A) 60% B) 70% C) 80% D) 90%

Answer: C Explanation: The 80/20 rule suggests spending 80% of study time on the 20% of content most likely to appear on your exam, which includes high-weight areas like E/M coding and major surgery sections.

Question 2: How long should each Pomodoro study block last for optimal focus?

A) 15 minutes B) 25 minutes C) 35 minutes D) 45 minutes

Answer: B Explanation: The Pomodoro Technique uses 25-minute focused study blocks followed by 5-minute breaks to maximize concentration and retention.

Question 3: What is the most effective way to build exam confidence?

A) Positive thinking alone B) Avoiding difficult questions C) Building genuine competence through practice D) Cramming the night before

Answer: C Explanation: True confidence comes from competence. Understanding concepts deeply and practicing until skills become automatic builds lasting confidence that performs under pressure.

Question 4: When should you spend more than 4 minutes on a single exam question?

A) When it's worth more points B) When you're sure you know the answer C) Never—make your best guess and move on D) Only on case study questions

Answer: C Explanation: Time management is crucial on the CPC exam. Spending more than 4 minutes on any question risks running out of time for questions you could answer correctly.

Question 5: What color should you use to highlight key guidelines in your books?

A) Blue B) Green C) Pink D) Yellow

Answer: D Explanation: The suggested highlighting system uses yellow for key guidelines and rules, making them easy to spot during the exam.

Chapter 3: Essential Resources and Code Books

"Give me six hours to chop down a tree and I will spend the first four sharpening the axe." - Abraham Lincoln

Your coding books aren't just reference materials—they're your primary tools for success on the CPC exam. This chapter teaches you how to transform these books from intimidating volumes into efficient, user-friendly resources that give you a competitive advantage on exam day.

You'll learn the structure and organization of each required code book, master navigation techniques that save precious time, and develop a systematic approach to finding information quickly and accurately. By the end of this chapter, your books will feel like extensions of your own knowledge.

Required Code Books: CPT®, ICD-10-CM, HCPCS Level II

The CPC exam allows you to bring three code books: CPT® (Current Procedural Terminology), ICD-10-CM (International Classification of Diseases, 10th Revision, Clinical Modification), and HCPCS Level II (Healthcare Common Procedure Coding System). Understanding each book's purpose, structure, and best uses is essential for exam success.

CPT® (Current Procedural Terminology)

Publisher: American Medical Association (AMA) **Purpose:** Codes for procedures, services, and supplies provided by healthcare professionals **Structure:** Numeric codes with five digits (e.g., 99213, 27447, 76700)

CPT® Categories:

- **Category I:** Most commonly used codes (10000-99000 series)
- **Category II:** Performance measurement codes (optional reporting)
- **Category III:** Temporary codes for emerging technologies

Main CPT® Sections:

1. **Evaluation and Management (99202-99499):** Office visits, consultations, hospital care
2. **Anesthesia (00100-01999):** Anesthesia services for surgical procedures
3. **Surgery (10000-69990):** All surgical procedures organized by body system
4. **Radiology (70010-79999):** Diagnostic imaging and radiation therapy

5. **Pathology and Laboratory (80047-89398):** Lab tests and pathological examinations
6. **Medicine (90281-99607):** Non-surgical services and procedures

Key CPT® Features:

- **Semicolon Convention:** Conserves space by avoiding repetitive text
- **Add-on Codes:** Used only with primary procedure codes
- **Modifier Appendix:** Critical for exam success—know your modifiers

ICD-10-CM (International Classification of Diseases, 10th Revision, Clinical Modification)

Publisher: Centers for Medicare & Medicaid Services (CMS) **Purpose:** Codes for diseases, injuries, symptoms, and external causes **Structure:** Alphanumeric codes, 3-7 characters (e.g., K21.9, S72.001A, Z51.11)

ICD-10-CM Organization:

- **Alphabetic Index:** Volume 1 - find terms alphabetically
- **Tabular List:** Volume 2 - verify and assign final codes
- **Official Guidelines:** Essential rules for proper code assignment

ICD-10-CM Chapter Structure:

1. A00-B99: Certain infectious and parasitic diseases
2. C00-D49: Neoplasms
3. D50-D89: Diseases of blood and blood-forming organs
4. E00-E89: Endocrine, nutritional and metabolic diseases
5. F01-F99: Mental, behavioral and neurodevelopmental disorders
6. G00-G99: Diseases of the nervous system
7. H00-H59: Diseases of the eye and adnexa
8. H60-H95: Diseases of the ear and mastoid process
9. I00-I99: Diseases of the circulatory system
10. J00-J99: Diseases of the respiratory system [Continues through Chapter 21: Z00-Z99]

Critical ICD-10-CM Features:

- **7th Character Extensions:** Required for certain conditions (initial, subsequent, sequela)
- **Combination Codes:** Single codes that identify multiple related conditions
- **Excludes Notes:** Help prevent incorrect code assignment

HCPCS Level II

Publisher: Centers for Medicare & Medicaid Services (CMS) **Purpose:** Codes for supplies, equipment, and services not covered in CPT® **Structure:** One letter followed by four digits (e.g., A4100, E0143, J7050)

HCPCS Level II Sections:

- **A Codes:** Transportation, medical supplies, administrative services
- **B Codes:** Enteral and parenteral therapy
- **C Codes:** Hospital outpatient prospective payment system
- **E Codes:** Durable medical equipment
- **G Codes:** Procedures/services temporarily assigned
- **H Codes:** Alcohol and drug abuse treatment
- **J Codes:** Drugs administered other than oral method
- **K Codes:** Temporary codes for DME regional carriers
- **L Codes:** Orthotic and prosthetic procedures
- **M Codes:** Medical services
- **P Codes:** Pathology and laboratory services
- **Q Codes:** Temporary codes
- **R Codes:** Diagnostic radiology services
- **S Codes:** Temporary national codes (non-Medicare)
- **T Codes:** Temporary national codes (state Medicaid agencies)
- **V Codes:** Vision services
- **Miscellaneous Codes:** Not otherwise classified

How to Navigate Your Code Books Efficiently

Efficient book navigation separates confident test-takers from those who struggle with time management. These techniques help you find information quickly and accurately.

The Two-Step Method for All Coding

Step 1: Start with the Alphabetic Index

- Always begin with the alphabetic section
- Never code directly from the tabular/numeric section
- Look up the main term, then subterms
- Note all code options provided

Step 2: Verify in Tabular/Numeric Section

- Go to each code suggested by the index
- Read the complete code description
- Check for additional instructions
- Assign the most specific code available

CPT® Navigation Strategies

Finding Procedures Efficiently:

1. **Identify the main term** (procedure, service, or anatomic site)
2. **Check the CPT® Index** for initial code ranges

3. **Go to the numeric section** and read complete descriptions
4. **Check for guidelines** at the section or subsection level

Example: Knee Arthroscopy

- Index lookup: "Arthroscopy, knee" → 29870-29887
- Numeric section: Review all codes 29870-29887
- Guidelines: Read knee arthroscopy guidelines
- Select most specific code for documented procedure

Common CPT® Index Terms:

- **Procedures:** Usually listed by procedure name
- **Anatomic sites:** Often listed by body part
- **Eponyms:** Listed by physician's name (e.g., "Whipple procedure")

ICD-10-CM Navigation Strategies

The STEP Method:

- **S**earch the Alphabetic Index
- **T**urn to the Tabular List
- **E**xamine all options and guidelines
- **P**ick the most specific code

Alphabetic Index Best Practices:

- Look up the **condition**, not the anatomic site
- Use **main terms**, not adjectives
- Check **"see" and "see also"** references
- Review **subterms** for specificity

Example: Acute Myocardial Infarction

- Main term: "Infarction"
- Subterm: "myocardial"
- Further subterm: "acute" → I21.-
- Tabular verification: Review I21 category for specificity

Tabular List Best Practices:

- Read the **three-character category** first
- Check for **inclusion and exclusion notes**
- Determine if **additional characters** are required
- Verify **7th character** requirements when applicable

HCPCS Level II Navigation

Quick Reference Method:

1. **Identify the type of item/service** (drug, supply, equipment)
2. **Determine the appropriate letter category**
3. **Use the index** to find specific items
4. **Verify in the tabular section**

Common HCPCS Scenarios:

- **Drugs:** Usually J codes, look up by generic name
- **Equipment:** Usually E codes, look up by equipment type
- **Supplies:** Usually A codes, look up by supply type

Tabbing and Marking Strategies

Proper book preparation can save 10-15 minutes on your exam—often the difference between passing and failing.

Professional Tabbing System

CPT® Book Tabs (Use different colors for easy identification):

Blue Tabs - Major Sections:

- Evaluation and Management (99202)
- Anesthesia (00100)
- Surgery Introduction (10000)
- Integumentary (10000)
- Musculoskeletal (20000)
- Respiratory (30000)
- Cardiovascular (33000)
- Digestive (40000)
- Urinary (50000)
- Reproductive (54000/55000)
- Nervous System (61000)
- Eye and Ocular (65000)
- Auditory (69000)
- Radiology (70000)
- Pathology/Laboratory (80000)
- Medicine (90000)

Red Tabs - Critical References:

- CPT® Guidelines (front of book)
- Appendix A (Modifiers)
- Appendix B (Summary of Additions, Deletions, Revisions)

ICD-10-CM Book Tabs:

Green Tabs - Structure:

- Official Guidelines (front)
- Alphabetic Index (Volume 1)
- Neoplasm Table
- Table of Drugs and Chemicals
- External Cause Index
- Tabular List (Volume 2)

Yellow Tabs - Common Chapters:

- A00-B99 (Infectious diseases)
- C00-D49 (Neoplasms)
- E00-E89 (Endocrine/metabolic)
- I00-I99 (Circulatory)
- J00-J99 (Respiratory)
- K00-K95 (Digestive)
- M00-M99 (Musculoskeletal)

- N00-N99 (Genitourinary)
- S00-T88 (Injury/poisoning)
- Z00-Z99 (Factors influencing health status)

HCPCS Level II Tabs:

Orange Tabs:

- Introduction and Guidelines
- A codes (Transportation/Supplies)
- E codes (DME)
- J codes (Drugs)
- L codes (Orthotics/Prosthetics)

Strategic Marking Techniques

Highlighting Strategy:

- **Yellow:** Key guidelines and instructions
- **Pink:** Modifiers and special notes
- **Green:** Code ranges and cross-references
- **Blue:** Exclusions and limitations

Margin Notes (Use abbreviations):

- **"CK GUIDE":** Check guidelines before coding
- **"MULT CODES":** Multiple codes may be needed
- **"MOD REQ":** Modifier typically required
- **"+ADD-ON":** Add-on code, use with primary
- **"BILAT":** Bilateral procedure considerations

Sticky Note System:

- **Page flags:** For frequently used references
- **Write-on flags:** For personal reminders
- **Color coding:** Different colors for different types of references

Using Guidelines and Conventions

Guidelines and conventions aren't just suggestions—they're rules that determine correct code assignment. Understanding and applying them accurately is essential for exam success.

CPT® Guidelines Hierarchy

1. Section Guidelines (Most Important)

- Apply to entire sections (e.g., all Surgery codes)
- Override general guidelines when conflicts arise
- Essential for understanding scope of codes

2. Subsection Guidelines

- Apply to subsections within larger sections
- More specific than section guidelines
- Often address modifier usage

3. Subheading Guidelines

- Apply to related groups of codes
- Very specific instructions
- Critical for accurate code selection

Essential CPT® Conventions

Semicolon Convention: The semicolon separates the common portion of a code description from the unique portion.

Example:

- 25600: Closed treatment of distal radial fracture (eg, Colles or Smith type) or epiphyseal separation, includes closed treatment of fracture of ulnar styloid, when performed; without manipulation
- 25605: ; with manipulation

Code 25605 includes everything before the semicolon in 25600, plus "with manipulation."

Add-on Codes (+):

- Cannot be reported alone
- Always used with a primary procedure code
- Exempt from modifier 51 (multiple procedures)

Modifier 51 Exempt (⊕):

- Multiple procedure modifier not required
- Usually add-on codes or procedures exempt by nature

FDA Approval Pending (◗):

- Procedure includes FDA approval pending status
- Important for new technology procedures

ICD-10-CM Guidelines and Conventions

Official Guidelines for Coding and Reporting: These guidelines, updated annually, provide binding instructions for code assignment. Major sections include:

Section I: Conventions, general coding guidelines, and chapter-specific guidelines Section II: Selection of principal diagnosis Section III: Reporting additional diagnoses Section IV: Diagnostic coding and reporting guidelines for outpatient services

Critical ICD-10-CM Conventions:

Includes Notes: Provide additional terms included in the code category.

Example: K21 Gastro-esophageal reflux disease **Includes:** newborn esophageal reflux

Excludes1 (∅): "Not coded here" - conditions that cannot be coded together.

Excludes2 (∅): "Not included here" - condition is not part of the condition represented by the code, but patient may have both conditions simultaneously.

Use Additional Code: Indicates that an additional code should be used to fully describe the condition.

Code First: Identifies conditions that should be sequenced before the current condition.

7th Character Requirements: Many injury codes and some disease codes require a 7th character:

- A: Initial encounter
- D: Subsequent encounter
- S: Sequela

HCPCS Level II Guidelines

General Principles:

- Use HCPCS when no CPT® code exists
- More specific codes take precedence
- Check for Medicare coverage limitations

Modifier Usage: HCPCS Level II has its own modifiers (e.g., -RT, -LT, -E1, -E2) that may be required for proper billing.

Understanding Code Updates for 2025-2026

Medical coding is dynamic, with annual updates reflecting advances in medical practice, technology, and healthcare delivery. Staying current with updates is crucial for exam success and professional practice.

CPT® Updates 2025-2026

New Codes: The AMA typically adds 200-300 new CPT® codes annually. Focus areas for recent updates include:

- **Digital health services** (remote patient monitoring)
- **Artificial intelligence applications** in healthcare

- **Advanced surgical techniques** (robotic-assisted procedures)
- **COVID-19 related services** (ongoing adaptations)

Revised Codes: Existing codes may be revised to:

- Clarify code descriptions
- Update technology references
- Reflect current medical practice
- Improve coding accuracy

Deleted Codes: Codes may be deleted due to:

- Obsolete procedures or technology
- Low utilization rates
- Consolidation with other codes
- Regulatory changes

Category III to Category I Migrations: Temporary Category III codes may become permanent Category I codes when:

- FDA approval is obtained
- Clinical efficacy is established
- Wide adoption occurs
- Long-term data supports usage

ICD-10-CM Updates 2025-2026

Annual Updates Include:

- **New codes** for emerging diseases and conditions
- **Code revisions** for improved specificity
- **Guideline updates** for better clarity
- **Index modifications** for easier navigation

Key Update Areas:

- **Mental health conditions** (expanded specificity)
- **Substance use disorders** (detailed classifications)
- **Injury codes** (improved anatomical specificity)
- **External cause codes** (new technology-related injuries)

HCPCS Level II Updates 2025-2026

Quarterly Updates: Unlike CPT® and ICD-10-CM, HCPCS Level II codes can be updated quarterly, reflecting:

- **New DME items**
- **Drug code additions**
- **Medicare policy changes**
- **Technology advancements**

Staying Current with Updates

Official Sources:

- **AMA (CPT®):** CPT® Network for latest updates
- **CMS (ICD-10-CM and HCPCS):** Official coding guidelines

- **AAPC:** Coding newsletters and updates
- **AHIMA:** Professional practice resources

Study Strategy:

- Focus on **high-frequency updates** (commonly used codes)
- Understand **reasoning behind changes** (improves retention)
- Practice with **updated code sets** during preparation
- Review **guideline changes** that affect multiple codes

Chapter 3 Summary

Your coding books are powerful tools when properly prepared and understood. Success requires:

Book Mastery: Understanding the structure, organization, and purpose of CPT®, ICD-10-CM, and HCPCS Level II

Navigation Skills: Using systematic approaches to find information quickly and accurately

Preparation Techniques: Strategic tabbing, marking, and organization that saves time during the exam

Guidelines Knowledge: Understanding and applying the rules that govern proper code assignment

Update Awareness: Staying current with annual code changes and guideline revisions

Remember: Your books contain all the answers to exam questions. The challenge isn't lack of information—it's finding the right information quickly. Proper preparation and practice transform your books from reference materials into competitive advantages.

Next, you'll build the foundation that makes all coding possible: mastering medical terminology.

Chapter 3 Practice Questions

Test your understanding of coding resources and navigation:

Question 1: What is the correct order for using your coding books?

A) Tabular section first, then alphabetic index B) Alphabetic index first, then tabular section C) Either order is acceptable D) Numeric section only

Answer: B Explanation: Always start with the alphabetic index to find potential codes, then verify in the tabular/numeric section. This prevents missed codes and ensures accuracy.

Question 2: What does the semicolon convention in CPT® indicate?

A) The code is deleted B) A modifier is required C) The common portion shared with indented codes D) The code is an add-on code

Answer: C Explanation: The semicolon separates the common portion of a code description from the unique portion that applies to indented codes below it.

Question 3: Which HCPCS Level II code category typically covers drugs administered by injection?

A) A codes B) E codes C) G codes D) J codes

Answer: D Explanation: J codes in HCPCS Level II cover drugs administered by methods other than oral, including injections and infusions.

Question 4: What do "Excludes1" notes in ICD-10-CM indicate?

A) The condition may be coded with other conditions B) The condition cannot be coded here C) Additional codes are required D) The code is being deleted

Answer: B Explanation: Excludes1 notes indicate "not coded here" - these conditions cannot be coded together as they represent mutually exclusive conditions.

Question 5: How often are HCPCS Level II codes typically updated?

A) Annually only B) Every two years C) Quarterly D) Monthly

Answer: C Explanation: HCPCS Level II codes can be updated quarterly to reflect new medical equipment, drugs, and Medicare policy changes, unlike CPT® and ICD-10-CM which are updated annually.

PART II: FOUNDATIONAL KNOWLEDGE

Chapter 4: Medical Terminology Mastery

"The beginning of wisdom is the definition of terms." - Socrates

Medical terminology is the universal language of healthcare, and fluency in this language is absolutely critical for CPC exam success. Every code description, every guideline, and every exam question assumes you understand the medical terms being used. This isn't just memorization—it's building the foundation that makes everything else possible.

This chapter transforms you from someone who recognizes medical terms to someone who truly understands their meaning, construction, and relationships. You'll learn to break down the most complex medical terms into understandable components and build your vocabulary systematically and efficiently.

Word Parts: Prefixes, Suffixes, and Root Words

Medical terminology follows logical construction patterns. Once you understand these patterns, you can decode thousands of terms you've never seen before. It's like learning the rules of a language—once you know them, you can understand words you've never encountered.

Understanding Word Construction

Medical terms are built like houses: they have foundations (root words), modifications (prefixes), and completions (suffixes). Understanding how these parts work together unlocks the meaning of complex terms.

Basic Construction Pattern: Prefix + Root + Suffix = Complete Medical Term

Examples:

- **Gastro** (stomach) + **enter** (intestine) + **itis** (inflammation) = Gastroenteritis
- **Hyper** (excessive) + **thyroid** (thyroid gland) + **ism** (condition) = Hyperthyroidism
- **Brady** (slow) + **card** (heart) + **ia** (condition) = Bradycardia

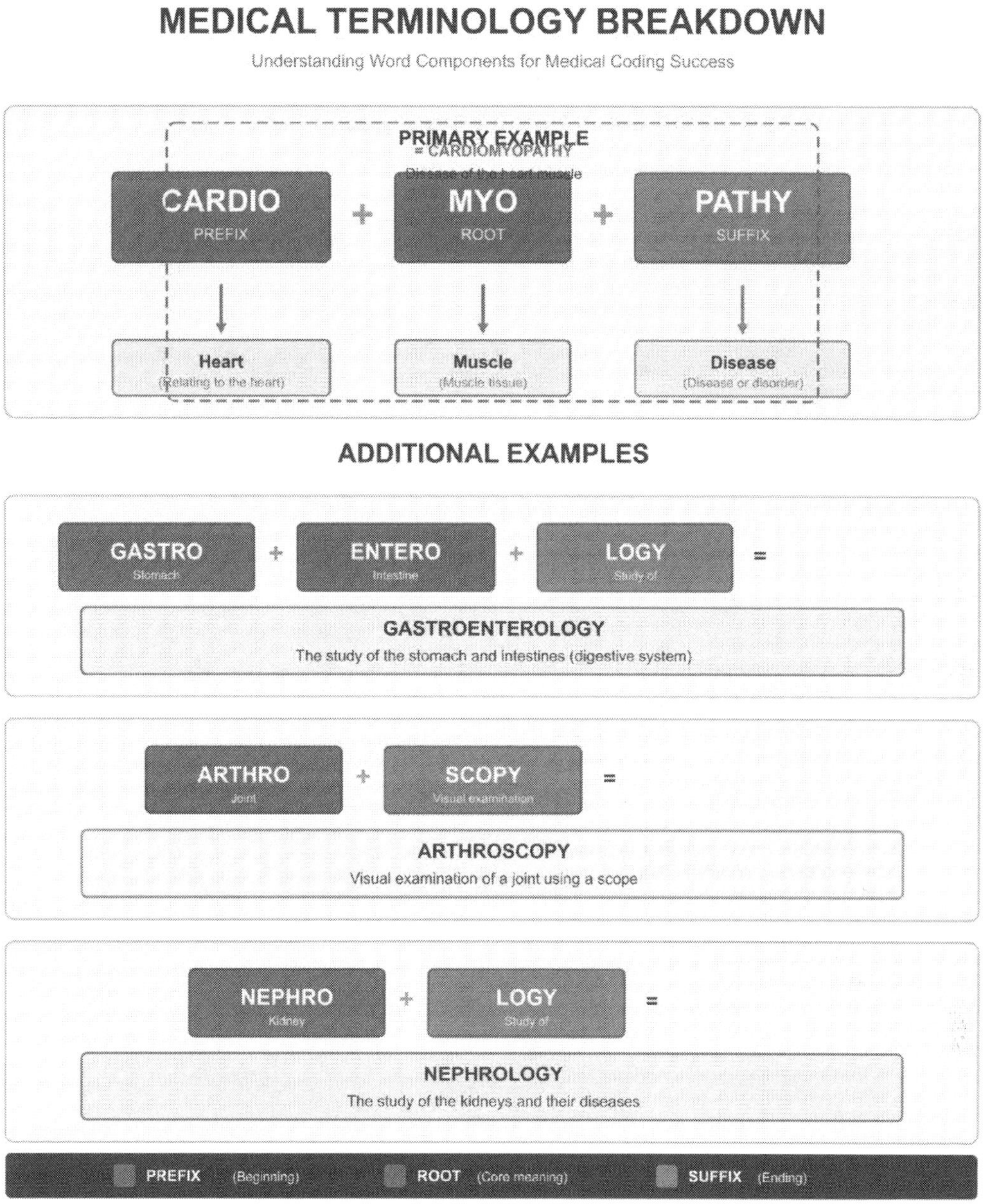

Essential Prefixes (Word Beginnings)

Prefixes modify the meaning of root words. Master these high-frequency prefixes that appear repeatedly on the CPC exam:

Quantity and Size Prefixes:

- **Mono-/Uni-:** One, single (monocyte = single cell type)
- **Bi-/Di-:** Two, double (bilateral = both sides)
- **Tri-:** Three (tricuspid = three flaps)
- **Multi-/Poly-:** Many, multiple (polyuria = excessive urination)
- **Micro-:** Small (microscopic = very small)

- **Macro-:** Large (macrocephalic = large head)
- **Mega-/Megalo-:** Enlarged, great (megacolon = enlarged colon)

Position and Direction Prefixes:

- **Ante-/Pre-:** Before, in front of (antepartum = before birth)
- **Post-:** After, behind (postoperative = after surgery)
- **Supra-:** Above, over (suprapubic = above the pubis)
- **Infra-/Sub-:** Below, under (infrarenal = below the kidney)
- **Inter-:** Between (intercostal = between ribs)
- **Intra-:** Within, inside (intramuscular = within muscle)
- **Extra-/Exo-:** Outside, beyond (extracellular = outside cells)
- **Endo-:** Within, inner (endoscopic = viewing inside)
- **Peri-:** Around, surrounding (pericardial = around the heart)

Condition and Quality Prefixes:

- **A-/An-:** Without, not (anemia = without blood)
- **Dys-:** Bad, difficult, painful (dyspnea = difficult breathing)
- **Hyper-:** Excessive, above normal (hypertension = high blood pressure)
- **Hypo-:** Below, under, decreased (hypotension = low blood pressure)
- **Tachy-:** Fast, rapid (tachycardia = fast heart rate)
- **Brady-:** Slow (bradycardia = slow heart rate)
- **Eu-:** Good, normal (eupnea = normal breathing)
- **Mal-:** Bad, poor (malnutrition = poor nutrition)

Negation Prefixes:

- **Anti-:** Against (antibiotic = against life/bacteria)
- **Contra-:** Against, opposite (contraindicated = against indication)
- **De-:** Away from, removal (dehydration = removal of water)
- **Dis-:** Apart, away from (dislocation = away from location)
- **Non-:** Not (non-invasive = not invasive)

Essential Root Words (Word Foundations)

Root words provide the core meaning of medical terms. These high-frequency roots appear in hundreds of medical terms:

Cardiovascular System Roots:

- **Cardi/o:** Heart (cardiology = study of heart)
- **Angi/o:** Vessel (angiogram = vessel image)
- **Vascul/o:** Blood vessel (vascular = relating to vessels)
- **Hemat/o, Hem/o:** Blood (hematology = study of blood)
- **Thromb/o:** Clot (thrombosis = clot condition)
- **Embol/o:** Plug, wedge (embolism = plug condition)

Respiratory System Roots:

- **Pneum/o, Pulmon/o:** Lung (pneumonia = lung inflammation)
- **Bronch/o:** Bronchus (bronchoscopy = viewing bronchus)
- **Trache/o:** Trachea (tracheostomy = trachea opening)
- **Laryng/o:** Larynx (laryngitis = larynx inflammation)
- **Rhin/o:** Nose (rhinoplasty = nose surgery)
- **Sinus/o:** Sinus (sinusitis = sinus inflammation)

Digestive System Roots:

- **Gastr/o:** Stomach (gastritis = stomach inflammation)
- **Enter/o:** Intestine (enteritis = intestine inflammation)
- **Col/o, Colon/o:** Colon (colostomy = colon opening)
- **Hepat/o:** Liver (hepatitis = liver inflammation)
- **Cholecyst/o:** Gallbladder (cholecystectomy = gallbladder removal)
- **Pancreat/o:** Pancreas (pancreatitis = pancreas inflammation)

Musculoskeletal System Roots:

- **Oste/o:** Bone (osteoporosis = bone porous condition)
- **Arthr/o:** Joint (arthritis = joint inflammation)
- **Myel/o:** Bone marrow, spinal cord (myelogram = marrow/cord image)
- **My/o, Muscul/o:** Muscle (myalgia = muscle pain)
- **Tend/o, Tendin/o:** Tendon (tendonitis = tendon inflammation)
- **Ligament/o:** Ligament (ligamentous = relating to ligaments)

Nervous System Roots:

- **Neur/o:** Nerve (neurology = study of nerves)
- **Encephalp/o:** Brain (encephalitis = brain inflammation)
- **Mening/o:** Meninges (meningitis = meninges inflammation)
- **Cerebell/o:** Cerebellum (cerebellar = relating to cerebellum)
- **Cerebr/o:** Cerebrum (cerebral = relating to cerebrum)

Genitourinary System Roots:

- **Nephr/o, Ren/o:** Kidney (nephrology = kidney study)
- **Ur/o, Urin/o:** Urine (urinalysis = urine analysis)
- **Cyst/o:** Bladder (cystoscopy = bladder viewing)
- **Ureter/o:** Ureter (ureterostomy = ureter opening)
- **Urethr/o:** Urethra (urethritis = urethra inflammation)

Essential Suffixes (Word Endings)

Suffixes complete medical terms and often indicate the type of condition, procedure, or study being described:

Condition/Disease Suffixes:

- **-itis:** Inflammation (appendicitis = appendix inflammation)
- **-osis:** Abnormal condition (cirrhosis = liver scarring condition)
- **-pathy:** Disease (neuropathy = nerve disease)
- **-emia:** Blood condition (anemia = blood deficiency condition)
- **-uria:** Urine condition (hematuria = blood in urine condition)
- **-pnea:** Breathing (dyspnea = difficult breathing)
- **-algia, -dynia:** Pain (neuralgia = nerve pain)
- **-phobia:** Fear (claustrophobia = fear of enclosed spaces)

Procedure/Treatment Suffixes:

- **-ectomy:** Surgical removal (appendectomy = appendix removal)
- **-otomy:** Surgical incision (tracheotomy = trachea incision)
- **-ostomy:** Surgical opening (colostomy = colon opening)
- **-plasty:** Surgical repair (rhinoplasty = nose repair)

- **-pexy:** Surgical fixation (gastropexy = stomach fixation)
- **-rrhaphy:** Suturing (herniorrhaphy = hernia suturing)
- **-centesis:** Surgical puncture (thoracentesis = chest puncture)
- **-clasis:** Breaking (osteoclasis = bone breaking)

Diagnostic/Study Suffixes:

- **-scopy:** Visual examination (colonoscopy = colon examination)
- **-graphy:** Process of recording (mammography = breast recording)
- **-gram:** Record/picture (electrocardiogram = heart electrical record)
- **-meter:** Measuring instrument (thermometer = heat measuring)
- **-metry:** Process of measuring (spirometry = breathing measuring)
- **-logy:** Study of (cardiology = heart study)
- **-logist:** Specialist in study (cardiologist = heart specialist)

Descriptive Suffixes:

- **-ic, -al, -ous:** Relating to, pertaining to (cardiac = relating to heart)
- **-ism:** Condition, process (hyperthyroidism = excessive thyroid condition)
- **-ist:** Specialist (radiologist = radiation specialist)
- **-ia, -y:** Condition (pneumonia = lung condition)
- **-ase:** Enzyme (lipase = fat-breaking enzyme)

Body Systems Terminology

Understanding terminology by body system helps you organize knowledge and improves code selection accuracy. Each system has characteristic terms that appear frequently on the CPC exam.

Integumentary System (Skin)

Key Anatomy Terms:

- **Epidermis:** Outer skin layer
- **Dermis:** Middle skin layer containing blood vessels and nerves
- **Subcutaneous:** Below skin layer (hypodermis)
- **Sebaceous:** Oil glands
- **Sudoriferous:** Sweat glands
- **Follicle:** Hair root structure
- **Keratin:** Protein in skin, hair, nails

Common Conditions:

- **Dermatitis:** Skin inflammation
- **Psoriasis:** Chronic skin scaling condition
- **Eczema:** Chronic itchy skin condition
- **Cellulitis:** Deep skin infection
- **Impetigo:** Superficial skin infection
- **Melanoma:** Malignant skin tumor
- **Basal cell carcinoma:** Common skin cancer
- **Acne vulgaris:** Common teenage skin condition

Common Procedures:

- **Biopsy:** Tissue sample removal for examination
- **Excision:** Surgical removal of skin lesion
- **Cryotherapy:** Freezing treatment
- **Electrocautery:** Electrical burning treatment
- **Dermabrasion:** Skin surface removal

- **Rhytidectomy:** Face lift surgery
- **Debridement:** Dead tissue removal

Musculoskeletal System

Key Anatomy Terms:

- **Cortical bone:** Dense outer bone layer
- **Cancellous bone:** Spongy inner bone
- **Periosteum:** Bone covering membrane
- **Epiphysis:** Bone end
- **Diaphysis:** Bone shaft
- **Metaphysis:** Area between shaft and end
- **Articular cartilage:** Joint surface cartilage
- **Synovial fluid:** Joint lubricating fluid

Directional Terms:

- **Proximal:** Closer to body center
- **Distal:** Farther from body center
- **Medial:** Toward midline
- **Lateral:** Away from midline
- **Superior:** Above
- **Inferior:** Below
- **Anterior:** Front
- **Posterior:** Back

Common Conditions:

- **Fracture types:** Closed, open, comminuted, spiral, greenstick
- **Osteoporosis:** Bone density loss
- **Osteoarthritis:** Joint degeneration
- **Rheumatoid arthritis:** Autoimmune joint inflammation
- **Fibromyalgia:** Chronic muscle pain syndrome
- **Tendonitis:** Tendon inflammation
- **Bursitis:** Bursa sac inflammation
- **Scoliosis:** Spinal curvature

Common Procedures:

- **ORIF:** Open reduction internal fixation
- **Arthroscopy:** Joint examination through scope
- **Arthroplasty:** Joint replacement surgery
- **Laminectomy:** Spinal bone removal
- **Discectomy:** Spinal disc removal
- **Meniscectomy:** Knee cartilage removal
- **Rotator cuff repair:** Shoulder muscle repair

Cardiovascular System

Key Anatomy Terms:

- **Myocardium:** Heart muscle
- **Pericardium:** Heart covering sac
- **Endocardium:** Heart inner lining
- **Atrium:** Heart upper chamber
- **Ventricle:** Heart lower chamber
- **Septum:** Heart dividing wall
- **Valve:** Heart blood flow controller
- **Coronary arteries:** Heart blood suppliers

Common Conditions:

- **Myocardial infarction:** Heart attack
- **Angina pectoris:** Chest pain from heart oxygen lack
- **Congestive heart failure:** Heart pumping weakness
- **Arrhythmia:** Irregular heartbeat
- **Hypertension:** High blood pressure
- **Atherosclerosis:** Artery hardening
- **Thrombosis:** Blood clot formation
- **Embolism:** Moving blood clot

Common Procedures:

- **Angioplasty:** Artery opening procedure
- **Stent placement:** Artery support device insertion
- **Bypass surgery:** Alternative blood path creation
- **Valve replacement:** Heart valve substitution
- **Pacemaker insertion:** Heart rhythm device placement
- **Catheterization:** Heart catheter insertion
- **Echocardiogram:** Heart ultrasound
- **Stress test:** Heart function under exercise

Respiratory System

Key Anatomy Terms:

- **Nares:** Nostrils
- **Nasopharynx:** Upper throat behind nose
- **Oropharynx:** Middle throat behind mouth
- **Laryngopharynx:** Lower throat
- **Epiglottis:** Airway covering flap
- **Trachea:** Windpipe
- **Bronchi:** Large airway branches
- **Bronchioles:** Small airway branches
- **Alveoli:** Air sacs for gas exchange

Common Conditions:

- **Asthma:** Airway constriction disease
- **COPD:** Chronic obstructive pulmonary disease
- **Pneumonia:** Lung infection
- **Bronchitis:** Airway inflammation
- **Emphysema:** Air sac destruction
- **Pneumothorax:** Collapsed lung
- **Pleural effusion:** Fluid around lung
- **Tuberculosis:** Chronic lung infection

Common Procedures:

- **Bronchoscopy:** Airway examination
- **Thoracentesis:** Chest fluid removal
- **Lobectomy:** Lung section removal
- **Tracheostomy:** Artificial airway creation
- **Spirometry:** Lung function testing
- **Intubation:** Breathing tube insertion
- **Mechanical ventilation:** Artificial breathing support

Common Medical Abbreviations

Medical abbreviations appear throughout exam questions and code descriptions. Knowing these saves time and prevents misinterpretation.

Frequency of Use Abbreviations (Know These Cold):

Anatomical Abbreviations:

- **CNS:** Central nervous system
- **PNS:** Peripheral nervous system
- **CVS:** Cardiovascular system
- **GI:** Gastrointestinal
- **GU:** Genitourinary
- **MSK:** Musculoskeletal
- **HEENT:** Head, eyes, ears, nose, throat
- **UE:** Upper extremity
- **LE:** Lower extremity

Directional Abbreviations:

- **AP:** Anteroposterior (front to back)
- **PA:** Posteroanterior (back to front)
- **LAT:** Lateral (side)
- **R:** Right
- **L:** Left
- **B/L:** Bilateral (both sides)
- **U/L:** Unilateral (one side)

Condition Abbreviations:

- **HTN:** Hypertension
- **DM:** Diabetes mellitus
- **MI:** Myocardial infarction
- **CVA:** Cerebrovascular accident (stroke)
- **CHF:** Congestive heart failure
- **COPD:** Chronic obstructive pulmonary disease
- **UTI:** Urinary tract infection
- **URI:** Upper respiratory infection
- **DVT:** Deep vein thrombosis
- **PE:** Pulmonary embolism

Procedure Abbreviations:

- **OR:** Operating room
- **ICU:** Intensive care unit
- **ER/ED:** Emergency room/department
- **Pre-op:** Preoperative
- **Post-op:** Postoperative
- **EKG/ECG:** Electrocardiogram
- **CXR:** Chest x-ray
- **CT:** Computed tomography
- **MRI:** Magnetic resonance imaging
- **US:** Ultrasound

Time and Frequency Abbreviations:

- **STAT:** Immediately
- **BID:** Twice daily
- **TID:** Three times daily
- **QID:** Four times daily
- **PRN:** As needed
- **QD:** Daily (once per day)
- **AC:** Before meals
- **PC:** After meals
- **HS:** At bedtime
- **AM:** Morning
- **PM:** Evening

Measurement Abbreviations:

- **mg:** Milligram
- **g:** Gram
- **kg:** Kilogram
- **mL:** Milliliter
- **L:** Liter
- **cm:** Centimeter
- **mm:** Millimeter
- **°C:** Celsius
- **°F:** Fahrenheit

Directional Terms and Anatomical Positions

Understanding spatial relationships is crucial for accurate coding, especially in surgery and radiology codes.

Standard Anatomical Position:

- Body standing upright
- Arms at sides
- Palms facing forward
- Feet pointing forward
- All directional terms reference this position

Primary Directional Terms:

Sagittal Plane (Divides body into right and left):

- **Medial:** Toward the midline (nose is medial to ears)
- **Lateral:** Away from the midline (ears are lateral to nose)
- **Ipsilateral:** Same side (right arm and right leg are ipsilateral)
- **Contralateral:** Opposite side (right arm and left leg are contralateral)

Frontal Plane (Divides body into front and back):

- **Anterior/Ventral:** Front of body (chest is anterior)
- **Posterior/Dorsal:** Back of body (spine is posterior)

Transverse Plane (Divides body into upper and lower):

- **Superior/Cranial:** Above, toward head (heart is superior to stomach)
- **Inferior/Caudal:** Below, toward feet (stomach is inferior to heart)
- **Cephalad:** Toward the head
- **Caudad:** Toward the tail/feet

Extremity-Specific Terms:

- **Proximal:** Closer to point of attachment (shoulder is proximal to wrist)
- **Distal:** Farther from point of attachment (wrist is distal to shoulder)
- **Radial:** Toward radius bone (thumb side of arm)
- **Ulnar:** Toward ulna bone (pinky side of arm)
- **Tibial:** Toward tibia bone (big toe side of leg)
- **Fibular:** Toward fibula bone (little toe side of leg)

Surface and Depth Terms:

- **Superficial:** Near surface (skin is superficial to muscle)
- **Deep:** Away from surface (bone is deep to skin)
- **External:** Outside (external ear)
- **Internal:** Inside (internal organs)

Movement Terms:

- **Flexion:** Decreasing joint angle (bending elbow)
- **Extension:** Increasing joint angle (straightening elbow)
- **Abduction:** Moving away from midline (raising arm sideways)
- **Adduction:** Moving toward midline (lowering raised arm)
- **Rotation:** Turning around axis (turning head)
- **Circumduction:** Circular movement (arm windmill)

Practice Exercises with Answer Explanations

Building terminology skills requires active practice. These exercises test your understanding and help identify areas needing additional study.

Exercise Set 1: Word Part Identification

Question 1: Break down the term "bradycardia" into its component parts and define each:

A) Brady- (slow) + cardi- (heart) + -ia (condition) B) Brad- (wide) + y- (with) + cardi- (heart) + -ia (condition)
C) Bradi- (brain) + card- (record) + -ia (condition) D) Brady- (bad) + cardi- (heart) + -ia (condition)

Answer: A Explanation: Bradycardia breaks down as brady- (slow) + cardi- (heart) + -ia (condition), meaning the condition of slow heart rate. This is a common term in cardiovascular coding.

Question 2: What does the prefix "hyper-" mean in medical terminology?

A) Below normal B) Above normal, excessive C) Between D) Around

Answer: B Explanation: The prefix "hyper-" means above normal or excessive, as in hypertension (high blood pressure) or hyperthyroidism (excessive thyroid function).

Question 3: The suffix "-ectomy" indicates:

A) Inflammation B) Study of C) Surgical removal D) Disease condition

Answer: C Explanation: The suffix "-ectomy" means surgical removal, as in appendectomy (appendix removal) or cholecystectomy (gallbladder removal). This is one of the most common surgical suffixes.

Exercise Set 2: Body System Terminology

Question 4: Which term refers to the windpipe?

A) Bronchus B) Trachea C) Larynx D) Pharynx

Answer: B Explanation: The trachea is the windpipe, the main airway that connects the larynx to the bronchi. This term appears frequently in respiratory system coding.

Question 5: The term "myocardial" refers to:

A) Heart covering B) Heart muscle C) Heart chamber D) Heart valve

Answer: B Explanation: Myocardial refers to the heart muscle (myocardium). This term is crucial for coding conditions like myocardial infarction (heart attack).

Exercise Set 3: Directional Terms

Question 6: The knee is _______ to the ankle:

A) Distal B) Proximal C) Medial D) Lateral

Answer: B Explanation: The knee is proximal to the ankle because it is closer to the point of attachment (hip). Proximal means closer to the center of the body or point of attachment.

Question 7: Which directional term means "toward the midline of the body"?

A) Lateral B) Medial C) Superior D) Anterior

Answer: B Explanation: Medial means toward the midline of the body. The nose is medial to the ears, for example. This is important for coding bilateral procedures and anatomical locations.

Exercise Set 4: Medical Abbreviations

Question 8: What does the abbreviation "COPD" stand for?

A) Chronic Obstructive Pulmonary Disease B) Coronary Occlusive Peripheral Disease C) Chronic Ongoing Pneumonia Disorder D) Complete Obstruction Pulmonary Defect

Answer: A Explanation: COPD stands for Chronic Obstructive Pulmonary Disease, a common respiratory condition that appears frequently in coding scenarios.

Question 9: The abbreviation "B/L" means:

A) Blood level B) Bilateral (both sides) C) Below limit D) Basic laboratory

Answer: B Explanation: B/L is the standard abbreviation for bilateral, meaning both sides. This appears in many procedure codes and documentation.

Exercise Set 5: Complex Term Analysis

Question 10: Analyze the term "gastroenterocolostomy" by breaking it into components:

A) Gastro- (stomach) + entero- (intestine) + colo- (colon) + -stomy (opening) B) Gas- (air) + entero- (intestine) + colo- (colon) + -stomy (opening) C) Gastro- (stomach) + enter- (enter) + colo- (color) + -stomy (study) D) Gastro- (stomach) + entero- (intestine) + colos- (large) + -tomy (cutting)

Answer: A Explanation: Gastroenterocolostomy breaks down as gastro- (stomach) + entero- (intestine) + colo- (colon) + -stomy (surgical opening/connection), referring to a surgical connection between stomach, intestine, and colon.

Chapter 4 Summary

Medical terminology mastery is your foundation for CPC exam success. Key achievements from this chapter:

Word Construction Understanding: You can now break down complex medical terms into prefixes, roots, and suffixes to understand their meaning.

Essential Vocabulary: You've learned high-frequency prefixes, roots, and suffixes that appear in hundreds of medical terms.

Body System Organization: You understand how terminology is organized by body system, making code selection more logical.

Abbreviation Recognition: You can interpret common medical abbreviations that appear throughout coding documentation.

Spatial Relationships: You understand directional terms essential for accurate anatomical coding.

Practice Application: You've tested your knowledge with realistic exam-style questions.

This terminology foundation makes everything else possible. As you move through subsequent chapters covering anatomy, diagnosis coding, and procedure coding, you'll find that your terminology mastery accelerates your learning and improves your accuracy.

Remember: Medical terminology isn't just memorization—it's pattern recognition. The patterns you've learned here will help you understand new terms throughout your coding career.

Next, you'll build on this foundation with a comprehensive anatomy and physiology review tailored specifically for medical coding success.

Additional Chapter 4 Practice Questions

Continue building your terminology skills:

Question 11: The term "rhinoplasty" means:

A) Nose inflammation B) Nose surgical repair C) Nose removal D) Nose examination

Answer: B Explanation: Rhinoplasty combines rhino- (nose) + -plasty (surgical repair), commonly known as a "nose job." The suffix -plasty always indicates surgical repair or reconstruction.

Question 12: What does "tachypnea" mean?

A) Slow breathing B) Difficult breathing C) Fast breathing D) No breathing

Answer: C Explanation: Tachypnea combines tachy- (fast) + -pnea (breathing), meaning rapid breathing. This term appears in respiratory condition coding.

Question 13: The prefix "intra-" means:

A) Between B) Around C) Within D) Outside

Answer: C Explanation: Intra- means within or inside, as in intramuscular (within muscle) or intravenous (within veins). This is important for distinguishing administration routes and surgical approaches.

Question 14: Which term means "surgical incision into the chest"?

A) Thoracentesis B) Thoracotomy C) Thoracoplasty D) Thoracoscopy

Answer: B Explanation: Thoracotomy combines thorac/o- (chest) + -otomy (surgical incision). Thoracentesis is puncturing, thoracoplasty is repair, and thoracoscopy is examination.

Question 15: The abbreviation "PRN" means:

A) Prior to now B) As needed C) Patient ready now D) Prescription number

Answer: B Explanation: PRN stands for "pro re nata" (Latin for "as needed"). This appears frequently in medication administration and treatment coding.

Chapter 5: Anatomy and Physiology Review

"The human body is the best work of art." - Jess C. Scott

Accurate medical coding requires more than recognizing anatomical terms—you must understand how body systems work together and how their functions relate to the procedures and conditions you'll code. This chapter provides the anatomical foundation necessary for CPC exam success, focusing on the structures and functions most relevant to medical coding.

You'll learn not just where structures are located, but how they function, how they connect to other systems, and why this knowledge matters for accurate code selection. This isn't a comprehensive anatomy course, but a targeted review designed specifically for coding professionals.

Integumentary System

The integumentary system—skin, hair, nails, and associated glands—represents the body's largest organ system and generates significant coding volume in medical practices.

Skin Structure and Layers

Epidermis (Outermost Layer):

- **Stratum corneum:** Dead, keratinized cells providing protection
- **Stratum lucidum:** Clear layer (only in thick skin like palms/soles)
- **Stratum granulosum:** Granular layer where cells begin dying
- **Stratum spinosum:** Spiny layer providing strength
- **Stratum basale:** Base layer where new cells are produced

Coding Relevance: Skin cancer and lesion codes require understanding of which layer is affected. Melanoma originates in the basal layer, while basal cell carcinoma affects the stratum basale.

Dermis (Middle Layer):

- **Papillary layer:** Upper dermis with blood vessels and nerve endings
- **Reticular layer:** Lower dermis with collagen and elastin fibers
- Contains hair follicles, sebaceous glands, sweat glands
- Houses blood vessels, lymphatic vessels, and sensory receptors

Coding Relevance: Many procedures (biopsies, excisions) specify depth. Understanding dermal involvement helps distinguish between simple and complex repairs.

11 BODY SYSTEMS

Anatomical Reference for Medical Coding

BODY SYSTEMS

1. INTEGUMENTARY
Skin, hair, nails

2. NERVOUS
Brain, spinal cord, nerves

3. CARDIOVASCULAR
Heart, blood vessels

4. RESPIRATORY
Lungs, airways, trachea

5. DIGESTIVE
Stomach, intestines, liver

6. URINARY
Kidneys, bladder, ureters

7. MUSCULOSKELETAL
Bones, muscles, joints

8. ENDOCRINE
Glands, hormones

9. LYMPHATIC
Lymph nodes, spleen

10. REPRODUCTIVE
Reproductive organs

11. SENSORY ORGANS
Eyes, ears, nose, tongue

CODING TIP:
Each system corresponds to specific ICD-10-CM code chapters

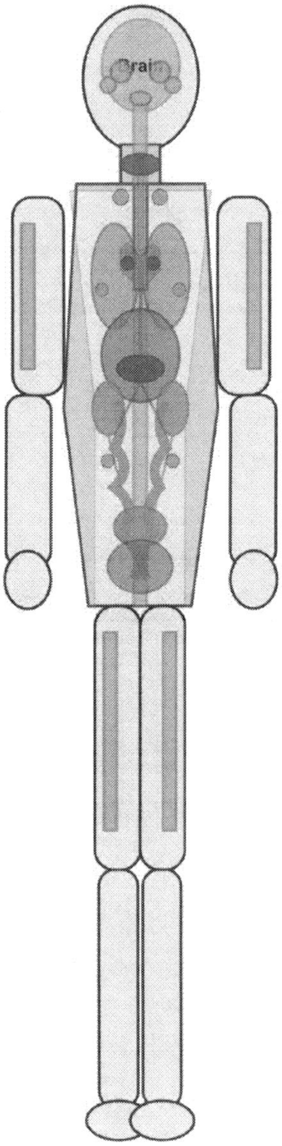

KEY FUNCTIONS

Integumentary:
Protection, temperature regulation

Nervous:
Control, coordination, sensation

Cardiovascular:
Blood circulation, oxygen transport

Respiratory:
Gas exchange, oxygen intake

Digestive:
Food breakdown, nutrient absorption

Urinary:
Waste filtration, fluid balance

Musculoskeletal:
Movement, support, protection

Endocrine:
Hormone production, regulation

Lymphatic:
Immunity, fluid balance

Reproductive:
Reproduction, hormone production

Sensory Organs:
Vision, hearing, taste, smell, touch

EXAM PREPARATION TIP

Understanding body systems helps you:

- Navigate ICD-10-CM chapters
- Identify correct CPT sections
- Understand medical reports
- Link diagnoses to procedures
- Answer scenario questions

Anatomical Position: Body facing forward, palms facing forward, feet slightly apart

Hypodermis/Subcutaneous Layer:

- Fatty tissue layer below dermis
- Provides insulation and energy storage
- Contains larger blood vessels and nerves
- Connects skin to underlying fascia

Coding Relevance: Subcutaneous injections, implant procedures, and deep tissue infections require understanding of this layer's extent and contents.

Skin Functions (Important for Pathology Understanding):

- **Protection:** Physical barrier against pathogens and trauma
- **Temperature regulation:** Through blood vessel dilation/constriction and sweating
- **Sensation:** Touch, pressure, temperature, pain reception
- **Synthesis:** Vitamin D production from sunlight
- **Excretion:** Waste elimination through sweat
- **Water regulation:** Prevents dehydration

Common Integumentary Conditions and Coding Implications:

Lesion Types:

- **Benign:** Non-cancerous (lipomas, cysts, moles)
- **Malignant:** Cancerous (melanoma, basal cell carcinoma, squamous cell carcinoma)
- **Pre-malignant:** Potentially cancerous (actinic keratosis)

Wound Classifications:

- **Superficial:** Epidermis only
- **Partial thickness:** Through epidermis into dermis
- **Full thickness:** Through all skin layers into subcutaneous tissue
- **Complex:** Involving muscle, bone, or organs

Repair Types:

- **Simple:** Superficial wounds requiring minimal closure
- **Intermediate:** Deeper wounds requiring layered closure
- **Complex:** Extensive wounds requiring complex reconstruction

Musculoskeletal System

The musculoskeletal system provides structure, support, and movement. Understanding bone and muscle anatomy is essential for coding fractures, surgeries, and therapeutic procedures.

Bone Tissue Types:

- **Cortical (compact) bone:** Dense outer layer providing strength
- **Cancellous (spongy) bone:** Inner trabecular network containing marrow
- **Periosteum:** Outer bone covering membrane containing blood vessels
- **Endosteum:** Inner bone lining

Bone Anatomy:

- **Diaphysis:** Shaft or main portion
- **Epiphysis:** Ends of long bones
- **Metaphysis:** Region between shaft and end
- **Epiphyseal plate:** Growth plate in developing bones
- **Medullary cavity:** Hollow center containing bone marrow

Coding Relevance: Fracture codes often specify anatomical location (shaft vs. end). Understanding epiphyseal involvement is crucial for pediatric fracture coding.

Bone Functions:

- **Support:** Framework for body structure
- **Protection:** Shield for vital organs (skull protects brain, ribs protect heart and lungs)

- **Movement:** Attachment points for muscles enabling locomotion
- **Mineral storage:** Calcium and phosphorus reservoir
- **Blood cell production:** Red marrow produces blood cells (hematopoiesis)

Joint Classifications:

By Structure:

- **Fibrous joints:** Connected by fibrous tissue (skull sutures)
- **Cartilaginous joints:** Connected by cartilage (vertebral discs)
- **Synovial joints:** Freely movable with joint cavity (knee, shoulder)

By Movement:

- **Immovable (synarthroses):** No movement (skull sutures)
- **Slightly movable (amphiarthroses):** Limited movement (vertebrae)
- **Freely movable (diarthroses):** Full range movement (ball and socket joints)

Coding Relevance: Joint replacement procedures require understanding of joint types. Arthroscopy procedures are limited to synovial joints.

Major Bone Groups and Coding Significance:

Axial Skeleton:

- **Skull:** 22 bones including cranium and facial bones
- **Vertebral column:** 26 bones (7 cervical, 12 thoracic, 5 lumbar, sacrum, coccyx)
- **Thoracic cage:** 12 pairs of ribs plus sternum

Appendicular Skeleton:

- **Upper extremities:** Arms, forearms, hands (64 bones)
- **Lower extremities:** Thighs, legs, feet (62 bones)
- **Pelvic and shoulder girdles:** Connect extremities to axial skeleton

Muscle Types and Functions

Skeletal Muscle:

- **Voluntary control:** Conscious movement
- **Striated appearance:** Organized contractile proteins
- **Multinucleated:** Multiple nuclei per cell
- **Function:** Body movement, posture maintenance

Cardiac Muscle:

- **Involuntary control:** Automatic rhythmic contraction
- **Striated appearance:** Like skeletal muscle
- **Single nucleus:** One nucleus per cell
- **Intercalated discs:** Specialized connections between cells
- **Function:** Heart pumping action

Smooth Muscle:

- **Involuntary control:** Automatic responses
- **Non-striated:** No visible striations
- **Single nucleus:** One nucleus per cell
- **Function:** Organ wall contractions (digestive tract, blood vessels, airways)

Coding Relevance: Understanding muscle types helps distinguish between procedures (cardiac muscle surgery vs. skeletal muscle repair).

Cardiovascular System

The cardiovascular system transports blood, nutrients, oxygen, and waste products throughout the body. Understanding heart anatomy and circulation is essential for coding cardiac procedures and conditions.

Heart Structure and Function

Heart Chambers:

- **Right atrium:** Receives deoxygenated blood from body
- **Right ventricle:** Pumps blood to lungs for oxygenation
- **Left atrium:** Receives oxygenated blood from lungs
- **Left ventricle:** Pumps oxygenated blood to body

Heart Valves:

- **Tricuspid valve:** Between right atrium and right ventricle
- **Pulmonary valve:** Between right ventricle and pulmonary artery
- **Mitral (bicuspid) valve:** Between left atrium and left ventricle
- **Aortic valve:** Between left ventricle and aorta

Coding Relevance: Valve procedures require precise identification. Understanding normal function helps code repair vs. replacement procedures.

Heart Wall Layers:

- **Epicardium:** Outer protective layer (visceral pericardium)
- **Myocardium:** Middle muscular layer (heart muscle)
- **Endocardium:** Inner smooth lining

Pericardium: Double-walled sac surrounding heart

- **Fibrous pericardium:** Tough outer layer
- **Serous pericardium:** Inner layer with parietal and visceral portions
- **Pericardial cavity:** Space between layers containing lubricating fluid

Coding Relevance: Pericardial procedures (pericardiocentesis, pericardial window) require understanding of these relationships.

Coronary Circulation

Coronary Arteries (Supply heart muscle):

- **Right coronary artery:** Supplies right ventricle and inferior left ventricle
- **Left main coronary artery:** Divides into left anterior descending and circumflex
- **Left anterior descending (LAD):** Supplies front wall of left ventricle
- **Left circumflex:** Supplies side and back walls of left ventricle

Coronary Veins:

- **Coronary sinus:** Main venous drainage into right atrium
- **Cardiac veins:** Return deoxygenated blood from heart muscle

Coding Relevance: Cardiac catheterization and bypass procedures require precise vessel identification. Understanding coronary anatomy helps code intervention procedures accurately.

Blood Vessel Types and Structure

Arteries:

- **Elastic arteries:** Large vessels near heart (aorta, pulmonary artery)
- **Muscular arteries:** Medium-sized distribution vessels
- **Arterioles:** Small vessels controlling blood flow to tissues

Veins:

- **Venules:** Small vessels collecting blood from capillaries
- **Medium veins:** Most veins in body with valves preventing backflow
- **Large veins:** Major return vessels to heart (vena cavae)

Capillaries:

- **Microscopic vessels:** Site of gas and nutrient exchange
- **Single cell layer:** Allows diffusion between blood and tissues

Coding Relevance: Vascular procedures specify vessel type and size. Understanding vessel hierarchy helps select appropriate codes.

Respiratory System

The respiratory system enables gas exchange—bringing oxygen into the body and removing carbon dioxide. Understanding airway anatomy is crucial for coding respiratory procedures.

Upper Respiratory Tract

Nasal Cavity:

- **Nares (nostrils):** External openings
- **Nasal septum:** Dividing wall between cavities
- **Turbinates (conchae):** Bony projections increasing surface area
- **Sinuses:** Air-filled cavities in skull bones
    - Frontal, ethmoid, sphenoid, maxillary sinuses

Pharynx (Throat):

- **Nasopharynx:** Upper portion behind nose
- **Oropharynx:** Middle portion behind mouth
- **Laryngopharynx:** Lower portion leading to esophagus and larynx

Larynx (Voice Box):

- **Epiglottis:** Flap covering airway during swallowing
- **Vocal cords:** Sound production structures
- **Cartilage framework:** Thyroid, cricoid, arytenoid cartilages

Coding Relevance: Many ENT procedures require precise anatomical identification. Understanding sinus relationships helps code endoscopic procedures.

Lower Respiratory Tract

Trachea (Windpipe):

- **Location:** From larynx to carina (T5 vertebral level)
- **Structure:** C-shaped cartilage rings maintaining patency
- **Carina:** Ridge where trachea divides into main bronchi

Bronchial Tree:

- **Main bronchi:** Right and left primary bronchi
- **Lobar bronchi:** Secondary bronchi to lung lobes
- **Segmental bronchi:** Tertiary bronchi to lung segments
- **Bronchioles:** Smallest airways without alveoli
- **Terminal bronchioles:** Final conducting airways
- **Respiratory bronchioles:** First airways with alveoli

Lungs:

- **Right lung:** Three lobes (upper, middle, lower)
- **Left lung:** Two lobes (upper, lower) with cardiac notch
- **Pleura:** Double membrane surrounding lungs
    - Visceral pleura: Covers lung surface
    - Parietal pleura: Lines chest cavity
    - Pleural cavity: Space between pleural layers

Coding Relevance: Lung procedures often specify lobe or segment. Understanding pleural relationships helps code thoracic procedures.

Gas Exchange Process:

- **Alveoli:** Microscopic air sacs where gas exchange occurs
- **Respiratory membrane:** Thin barrier between air and blood
- **Surfactant:** Substance reducing surface tension in alveoli
- **Diffusion:** Movement of gases across respiratory membrane

Nervous System

The nervous system controls body functions through electrical and chemical signals. Understanding neurological anatomy is essential for coding neurosurgical and neurological procedures.

Central Nervous System (CNS)

Brain Structure:

- **Cerebrum:** Largest part with four lobes
    - Frontal lobe: Motor control, personality, decision-making
    - Parietal lobe: Sensory processing, spatial awareness
    - Temporal lobe: Hearing, memory, language comprehension
    - Occipital lobe: Visual processing

- **Cerebellum:** Coordination, balance, fine motor control
- **Brainstem:** Vital functions control
    - Midbrain: Eye movement, reflexes
    - Pons: Sleep, arousal, facial sensation
    - Medulla oblongata: Breathing, heart rate, blood pressure

Brain Protection:

- **Skull:** Bony protection
- **Meninges:** Three protective membranes
    - Dura mater: Tough outer layer
    - Arachnoid mater: Middle web-like layer
    - Pia mater: Delicate inner layer adhering to brain
- **Cerebrospinal fluid (CSF):** Cushioning fluid in ventricles and subarachnoid space

Coding Relevance: Neurosurgical procedures require precise location identification. Understanding meningeal layers helps code procedures like subdural hematoma evacuation.

Spinal Cord:

- **Location:** From medulla to L1-L2 vertebral level
- **Gray matter:** Nerve cell bodies in H-shaped central area
- **White matter:** Myelinated axons in surrounding areas
- **Central canal:** CSF-filled cavity
- **Spinal nerves:** 31 pairs exiting through intervertebral foramina
    - 8 cervical, 12 thoracic, 5 lumbar, 5 sacral, 1 coccygeal

Peripheral Nervous System (PNS)

Cranial Nerves (12 pairs):

1. **Olfactory:** Smell
2. **Optic:** Vision
3. **Oculomotor:** Eye movement, pupil control
4. **Trochlear:** Superior oblique eye muscle
5. **Trigeminal:** Facial sensation, chewing muscles
6. **Abducens:** Lateral rectus eye muscle
7. **Facial:** Facial muscles, taste
8. **Vestibulocochlear:** Hearing, balance
9. **Glossopharyngeal:** Swallowing, taste
10. **Vagus:** Parasympathetic control of organs
11. **Accessory:** Neck and shoulder muscles
12. **Hypoglossal:** Tongue muscles

Spinal Nerves:

- **Sensory (afferent):** Carry sensory information to CNS
- **Motor (efferent):** Carry motor commands from CNS
- **Mixed nerves:** Contain both sensory and motor fibers
- **Dermatomes:** Skin areas supplied by specific spinal nerves
- **Myotomes:** Muscle groups supplied by specific spinal nerves

Coding Relevance: Nerve procedures require specific nerve identification. Understanding distribution patterns helps code nerve blocks and repairs.

Digestive System

The digestive system processes food, absorbs nutrients, and eliminates waste. Understanding GI anatomy is crucial for coding endoscopic and surgical procedures.

Upper GI Tract

Mouth (Oral Cavity):

- **Teeth:** Mechanical food breakdown
- **Tongue:** Taste, swallowing assistance
- **Salivary glands:** Parotid, submandibular, sublingual

Pharynx and Esophagus:

- **Pharynx:** Shared pathway for digestive and respiratory systems
- **Esophagus:** Muscular tube connecting pharynx to stomach
- **Lower esophageal sphincter:** Prevents stomach acid reflux

Stomach:

- **Regions:** Fundus, body, antrum, pylorus
- **Functions:** Food storage, protein digestion initiation, acid production
- **Pyloric sphincter:** Controls emptying into duodenum

Coding Relevance: Upper endoscopy procedures require understanding of anatomical landmarks. Stomach procedures often specify region.

Lower GI Tract

Small Intestine:

- **Duodenum:** First 10 inches, receives bile and pancreatic enzymes
- **Jejunum:** Middle portion, major nutrient absorption
- **Ileum:** Final portion, B12 and bile salt absorption
- **Ileocecal valve:** Prevents backflow into small intestine

Large Intestine (Colon):

- **Cecum:** First portion with appendix
- **Ascending colon:** Right side, ascending toward liver
- **Transverse colon:** Crosses abdomen below stomach
- **Descending colon:** Left side, descending toward pelvis
- **Sigmoid colon:** S-shaped portion leading to rectum
- **Rectum:** Final 6 inches before anus
- **Anal canal:** Terminal portion with internal and external sphincters

Coding Relevance: Colonoscopy and surgical procedures require precise anatomical identification. Understanding colon segments helps code partial colectomies.

Accessory Organs

Liver:

- **Lobes:** Right (larger), left, quadrate, caudate
- **Functions:** Bile production, protein synthesis, detoxification
- **Blood supply:** Dual supply from hepatic artery and portal vein

Gallbladder:

- **Location:** Under right liver lobe
- **Function:** Bile storage and concentration
- **Connections:** Cystic artery, cystic duct leading to common bile duct

Pancreas:

- **Regions:** Head, neck, body, tail
- **Functions:** Digestive enzyme production, hormone production (insulin, glucagon)
- **Ducts:** Main pancreatic duct joins common bile duct

Coding Relevance: Biliary procedures require understanding of ductal anatomy. Pancreatic procedures often specify anatomical region.

Genitourinary System

The genitourinary system eliminates waste and enables reproduction. Understanding these structures is essential for coding urological and gynecological procedures.

Urinary System

Kidneys:

- **Location:** Retroperitoneal, T12-L3 vertebral levels
- **Structure:** Cortex (outer), medulla (inner), pelvis (collection area)
- **Nephron:** Functional unit consisting of glomerulus and tubules
- **Functions:** Filtration, reabsorption, secretion, hormone production

Ureters:

- **Structure:** Muscular tubes connecting kidneys to bladder
- **Length:** Approximately 25 cm each
- **Narrowed areas:** Ureteropelvic junction, crossing iliac vessels, ureterovesical junction

Bladder:

- **Location:** Pelvic cavity behind pubic symphysis

- **Structure:** Muscular wall (detrusor muscle) with urothelial lining
- **Capacity:** 400-500 mL normal capacity
- **Trigone:** Triangular area between ureteral orifices and internal urethral orifice

Urethra:

- **Female:** Short (4 cm), straight path to external opening
- **Male:** Longer (20 cm), passes through prostate and penis
    - Prostatic urethra: Through prostate
    - Membranous urethra: Through urogenital diaphragm
    - Penile urethra: Through corpus spongiosum

Coding Relevance: Urological procedures require precise anatomical identification. Understanding urethral anatomy helps distinguish male vs. female procedures.

Male Reproductive System

Testes:

- **Location:** Scrotum (external for temperature regulation)
- **Functions:** Sperm production, testosterone production
- **Structure:** Seminiferous tubules, interstitial cells

Ductal System:

- **Epididymis:** Sperm maturation and storage
- **Vas deferens:** Sperm transport to urethra
- **Ejaculatory ducts:** Join vas deferens with seminal vesicle ducts

Accessory Glands:

- **Prostate:** Surrounds urethra, produces alkaline fluid
- **Seminal vesicles:** Produce fructose-rich fluid
- **Bulbourethral glands:** Produce pre-ejaculatory fluid

External Structures:

- **Penis:** Corpus cavernosum (2), corpus spongiosum (1)
- **Scrotum:** Contains testes and epididymides

Female Reproductive System

Ovaries:

- **Location:** Lateral to uterus in pelvic cavity
- **Functions:** Egg production, hormone production (estrogen, progesterone)
- **Structure:** Follicles in various stages of development

Fallopian Tubes:

- **Regions:** Infundibulum (fimbriae), ampulla, isthmus, interstitial

- **Function:** Egg transport, fertilization site
- **Length:** Approximately 10 cm each

Uterus:

- **Regions:** Fundus, body, cervix
- **Layers:** Endometrium (lining), myometrium (muscle), perimetrium (covering)
- **Support:** Ligaments maintaining position

Vagina:

- **Structure:** Muscular canal connecting cervix to external opening
- **Fornices:** Recesses around cervix (anterior, posterior, lateral)

Coding Relevance: Gynecological procedures require understanding of anatomical relationships. Cesarean section codes specify approach (lower segment vs. classical).

Practice Questions for Each System

Test your anatomical knowledge with these CPC-style questions:

Question 1: Which layer of skin contains the hair follicles and sweat glands?

A) Epidermis B) Dermis
C) Hypodermis D) Subcutaneous tissue

Answer: B Explanation: The dermis contains hair follicles, sebaceous glands, and sweat glands. The epidermis is the outer protective layer, while the hypodermis (subcutaneous tissue) is primarily fatty tissue.

Question 2: The epiphysis refers to which part of a long bone?

A) The shaft B) The end C) The growth plate D) The marrow cavity

Answer: B Explanation: The epiphysis is the end of a long bone. The diaphysis is the shaft, the epiphyseal plate is the growth plate, and the medullary cavity contains bone marrow.

Question 3: Which heart valve is located between the left atrium and left ventricle?

A) Tricuspid valve B) Pulmonary valve C) Mitral valve D) Aortic valve

Answer: C Explanation: The mitral (bicuspid) valve is located between the left atrium and left ventricle. The tricuspid valve is between the right atrium and right ventricle.

Question 4: The carina is located at which anatomical landmark?

A) Where the trachea divides into main bronchi B) The opening between vocal cords C) The junction of the pharynx and larynx D) The entrance to the nasal cavity

Answer: A Explanation: The carina is the ridge where the trachea bifurcates into the right and left main bronchi, typically at the T5 vertebral level.

Question 5: Which part of the brain controls balance and coordination?

A) Cerebrum B) Cerebellum C) Brainstem D) Diencephalon

Answer: B Explanation: The cerebellum controls balance, coordination, and fine motor movements. The cerebrum handles higher cognitive functions, while the brainstem controls vital functions.

Question 6: The duodenum is part of which organ?

A) Large intestine B) Small intestine C) Stomach D) Pancreas

Answer: B Explanation: The duodenum is the first portion of the small intestine, approximately 10 inches long, where most chemical digestion occurs.

Question 7: Which structure connects the kidney to the bladder?

A) Urethra B) Ureter C) Renal pelvis D) Collecting duct

Answer: B Explanation: The ureter is the muscular tube that transports urine from the kidney to the bladder. The urethra carries urine from the bladder to outside the body.

Question 8: In males, which gland surrounds the urethra?

A) Seminal vesicle B) Bulbourethral gland C) Prostate gland D) Testicle

Answer: C Explanation: The prostate gland surrounds the urethra in males and produces alkaline fluid that neutralizes acidic vaginal secretions during reproduction.

Chapter 5 Summary

Understanding anatomy and physiology provides the foundation for accurate medical coding. Key achievements from this chapter:

System Integration: You understand how body systems work together and affect coding decisions.

Anatomical Precision: You can identify specific structures referenced in code descriptions and medical documentation.

Functional Relationships: You understand how structure relates to function, helping you select appropriate codes for procedures and conditions.

Clinical Context: You can connect anatomical knowledge to common medical conditions and procedures.

Coding Applications: You see how anatomical understanding directly impacts code selection accuracy.

This anatomical foundation supports everything that follows. As you learn ICD-10-CM diagnosis coding, you'll understand why codes are organized by body system. As you study CPT® procedure coding, you'll recognize anatomical references in code descriptions. Your investment in anatomical knowledge pays dividends throughout your coding career.

Remember: Medical coding isn't just about memorizing code numbers—it's about understanding the medicine behind the codes. Your anatomical knowledge makes you a more accurate, confident, and valuable coding professional.

Next, you'll apply this foundation to master ICD-10-CM diagnosis coding, where anatomical precision becomes critical for accurate code assignment.

Additional Chapter 5 Practice Questions

Continue testing your anatomical knowledge:

Question 9: Which bone is commonly called the "collarbone"?

A) Scapula B) Humerus C) Clavicle D) Sternum

Answer: C Explanation: The clavicle is commonly called the collarbone. It connects the arm to the trunk and is frequently fractured in falls and sports injuries.

Question 10: The myocardium refers to which layer of the heart?

A) Outer protective layer B) Middle muscular layer C) Inner smooth lining D) External covering sac

Answer: B Explanation: The myocardium is the middle muscular layer of the heart that contracts to pump blood. The epicardium is the outer layer, and the endocardium is the inner lining.

Question 11: Which structure prevents food from entering the trachea during swallowing?

A) Uvula B) Epiglottis C) Vocal cords D) Soft palate

Answer: B Explanation: The epiglottis is a flap of tissue that covers the airway opening during swallowing, preventing food and liquids from entering the trachea and lungs.

Question 12: The cerebral cortex is part of which major brain division?

A) Brainstem B) Cerebellum C) Cerebrum D) Diencephalon

Answer: C Explanation: The cerebral cortex is the outer gray matter layer of the cerebrum, responsible for higher cognitive functions like thought, memory, and consciousness.

Question 13: Which part of the colon is located in the right lower abdomen?

A) Ascending colon B) Descending colon C) Transverse colon D) Sigmoid colon

Answer: A Explanation: The ascending colon is located in the right side of the abdomen, extending upward from the cecum toward the liver, where it becomes the transverse colon.

Question 14: The glomerulus is found in which organ?

A) Liver B) Kidney C) Spleen D) Pancreas

Answer: B Explanation: The glomerulus is a cluster of tiny blood vessels in the kidney where blood filtration begins. It's part of the nephron, the kidney's functional unit.

Question 15: Which female reproductive structure is the site of fertilization?

A) Ovary B) Uterus C) Fallopian tube D) Vagina

Answer: C Explanation: Fertilization typically occurs in the ampulla of the fallopian tube, where the egg and sperm meet after ovulation.

PART III: ICD-10-CM DIAGNOSIS CODING

Chapter 6: ICD-10-CM Fundamentals

"The beginning of knowledge is the discovery of something we do not understand." - Frank Herbert

Welcome to the heart of medical coding. ICD-10-CM diagnosis coding isn't just about looking up codes in a book—it's about understanding the language of disease and translating clinical documentation into standardized codes that tell the complete story of a patient's health status.

This chapter transforms you from someone who recognizes diagnosis codes to someone who truly understands how to assign them accurately and completely. You'll master the structure that governs over 70,000 diagnosis codes and learn the systematic approach that ensures coding accuracy every time.

The skills you build here directly impact your CPC exam score and your future career success. Every claim, every quality measure, and every healthcare statistic begins with accurate diagnosis coding. You're about to become fluent in the most important coding system in healthcare.

ICD-10-CM Structure and Organization

ICD-10-CM follows a logical hierarchical structure that becomes intuitive once you understand its organization. Think of it as a sophisticated filing system where every condition has its precise place, with increasingly specific categories narrowing down to the exact diagnosis.

The Three-Volume Structure

Volume 1: Tabular List

- Contains all diagnosis codes organized numerically by chapter
- Provides complete code descriptions and instructions
- Includes inclusion notes, exclusion notes, and coding guidelines
- Used for final code verification and selection

Volume 2: Alphabetic Index

- Alphabetical listing of conditions, injuries, and reasons for healthcare encounters
- Provides initial code references for conditions
- Includes cross-references and "see also" notations
- Never used for final code assignment—always verify in tabular list

Volume 3: Procedures (Not used for CPC exam)

- Hospital inpatient procedure codes
- Not tested on CPC exam since it focuses on outpatient coding

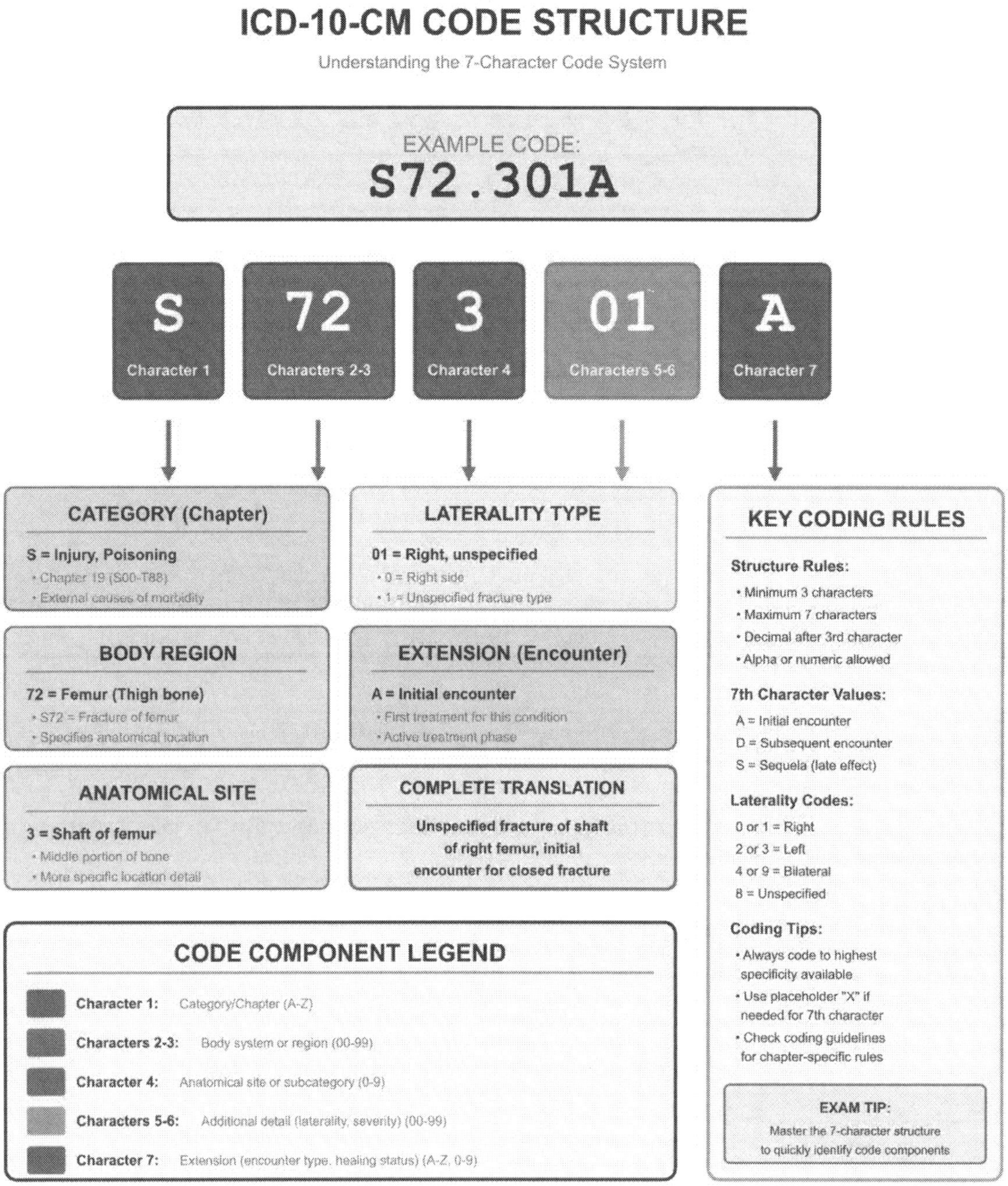

Code Structure and Format

ICD-10-CM codes follow a specific alphanumeric pattern that provides systematic organization:

Basic Format: Letter + 2 Numbers + Up to 4 Additional Characters

First Character (Category): Always a letter (A-Z)

- Indicates the chapter and broad disease category

- Example: K = Diseases of the digestive system

Second and Third Characters (Categories): Always numbers (00-99)

- Provide more specific disease classification within the chapter
- Example: K21 = Gastro-esophageal reflux disease

Fourth Character (Subcategory): Number or letter

- Adds specificity to the three-character category
- Required when available for complete coding
- Example: K21.0 = Gastro-esophageal reflux disease with esophagitis

Fifth, Sixth, Seventh Characters (Sub-classification): Numbers or letters

- Provide maximum specificity available
- Must be used when available
- Example: K21.00 = Gastro-esophageal reflux disease with esophagitis, without bleeding

Understanding Code Hierarchy

ICD-10-CM follows a tree-like structure where each level adds specificity:

Level 1 (Chapter): K00-K95 Diseases of the digestive system **Level 2 (Block):** K20-K31 Diseases of esophagus, stomach and duodenum
Level 3 (Category): K21 Gastro-esophageal reflux disease **Level 4 (Subcategory):** K21.0 Gastro-esophageal reflux disease with esophagitis **Level 5 (Sub-classification):** K21.00 GERD with esophagitis, without bleeding

Coding Rule: Always assign the most specific code available. Using K21 when K21.00 is available would be incorrect and incomplete coding.

Chapter Organization

ICD-10-CM organizes diseases and conditions into 21 chapters based on etiology (cause) or anatomical system:

Chapter 1 (A00-B99): Certain infectious and parasitic diseases **Chapter 2 (C00-D49):** Neoplasms
Chapter 3 (D50-D89): Diseases of blood and blood-forming organs and certain disorders involving immune mechanism **Chapter 4 (E00-E89):** Endocrine, nutritional and metabolic diseases **Chapter 5 (F01-F99):** Mental, behavioral and neurodevelopmental disorders **Chapter 6 (G00-G99):** Diseases of the nervous system **Chapter 7 (H00-H59):** Diseases of the eye and adnexa **Chapter 8 (H60-H95):** Diseases of the ear and mastoid process **Chapter 9 (I00-I99):** Diseases of the circulatory system **Chapter 10 (J00-J99):** Diseases of the respiratory system **Chapter 11 (K00-K95):** Diseases of the digestive system **Chapter 12 (L00-L99):** Diseases of the skin and subcutaneous tissue **Chapter 13 (M00-M99):** Diseases of the musculoskeletal system and connective tissue **Chapter 14 (N00-N99):** Diseases of the

genitourinary system **Chapter 15 (O00-O9A):** Pregnancy, childbirth and the puerperium **Chapter 16 (P00-P96):** Certain conditions originating in the perinatal period **Chapter 17 (Q00-Q99):** Congenital malformations, deformations and chromosomal abnormalities **Chapter 18 (R00-R99):** Symptoms, signs and abnormal clinical and laboratory findings, not elsewhere classified **Chapter 19 (S00-T88):** Injury, poisoning and certain other consequences of external causes **Chapter 20 (V00-Y99):** External causes of morbidity **Chapter 21 (Z00-Z99):** Factors influencing health status and contact with health services

Coding Conventions and Guidelines

ICD-10-CM conventions are standardized rules that ensure consistent code assignment. These aren't suggestions—they're binding requirements that determine correct coding.

Essential Coding Conventions

Includes Notes Provide additional terms that are included in the code category, even if not specifically mentioned in the code title.

Example:

K21 Gastro-esophageal reflux disease
  Includes: newborn esophageal reflux

Coding Application: Even though "newborn esophageal reflux" isn't in the code title, it's included in K21 categories.

Excludes Notes Critical for preventing incorrect code assignment. Two types exist:

Excludes1 (∅): "Not coded here"

- Conditions that cannot be coded together
- Mutually exclusive conditions

Example:

F10 Alcohol related disorders
  Excludes1: alcohol use, unspecified (Z72.1)

Coding Application: You cannot use both F10.- codes and Z72.1 for the same patient encounter.

Excludes2 (∅): "Not included here"

- Condition is not part of the current code but may be coded additionally
- Can be used together if both conditions are present

Example:

K21 Gastro-esophageal reflux disease
Excludes2: newborn esophageal reflux (P78.83)

Coding Application: For newborns, use P78.83 instead of K21, but other conditions may be coded with K21.

Use Additional Code Notes Indicate when additional codes are required to fully describe the condition.

Example:

F10.1 Alcohol abuse
Use additional code for blood alcohol level, if applicable (Y90.-)

Coding Application: Always assign the additional code when documentation supports it.

Code First Notes Indicate that another condition should be sequenced before the current condition.

Example:

G20 Parkinson's disease
Code first underlying disease, such as:
dementia with Parkinsonism (F02.80-F02.81)

Coding Application: List the underlying condition first, followed by the manifestation.

And/Or Conventions

"And": Can be interpreted as "and" or "or"

- N18.6 End stage renal disease includes conditions described as "end stage renal disease" AND/OR "chronic kidney disease requiring chronic dialysis"

"With": Indicates association

- When documentation doesn't specify relationship, assume the conditions are related
- K72.00 Acute and subacute hepatic failure with coma

"See" and "Scc Also" References

"See": Mandatory cross-reference

- Must follow the instruction to find the correct code
- "Heart—see condition" directs you to look under the specific heart condition

"See also": Provides additional information

- May provide alternative or additional code options
- "Abnormal, abnormality—see also Anomaly"

Abbreviations and Symbols

NEC (Not Elsewhere Classified):

- Used when information is available but no specific category exists
- Always check if more specific codes are available

NOS (Not Otherwise Specified):

- Used when information is insufficient for more specific code assignment
- Often indicates incomplete documentation

Brackets [ ]: Provide synonyms, alternative wording, or explanatory phrases **Parentheses ( ):** Contain supplementary words that may be present or absent

Official Guidelines for Coding and Reporting

The ICD-10-CM Official Guidelines for Coding and Reporting provide authoritative instructions for accurate code assignment. These guidelines are updated annually and are legally binding for all healthcare settings.

Section I: Conventions, General Coding Guidelines and Chapter-Specific Guidelines

A. Conventions for ICD-10-CM Reviews the format and structure conventions described above.

B. General Coding Guidelines Establishes fundamental coding principles applicable to all chapters.

Level of Detail in Coding:

- Use highest level of specificity available
- Three-character codes only when no fourth character exists
- Fourth and subsequent characters mandatory when available

Code Assignment:

- Assign codes to highest level of specificity supported by documentation
- Cannot assume conditions not documented
- Query providers for clarification when documentation is unclear

Multiple Coding for Single Condition: Some conditions require multiple codes:

- **Etiology/manifestation:** Underlying condition plus manifestation
- **Use additional code:** Primary condition plus secondary characteristics

- **Code also:** Related conditions that may occur together

Same Diagnosis Code Multiple Times: Generally assign once per encounter unless:

- Different anatomical sites
- Bilateral conditions requiring separate codes
- Different stages or types of same condition

C. Chapter-Specific Guidelines Each chapter has specific rules that override general guidelines when conflicts occur.

Section II: Selection of Principal Diagnosis (Hospital Focus) Primarily applies to inpatient coding but understanding helps with complex outpatient scenarios.

Section III: Reporting Additional Diagnoses (Hospital Focus) Guidelines for reporting secondary diagnoses in hospital settings.

Section IV: Diagnostic Coding and Reporting Guidelines for Outpatient Services

First-Listed Diagnosis:

- Primary reason for encounter
- Condition chiefly responsible for services provided
- May differ from chief complaint

Uncertain Diagnosis:

- Don't code "rule out," "suspected," "probable," or "questionable" diagnoses
- Code symptoms or signs instead
- Exception: Inpatient settings may code uncertain diagnoses as if confirmed

Chronic Diseases:

- Code chronic conditions being managed during encounter
- Include even if not the primary reason for visit

Multiple Diagnoses:

- Sequence according to reason for encounter
- List additional diagnoses that affect patient care

Level of Detail:

- Assign most specific diagnosis code available
- Use appropriate level of specificity for documentation provided

Using the Alphabetic Index

The Alphabetic Index is your starting point for all diagnosis coding, but it requires systematic approach and careful attention to detail.

Index Structure and Organization

Main Terms:

- Listed in alphabetical order
- Usually the condition, disease, or diagnostic term
- Never anatomical sites (except for neoplasms)

Subterms:

- Indented under main terms
- Provide specificity to the main term
- Multiple levels of indentation possible

Example Structure:

Pneumonia J18.9
  aspiration J69.0
    due to
      blood J69.8
      food (regurgitated) J69.0
      gastric secretions J69.0
  bacterial J15.9
    Friedländer's bacillus J15.0
    Hemophilus influenzae J14
    Klebsiella J15.0
  broncho-, bronchial (confluent) (croupous) (diffuse) J18.0

Reading Index Entries

Following the Indentation:

- Each level of indentation adds specificity
- Read main term plus all applicable subterms
- Combine terms to create complete description

Example: "Pneumonia due to Klebsiella" requires:

- Main term: "Pneumonia"
- First subterm: "bacterial"
- Second subterm: "Klebsiella" → J15.0

Cross-References in Index

"See" References:

- Mandatory direction to another main term
- Follow instruction completely before looking up codes

"See also" References:

- Provides additional information
- May offer alternative coding paths

"See category" References:

- Directs to specific category in tabular list
- Review entire category for appropriate code

Special Index Sections

Neoplasm Table:

- Separate table for cancer and tumor codes
- Organized by anatomical site
- Columns for behavior type (malignant, benign, uncertain, unspecified)

Table of Drugs and Chemicals:

- Poisoning and adverse effect codes
- Organized by substance name
- Multiple columns for different circumstances

External Causes Index:

- Injury and poisoning external cause codes
- Describes how injury occurred
- Supplements main injury codes

Common Index Navigation Mistakes

Mistake 1: Coding Directly from Index

- Never assign codes directly from alphabetic index
- Always verify in tabular list
- Index may not show complete code

Mistake 2: Using Anatomical Sites as Main Terms

- Anatomical sites rarely serve as main terms
- Look up the condition affecting the anatomical site
- Exception: Neoplasm table uses anatomical sites

Mistake 3: Ignoring Cross-References

- Always follow "see" references completely
- Consider "see also" references for addiional options
- Cross-references prevent coding errors

Mistake 4: Incomplete Subterm Review

- Review all applicable subterms before selecting code
- More specific subterms take precedence over general ones
- Don't stop at first code that seems appropriate

Using the Tabular List

The tabular list provides complete code descriptions, instructions, and guidelines necessary for final code assignment. This is where coding accuracy is confirmed or corrected.

Tabular List Structure

Code Categories:

- Three-character codes representing general disease categories
- Example: K21 Gastro-esophageal reflux disease

Subcategories:

- Four-character codes providing increased specificity
- Example: K21.0 Gastro-esophageal reflux disease with esophagitis

Sub-classifications:

- Five, six, or seven-character codes providing maximum specificity
- Example: K21.00 GERD with esophagitis, without bleeding

Essential Tabular List Elements

Code Descriptions:

- Complete, official description of the condition
- May differ from abbreviated index descriptions
- Includes all terms covered by the code

Inclusion Notes:

- List conditions included in the code category
- Apply to category and all subcategories unless specifically excluded
- Help clarify code usage

Exclusion Notes:

- Prevent incorrect code assignment

- Excludes1: Mutually exclusive conditions
- Excludes2: Conditions coded elsewhere but may coexist

Instructional Notes:

- "Use additional code" directives
- "Code first" requirements
- "Code also" suggestions

Reading Tabular Entries Systematically

Step 1: Locate the Category

- Find three-character category from index reference
- Read category title and any notes

Step 2: Review Subcategories

- Examine all subcategories within the category
- Identify most specific option for documented condition

Step 3: Check for Required Characters

- Determine if fourth, fifth, sixth, or seventh characters are required
- Assign most specific code supported by documentation

Step 4: Apply All Instructions

- Follow all "use additional code" instructions
- Apply "code first" requirements
- Consider "code also" suggestions

Step 5: Verify Against Documentation

- Ensure selected code matches documented condition
- Confirm all elements of code description are supported

Understanding Code Specificity Requirements

Three-Character Categories:

- Used only when no fourth character subcategory exists
- Rare in ICD-10-CM due to increased specificity requirements

Four-Character Subcategories:

- Minimum specificity for most conditions
- Required when subcategories exist within category

Five+ Character Sub-classifications:

- Maximum available specificity
- Must be used when available and supported by documentation

Example of Specificity Requirements:

Documentation: "Type 2 diabetes mellitus with diabetic nephropathy"

Incorrect: E11 Type 2 diabetes mellitus (too general) **Incorrect:** E11.2 Type 2 diabetes mellitus with kidney complications (insufficient specificity) **Correct:** E11.21 Type 2 diabetes mellitus with diabetic nephropathy (appropriate specificity)

Common Coding Scenarios

Real-world coding requires applying conventions and guidelines to complex clinical scenarios. These common situations test your understanding of ICD-10-CM fundamentals.

Scenario 1: Combination Codes

Documentation: "Acute cholangitis due to choledocholithiasis"

Coding Process:

1. **Index lookup:** "Cholangitis" → K83.09
2. **Tabular verification:** K83.09 Other cholangitis
3. **Check for combination codes:** Look for codes that include both conditions
4. **Better option found:** K80.32 Calculus of bile duct with acute cholangitis, without obstruction

Key Learning: Always check for combination codes that capture multiple related conditions with a single code.

Scenario 2: Etiology and Manifestation

Documentation: "Dementia due to Alzheimer's disease with behavioral disturbance"

Coding Process:

1. **Primary condition:** G30.9 Alzheimer's disease, unspecified
2. **Manifestation:** F02.81 Dementia in other diseases classified elsewhere with behavioral disturbance
3. **Sequencing:** List etiology first (G30.9), manifestation second (F02.81)

Key Learning: Some conditions require dual coding with specific sequencing rules.

Scenario 3: Signs and Symptoms

Documentation: "Chest pain, rule out myocardial infarction. EKG normal, cardiac enzymes normal."

Coding Process:

1. **Don't code:** "Rule out myocardial infarction" (uncertain diagnosis)
2. **Do code:** R06.02 Shortness of breath (documented symptom)
3. **Additional codes:** Any other documented signs/symptoms

Key Learning: In outpatient settings, never code uncertain diagnoses. Code confirmed conditions and documented signs/symptoms.

Scenario 4: External Causes

Documentation: "Closed fracture of right wrist sustained in fall from ladder at home"

Coding Process:

1. **Primary diagnosis:** S62.101A Fracture of unspecified carpal bone, right wrist, initial encounter
2. **External cause:** W11.XXXA Fall on and from ladder, initial encounter
3. **Place of occurrence:** Y92.009 Unspecified place in unspecified non-institutional (private) residence

Key Learning: Injury codes often require external cause codes to provide complete picture.

Chapter 6 Practice Questions

Test your understanding of ICD-10-CM fundamentals:

Question 1: What is the correct order for using ICD-10-CM code books?

A) Tabular list first, then alphabetic index B) Alphabetic index first, then tabular list C) Either order is acceptable D) Only the tabular list is needed

Answer: B Explanation: Always start with the alphabetic index to find potential codes, then verify in the tabular list. The alphabetic index provides initial code references, but final code assignment must be confirmed in the tabular list.

Question 2: An "Excludes1" note means:

A) The condition may be coded with other conditions B) The condition cannot be coded here C) Additional codes are required D) The condition is being deleted

Answer: B Explanation: Excludes1 notes indicate "not coded here" - these are mutually exclusive conditions that cannot be coded together. This prevents inappropriate dual coding of related conditions.

Question 3: Which character in an ICD-10-CM code indicates the chapter?

A) First character (letter) B) Second character (number) C) Third character (number) D) Fourth character (letter or number)

Answer: A Explanation: The first character is always a letter (A-Z) that indicates the chapter and broad disease category. For example, K indicates diseases of the digestive system.

Question 4: When should you assign a three-character category code?

A) When more specific codes are available B) When no fourth character subcategory exists C) When documentation is incomplete D) Never - always use the most specific code available

Answer: B Explanation: Three-character codes should only be used when no fourth character subcategory exists within that category. If more specific codes are available, they must be used.

Question 5: "NOS" in ICD-10-CM means:

A) Not Otherwise Specified B) Not Elsewhere Classified C) New Official Standard D) No Other Symptoms

Answer: A Explanation: NOS stands for "Not Otherwise Specified" and is used when information in the documentation is insufficient for assignment of a more specific code.

Question 6: Which section of the Official Guidelines applies specifically to outpatient coding?

A) Section I B) Section II C) Section III D) Section IV

Answer: D Explanation: Section IV provides "Diagnostic Coding and Reporting Guidelines for Outpatient Services," including rules for first-listed diagnosis, uncertain diagnoses, and chronic conditions.

Question 7: In outpatient coding, how should you handle a "rule out" diagnosis?

A) Code it as if confirmed B) Use the appropriate "rule out" code C) Code the documented signs and symptoms instead D) Do not code anything for that condition

Answer: C Explanation: In outpatient settings, uncertain diagnoses like "rule out," "suspected," or "probable" conditions should not be coded. Instead, code the documented signs, symptoms, or test results.

Question 8: What does a "Use additional code" instruction indicate?

A) The condition is optional to code B) An additional code is required to fully describe the condition C) Multiple codes cannot be used together D) The primary code is incorrect

Answer: B Explanation: "Use additional code" instructions indicate that an additional code is required to fully describe the condition or provide additional important information about the patient's status.

Question 9: Which index should you use to find codes for cancer?

A) Alphabetic Index main entries B) Neoplasm Table C) External Causes Index D) Table of Drugs and Chemicals

Answer: B Explanation: The Neoplasm Table is a separate section of the alphabetic index specifically organized by anatomical site for coding cancers, tumors, and neoplasms of various behaviors.

Question 10: When coding "Type 2 diabetes with diabetic nephropathy," which represents the most appropriate code selection?

A) E11 Type 2 diabetes mellitus B) E11.2 Type 2 diabetes mellitus with kidney complications C) E11.21 Type 2 diabetes mellitus with diabetic nephropathy D) E11 + N18.6 Type 2 diabetes + chronic kidney disease

Answer: C Explanation: E11.21 provides the most specific code available for the documented condition. Always assign codes to the highest level of specificity supported by the documentation.

Chapter 6 Summary

ICD-10-CM fundamentals provide the foundation for accurate diagnosis coding. Key achievements from this chapter:

Structure Mastery: You understand the hierarchical organization of ICD-10-CM and can navigate between the alphabetic index and tabular list effectively.

Convention Application: You can interpret and apply coding conventions including includes notes, excludes notes, and instructional notes to ensure accurate code assignment.

Guideline Knowledge: You understand the Official Guidelines for Coding and Reporting and can apply them to common outpatient coding scenarios.

Systematic Approach: You've learned the step-by-step process for accurate code assignment: index lookup, tabular verification, specificity confirmation, and instruction application.

Common Scenarios: You can handle typical coding situations including combination codes, etiology/manifestation pairs, signs and symptoms, and external causes.

This foundation makes everything else possible. You're now ready to apply these fundamentals systematically to specific disease categories and complex coding scenarios.

The next chapter will take you through ICD-10-CM coding organized by body system, where you'll see these fundamentals applied to real-world diagnostic coding challenges.

Question 11: The abbreviation "NEC" means:

A) Not Elsewhere Classified B) Not Otherwise Specified C) New Electronic Code D) No External Cause

Answer: A Explanation: NEC stands for "Not Elsewhere Classified" and is used when the information is available but there is no specific category for the condition in the classification system.

Question 12: Which type of note indicates mutually exclusive conditions?

A) Includes notes B) Excludes2 notes C) Excludes1 notes D) Use additional code notes

Answer: C Explanation: Excludes1 notes indicate mutually exclusive conditions that cannot be coded together because they represent different manifestations of the same condition or are otherwise incompatible.

Question 13: When you see "Code first underlying disease" in the tabular list, this means:

A) This code should always be listed first B) Another condition should be sequenced before this code C) This code requires an additional code D) This code is the most important diagnosis

Answer: B Explanation: "Code first" instructions indicate that another condition (usually the underlying disease) should be sequenced before the current code, which typically represents a manifestation.

Question 14: In the alphabetic index, what do brackets [ ] contain?

A) Mandatory cross-references B) Synonyms, alternative wording, or explanatory phrases C) Exclusion notes D) Required additional codes

Answer: B Explanation: Brackets [ ] contain synonyms, alternative wording, or explanatory phrases that help clarify the meaning of terms but do not affect code assignment.

Question 15: How should you handle a diagnosis documented as "possible pneumonia" in an outpatient setting?

A) Code J18.9 Pneumonia, unspecified B) Code Z87.01 Personal history of pneumonia C) Code the signs and symptoms present D) Do not assign any code

Answer: C Explanation: In outpatient settings, uncertain diagnoses like "possible," "probable," or "rule out" conditions should not be coded. Instead, code any documented signs, symptoms, abnormal test results, or other definitive findings.

Chapter 7: ICD-10-CM by Body System

"Excellence is never an accident. It is always the result of high intention, sincere effort, and intelligent execution." - Aristotle

Now that you've mastered ICD-10-CM fundamentals, it's time to apply that knowledge systematically across all body systems. This chapter organizes diagnosis coding by anatomical system, showing you how diseases and conditions are classified, coded, and sequenced within each specialty area.

You'll discover patterns within each chapter that make coding more intuitive, learn system-specific guidelines that override general rules, and master the complex conditions that frequently appear on the CPC exam. This isn't just a code list—it's your roadmap to confident, accurate coding across all medical specialties.

Each section builds your expertise with real-world examples, common pitfalls, and strategic insights that separate successful coders from those who struggle. By the end of this chapter, you'll think like the system architects who designed ICD-10-CM.

Certain Infectious and Parasitic Diseases (A00-B99)

Infectious disease coding requires understanding disease processes, causative organisms, and complex relationships between infections and other conditions. This chapter sets important precedents for combination coding and sequencing rules used throughout ICD-10-CM.

Chapter Organization and Key Concepts

Block Structure:

- A00-A09: Intestinal infectious diseases
- A15-A19: Tuberculosis
- A20-A28: Certain zoonotic bacterial diseases
- A30-A49: Other bacterial diseases
- A50-A64: Infections with a predominantly sexual mode of transmission
- A65-A69: Other spirochetal diseases
- A70-A74: Other diseases caused by chlamydiae
- A75-A79: Rickettsioses
- A80-A89: Viral and prion infections of the central nervous system
- A90-A99: Arthropod-borne viral fevers and viral hemorrhagic fevers
- B00-B09: Viral infections characterized by skin and mucous membrane lesions
- B10: Other human herpesviruses
- B15-B19: Viral hepatitis
- B20: Human immunodeficiency virus [HIV] disease
- B25-B34: Other viral diseases
- B35-B49: Mycoses (fungal infections)
- B50-B64: Protozoal diseases

- B65-B83: Helminthiases (worm infections)
- B85-B89: Pediculosis, acariasis and other infestations
- B90-B94: Sequelae of infectious and parasitic diseases
- B95-B97: Bacterial and viral infectious agents
- B99: Other infectious diseases

ICD-10-CM CHAPTER REFERENCE CHART

Complete Guide to All 21 Diagnosis Code Chapters

CHAPTER	CODE RANGE	DESCRIPTION
1	A00-B99	Certain Infectious and Parasitic Diseases
2	C00-D49	Neoplasms (Tumors, Cancer)
3	D50-D89	Diseases of the Blood and Blood-Forming Organs
4	E00-E89	Endocrine, Nutritional and Metabolic Diseases
5	F01-F99	Mental, Behavioral and Neurodevelopmental Disorders
6	G00-G99	Diseases of the Nervous System
7	H00-H59	Diseases of the Eye and Adnexa
8	H60-H95	Diseases of the Ear and Mastoid Process
9	I00-I99	Diseases of the Circulatory System
10	J00-J99	Diseases of the Respiratory System
11	K00-K95	Diseases of the Digestive System
12	L00-L99	Diseases of the Skin and Subcutaneous Tissue
13	M00-M99	Diseases of the Musculoskeletal System and Connective Tissue
14	N00-N99	Diseases of the Genitourinary System
15	O00-O9A	Pregnancy, Childbirth and the Puerperium
16	P00-P96	Certain Conditions Originating in the Perinatal Period
17	Q00-Q99	Congenital Malformations, Deformations and Chromosomal Abnormalities
18	R00-R99	Symptoms, Signs and Abnormal Clinical and Laboratory Findings
19	S00-T88	Injury, Poisoning and Certain Other Consequences of External Causes
20	V00-Y99	External Causes of Morbidity
21	Z00-Z99	Factors Influencing Health Status and Contact with Health Services
U	U00-U85	Codes for Special Purposes (Emergency use, e.g., COVID-19)

MEMORIZATION TIPS

✓ **Use the alphabet pattern:**
A-B = Infectious, C-D = Neoplasms, E = Endocrine

✓ **Associate icons with chapters:**
Visual memory helps recall chapter content faster

✓ **Focus on high-frequency chapters:**
Chapters 9, 10, 13, 19, and 21 appear most often

CODING NOTES

! Chapter U codes (U00-U85):
Reserved for emergency use and provisional assignments

! Always code to highest specificity:
Use 4th, 5th, 6th, or 7th characters when available

! Refer to coding guidelines:
Each chapter has specific coding conventions and rules

Organism Identification: Many infectious disease codes include the specific causative organism. When documented, assign the most specific code available.

Example:

- J15.9 Unspecified bacterial pneumonia (organism not specified)
- J15.0 Pneumonia due to Klebsiella pneumoniae (organism specified)

Combination vs. Multiple Codes: Some infections require combination codes, others need separate codes for infection and organism.

Combination Code Example: A41.01 Sepsis due to Methicillin susceptible Staphylococcus aureus *(Single code captures both condition and organism)*

Multiple Code Example: A41.9 Sepsis, unspecified organism B95.61 Methicillin susceptible Staphylococcus aureus as cause of disease classified elsewhere *(Two codes needed when organism is specified separately)*

Important Infectious Disease Categories

Sepsis and Severe Sepsis (A40-A41)

Sepsis coding involves complex sequencing rules and multiple code requirements:

Basic Sepsis:

- A40.- Streptococcal sepsis
- A41.- Other sepsis

Severe Sepsis:

- Requires two codes:
    1. Underlying sepsis code (A40.- or A41.-)
    2. R65.2- Severe sepsis

Septic Shock:

- Requires three codes:
    1. Underlying sepsis code
    2. R65.21 Severe sepsis with septic shock
    3. Additional codes for organ dysfunction

Coding Guidelines:

- Never assign code R65.1- (systemic inflammatory response syndrome of non-infectious origin) with sepsis codes
- Code underlying systemic infection when known
- Assign additional codes for associated organ dysfunction

HIV Disease (B20)

HIV coding follows specific guidelines that differ from other conditions:

Confirmed HIV:

- B20 Human immunodeficiency virus [HIV] disease (for symptomatic HIV)
- Z21 Asymptomatic human immunodeficiency virus [HIV] infection status (for asymptomatic HIV)

HIV Testing:

- Z11.4 Encounter for screening for human immunodeficiency virus [HIV]
- Z71.7 Human immunodeficiency virus [HIV] counseling

Special Guidelines:

- Only assign HIV codes when HIV status is confirmed by provider documentation
- Never code HIV based solely on positive lab results without provider confirmation
- Code HIV-related conditions as additional diagnoses when present

Viral Hepatitis (B15-B19)

Hepatitis coding requires attention to type, acuity, and complications:

Acute Hepatitis:

- B15.- Acute hepatitis A
- B16.- Acute hepatitis B
- B17.- Other acute viral hepatitis

Chronic Hepatitis:

- B18.- Chronic viral hepatitis

Key Coding Guidelines:

- Distinguish between acute and chronic forms
- Some codes capture both hepatitis and associated complications
- Delta hepatitis (B17.0) requires coexisting hepatitis B infection

Tuberculosis (A15-A19)

TB coding requires understanding of anatomical sites and disease activity:

Active Tuberculosis:

- A15.- Respiratory tuberculosis
- A17.- Tuberculosis of nervous system
- A18.- Tuberculosis of other organs

Latent Tuberculosis:

- Z87.891 Personal history of nicotine dependence

Coding Guidelines:

- Active TB requires confirmation by provider
- Code anatomical site when specified
- Use additional codes for HIV if present

Neoplasms (C00-D49)

Neoplasm coding involves complex decision-making about behavior, morphology, and anatomical sites. The Neoplasm Table is your primary tool, but understanding underlying principles prevents costly mistakes.

Understanding Neoplasm Behavior

Malignant Primary (C00-C96):

- Original cancer site
- Most specific anatomical location
- Includes metastatic cancer originating from this site

Malignant Secondary (C77-C79):

- Cancer that has spread to this site
- Always indicates metastasis from another site
- Requires primary site coding when known

Ca in situ (D00-D09):

- Abnormal cells confined to original location
- Not yet invasive but pre-malignant
- Different treatment and prognosis than invasive cancer

Benign (D10-D36):

- Non-cancerous growths
- Don't spread to other locations
- Generally good prognosis with treatment

Uncertain Behavior (D37-D48):

- Pathologist cannot determine if benign or malignant
- Requires additional testing or monitoring
- Use only when specifically documented

Unspecified Behavior (D49.-):

- Insufficient information for behavior determination
- Use sparingly and only when no additional information available

Using the Neoplasm Table Effectively

Table Organization:

- Anatomical sites listed alphabetically
- Six columns for different behaviors:
  - Malignant Primary
  - Malignant Secondary
  - Ca in situ
  - Benign
  - Uncertain Behavior
  - Unspecified Behavior

Reading Table Entries:

Example: Lung, upper lobe

```
              Malignant
             Primary  Secondary  Ca in situ  Benign  Uncertain  Unspecified
lung, upper   C34.1-    C78.0-     D02.2-    D14.3-  D38.1      D49.1
lobe
```

Selecting Appropriate Column:

- Documentation: "Primary adenocarcinoma, right upper lobe of lung"
- Selection: Malignant Primary column → C34.10
- Additional: Need 5th character for laterality → C34.11

Common Neoplasm Coding Scenarios

Scenario 1: Primary with Metastasis

Documentation: "Primary lung cancer with liver metastases"

Coding:

1. **Primary site:** C34.10 Malignant neoplasm of unspecified part of unspecified bronchus or lung
2. **Metastatic site:** C78.02 Secondary malignant neoplasm of liver and intrahepatic bile duct

Sequencing: List primary first, then secondary sites

Scenario 2: Metastatic Cancer, Primary Unknown

Documentation: "Metastatic liver cancer, primary site unknown"

Coding:

1. **Secondary site:** C78.02 Secondary malignant neoplasm of liver and intrahepatic bile duct
2. **Unknown primary:** C80.1 Malignant neoplasm, unspecified

Sequencing: May sequence either first depending on focus of treatment

Scenario 3: History of Cancer

Documentation: "Personal history of breast cancer, currently cancer-free"

Coding:

- **Z85.3** Personal history of malignant neoplasm of breast
- **Do NOT use:** Active cancer codes for resolved conditions

Important Neoplasm Guidelines

Primary vs Secondary Determination:

- Primary: Original tumor site
- Secondary: Site where primary tumor has spread
- When documentation states "metastatic to," the site mentioned is secondary
- When documentation states "metastatic from," the site mentioned is primary

Admission for Complications:

- When patient admitted for complication of malignancy, sequence complication first
- Follow with appropriate neoplasm code

Chemotherapy/Radiation Encounters:

- Z51.11 Encounter for antineoplastic chemotherapy
- Z51.0 Encounter for antineoplastic radiation therapy
- Sequence Z-code first, then neoplasm code

Diseases of Blood and Blood-Forming Organs (D50-D89)

This chapter covers anemias, coagulation disorders, and immune system conditions. Understanding pathophysiology helps with accurate code selection.

Anemia Categories (D50-D64)

Iron Deficiency Anemia (D50):

- D50.0 Iron deficiency anemia secondary to blood loss (chronic)
- D50.9 Iron deficiency anemia, unspecified

Other Nutritional Anemias (D51-D53):

- D51.- Vitamin B12 deficiency anemia
- D52.- Folate deficiency anemia
- D53.- Other nutritional anemias

Hemolytic Anemias (D55-D59):

- D55.- Anemia due to enzyme disorders
- D56.- Thalassemia
- D57.- Sickle-cell disorders
- D58.- Other hereditary hemolytic anemias
- D59.- Acquired hemolytic anemia

Aplastic Anemias (D60-D61):

- D60.- Acquired pure red cell aplasia
- D61.- Other aplastic anemias

Coding Guidelines:

- Identify underlying cause when documented
- Use additional codes for associated conditions
- Distinguish between acute and chronic forms

Coagulation Disorders (D65-D69)

Key Conditions:

- D65 Disseminated intravascular coagulation
- D66 Hereditary factor VIII deficiency (Classic hemophilia)
- D67 Hereditary factor IX deficiency (Christmas disease)
- D68.- Other coagulation defects
- D69.- Purpura and other hemorrhagic conditions

Clinical Applications:

- Important for surgical planning
- Affects medication choices
- May require special precautions

Endocrine, Nutritional and Metabolic Diseases (E00-E89)

Endocrine conditions often involve complex relationships between multiple glands and systems. This chapter requires understanding of normal physiology and disease interactions.

Diabetes Mellitus (E08-E13)

Diabetes coding involves understanding type, complications, and management status.

Diabetes Types:

- **E08.-** Diabetes mellitus due to underlying condition
- **E09.-** Drug or chemical induced diabetes mellitus
- **E10.-** Type 1 diabetes mellitus
- **E11.-** Type 2 diabetes mellitus
- **E13.-** Other specified diabetes mellitus

Fourth Character Complications:

- **.0** With hyperosmolarity
- **.1** With ketoacidosis
- **.2** With kidney complications
- **.3** With ophthalmic complications
- **.4** With neurological complications
- **.5** With circulatory complications
- **.6** With other specified complications
- **.8** With unspecified complications
- **.9** Without complications

Fifth Character Specificity: Each complication category has specific fifth characters for detailed complications.

Example: E11.21 Type 2 diabetes mellitus with diabetic nephropathy

Coding Guidelines:

- Type 1 vs Type 2 determination based on provider documentation
- Code all documented complications
- Use additional codes for insulin use when applicable (Z79.4)
- Don't assume type based on age or treatment

Thyroid Disorders (E00-E07)

Hypothyroidism:

- E00.- Congenital iodine-deficiency syndrome
- E01.- Iodine-deficiency related thyroid disorders
- E02 Subclinical iodine-deficiency hypothyroidism
- E03.- Other hypothyroidism

Hyperthyroidism:

- E05.- Thyrotoxicosis [hyperthyroidism]

Other Thyroid Conditions:

- E06.- Thyroiditis
- E07.- Other disorders of thyroid

Nutritional Deficiencies (E40-E64)

Protein-Energy Malnutrition:

- E40 Kwashiorkor
- E41 Nutritional marasmus
- E42 Marasmic kwashiorkor
- E43 Unspecified severe protein-energy malnutrition
- E44.- Protein-energy malnutrition of moderate and mild degree
- E45 Retarded development following protein-energy malnutrition
- E46 Unspecified protein-energy malnutrition

Vitamin Deficiencies:

- E50.- Vitamin A deficiency
- E51.- Thiamine deficiency
- E52 Niacin deficiency
- E53.- Deficiency of other B group vitamins
- E54 Ascorbic acid deficiency
- E55.- Vitamin D deficiency
- E56.- Other vitamin deficiencies
- E58 Dietary calcium deficiency
- E59 Dietary selenium deficiency
- E60 Dietary zinc deficiency
- E61.- Deficiency of other nutrient elements

Mental, Behavioral and Neurodevelopmental Disorders (F01-F99)

Mental health coding requires sensitivity to documentation practices and understanding of complex conditions that often present with multiple symptoms.

Organic Mental Disorders (F01-F09)

Dementia:

- F01.- Vascular dementia
- F02.- Dementia in other diseases classified elsewhere
- F03.- Unspecified dementia

Coding Guidelines:

- Code underlying condition first when applicable
- Use behavioral disturbance codes when documented
- Example: F02.81 Dementia in other diseases classified elsewhere with behavioral disturbance

Substance Use Disorders (F10-F19)

Pattern Recognition: All substance categories follow similar structure:

- **.1** Abuse
- **.2** Dependence
- **.9** Unspecified use

Example Categories:

- F10.- Alcohol related disorders
- F11.- Opioid related disorders
- F12.- Cannabis related disorders
- F13.- Sedative, hypnotic, or anxiolytic related disorders
- F14.- Cocaine related disorders
- F15.- Other stimulant related disorders
- F16.- Hallucinogen related disorders
- F17.- Nicotine dependence
- F18.- Inhalant related disorders
- F19.- Other psychoactive substance related disorders

Fourth Character Specificity:

- **.10/.20** Uncomplicated
- **.11/.21** In remission
- **.12-.19/.22-.29** With various complications (intoxication, withdrawal, psychotic features, etc.)

Mood Disorders (F30-F39)

Major Categories:

- F30.- Manic episode
- F31.- Bipolar disorder
- F32.- Depressive episode
- F33.- Recurrent depressive disorder
- F34.- Persistent mood [affective] disorders
- F39 Unspecified mood [affective] disorder

Coding Considerations:

- Current episode severity when documented
- Psychotic features when present
- Remission status

Anxiety and Stress-Related Disorders (F40-F48)

Common Conditions:

- F40.- Phobic anxiety disorders
- F41.- Other anxiety disorders
- F42.- Obsessive-compulsive disorder
- F43.- Reaction to severe stress, and adjustment disorders
- F44.- Dissociative and conversion disorders
- F45.- Somatoform disorders
- F48.- Other nonpsychotic mental disorders

Practice Questions - Body Systems

Test your understanding of system-specific coding:

Question 1: A patient has acute hepatitis B with hepatic coma. What is the correct code assignment?

A) B16.2 Acute hepatitis B with hepatic coma, without delta-agent B) B16.9 Acute hepatitis B without delta-agent and without hepatic coma C) B18.1 Chronic viral hepatitis B without delta-agent D) K72.90 Hepatic failure, unspecified without coma

Answer: A Explanation: B16.2 specifically identifies acute hepatitis B with hepatic coma. The code includes both the infection and the complication in a single code, demonstrating the combination coding principle in infectious diseases.

Question 2: For a patient with primary lung cancer that has metastasized to the brain, what is the correct sequencing?

A) C78.00 (brain metastases) first, then C34.10 (lung primary) B) C34.10 (lung primary) first, then C78.00 (brain metastases) C) C80.1 (unknown primary) first, then C78.00 (brain metastases) D) Only code C34.10 (lung primary)

Answer: B Explanation: When both primary and secondary sites are known and documented, sequence the primary malignancy first, followed by the secondary (metastatic) sites. This follows standard neoplasm sequencing guidelines.

Question 3: A patient with iron deficiency anemia due to chronic blood loss from gastric ulcer should be coded as:

A) D50.9 Iron deficiency anemia, unspecified only B) D50.0 Iron deficiency anemia secondary to blood loss (chronic) only C) D50.0 and K25.4 Chronic gastric ulcer with hemorrhage D) K25.4 Chronic gastric ulcer with hemorrhage only

Answer: C Explanation: Code both the anemia (D50.0) and its underlying cause (K25.4). The "use additional code" instruction under D50.0 requires coding the source of blood loss when known.

Question 4: For Type 2 diabetes with diabetic nephropathy in a patient using insulin, the correct coding is:

A) E11.9 Type 2 diabetes without complications and Z79.4 insulin use B) E11.21 Type 2 diabetes with diabetic nephropathy only C) E11.21 Type 2 diabetes with diabetic nephropathy and Z79.4 long-term insulin use D) E10.21 Type 1 diabetes with diabetic nephropathy

Answer: C Explanation: Code the diabetes with its specific complication (E11.21) and add Z79.4 for long-term insulin use. The insulin use doesn't change the diabetes type but should be documented with the additional Z-code.

Question 5: A patient in early remission from alcohol dependence should be coded as:

A) F10.10 Alcohol abuse, uncomplicated B) F10.20 Alcohol dependence, uncomplicated
C) F10.21 Alcohol dependence, in remission D) Z87.891 Personal history of nicotine dependence

Answer: C Explanation: F10.21 specifically addresses alcohol dependence in remission. Early remission is still considered active dependence status, not history, so Z-codes for personal history would be inappropriate.

Chapter 7 Summary: Building System Expertise

You've now developed systematic expertise in ICD-10-CM diagnosis coding across multiple body systems. Your achievements include:

Pattern Recognition: You understand how similar conditions are organized within and across chapters, making code location more intuitive.

System-Specific Rules: You've mastered guidelines that apply to specific conditions like sepsis, neoplasms, diabetes, and mental health disorders.

Complex Relationships: You can handle conditions requiring multiple codes, proper sequencing, and combination code selection.

Clinical Context: You understand how disease processes affect coding decisions and documentation requirements.

Practical Application: You can apply this knowledge to real-world scenarios that mirror CPC exam questions and professional practice.

Remember: Every diagnosis tells a story about the patient's health status. Your role as a coder is to translate that story accurately using the standardized language of ICD-10-CM. The patterns and principles you've learned here apply to all remaining body systems and prepare you for the complex scenarios in Chapter 8.

Next, you'll tackle the most challenging aspect of ICD-10-CM: complex coding scenarios that combine multiple systems, sequencing decisions, and special circumstances that separate expert coders from average ones.

Additional Chapter 7 Practice Questions

Continue building your system-specific expertise:

Question 6: Which code represents latent tuberculosis infection?

A) A15.9 Respiratory tuberculosis unspecified B) Z87.01 Personal history of tuberculosis
C) Z22.7 Latent tuberculosis D) A19.9 Miliary tuberculosis, unspecified

Answer: C Explanation: Z22.7 identifies latent tuberculosis infection, where the patient has been infected but doesn't have active disease. This is different from active TB (A15-A19) or personal history of resolved TB (Z87.01).

Question 7: For malignant neoplasm described as "metastatic prostate cancer," the correct interpretation is:

A) Primary prostate cancer only B) Secondary prostate cancer only
C) Primary prostate cancer with unspecified metastases D) Cannot determine without more information

Answer: C Explanation: "Metastatic prostate cancer" indicates primary prostate cancer that has spread elsewhere. Code C61 (primary prostate) plus C79.9 (secondary site unspecified) unless specific metastatic sites are documented.

Question 8: A patient with pernicious anemia should be coded as:

A) D50.9 Iron deficiency anemia, unspecified B) D51.0 Vitamin B12 deficiency anemia due to intrinsic factor deficiency C) D64.9 Anemia, unspecified D) E53.8 Deficiency of other specified B group vitamins

Answer: B Explanation: Pernicious anemia is specifically vitamin B12 deficiency anemia due to intrinsic factor deficiency, which is accurately captured by D51.0.

Question 9: For gestational diabetes in a currently pregnant patient at 28 weeks, use:

A) E11.9 Type 2 diabetes mellitus without complications B) O24.419 Gestational diabetes mellitus, unspecified control C) O99.810 Abnormal glucose complicating pregnancy D) Z87.59 Personal history of other endocrine disorders

Answer: B Explanation: Gestational diabetes in a currently pregnant patient requires an O-code from Chapter 15 (Pregnancy). O24.419 specifically addresses gestational diabetes with unspecified control method.

Question 10: Major depressive disorder, recurrent episode, severe without psychotic features should be coded as:

A) F32.2 Major depressive disorder, single episode, severe without psychotic features B) F33.2 Major depressive disorder, recurrent severe without psychotic features
C) F31.4 Bipolar disorder, current episode depressed, severe, without psychotic features D) F39 Unspecified mood disorder

Answer: B Explanation: F33.2 specifically captures recurrent major depressive disorder, severe episode, without psychotic features. The "recurrent" terminology is key for selecting F33.- rather than F32.- (single episode).

Chapter 8: Complex ICD-10-CM Coding Scenarios

"The expert in anything was once a beginner who refused to give up." - Helen Hayes

You've mastered individual body systems—now it's time to tackle the complex scenarios that separate competent coders from coding experts. Real-world patients don't fit neatly into single categories. They present with multiple conditions, unclear documentation, and situations requiring advanced decision-making skills.

This chapter challenges you with the types of scenarios you'll encounter on the CPC exam and in professional practice. You'll learn to navigate ambiguous documentation, apply complex sequencing rules, and make coding decisions that affect patient care and organizational outcomes.

These aren't just coding exercises—they're the situations where your expertise truly matters. Master these concepts, and you'll approach even the most challenging coding scenarios with confidence and accuracy.

Multiple Diagnoses and Sequencing Rules

Healthcare is rarely simple, and neither is coding multiple conditions. Understanding when and how to sequence diagnoses affects reimbursement, quality reporting, and clinical documentation integrity.

Fundamental Sequencing Principles

Principal/First-Listed Diagnosis: The condition established after study to be chiefly responsible for occasioning the encounter.

Secondary Diagnoses: All other conditions that coexist at the time of admission/encounter, develop subsequently, or affect the treatment received and/or length of stay.

Sequencing Hierarchy (in order of precedence):

1. **Official Guidelines** (most authoritative)
2. **Alphabetic Index** (provides initial guidance)
3. **Tabular List** (includes specific instructions)
4. **Chapter-specific guidelines** (override general rules)
5. **Clinical judgment** (when guidelines don't provide specific direction)

Complex Sequencing Scenarios

Scenario 1: Symptoms vs. Definitive Diagnosis

Documentation: "Patient presents with severe chest pain. EKG shows acute ST-elevation MI."

Analysis:

- Chest pain (R06.02) was presenting symptom
- Acute STEMI (I21.-) is definitive diagnosis
- Sequencing: List definitive diagnosis first

Correct Coding:

- First-listed: I21.9 Acute myocardial infarction, unspecified
- Chest pain not coded separately (integral to MI)

Rule: When symptom is integral to definitive diagnosis, don't code symptom separately.

Scenario 2: Acute Exacerbation of Chronic Condition

Documentation: "COPD with acute exacerbation due to pneumonia"

Analysis:

- Chronic condition (COPD) with acute worsening
- External trigger (pneumonia) identified
- Multiple coding required

Correct Coding:

- First-listed: J44.1 Chronic obstructive pulmonary disease with acute exacerbation
- Additional: J18.9 Pneumonia, unspecified organism

Rule: Code both the exacerbated chronic condition and the precipitating cause when documented.

Scenario 3: Complications of Care

Documentation: "Post-operative wound infection following appendectomy"

Analysis:

- Complication occurred after surgical procedure
- Relationship between procedure and complication established
- Complication sequencing rules apply

Correct Coding:

- First-listed: T81.4XXA Infection following a procedure, initial encounter
- Additional: K35.9 Acute appendicitis, unspecified (if reason for original surgery relevant to current encounter)

Rule: Complications of medical and surgical care are sequenced according to the reason for the encounter.

Combination Codes

ICD-10-CM frequently uses single codes to capture multiple related conditions, reducing coding burden and improving data quality. Recognizing when combination codes exist prevents overcoding.

Types of Combination Codes

Etiology/Manifestation Combinations: Single codes that capture both underlying cause and resulting condition.

Example:

- I25.119 Atherosclerotic heart disease of native coronary artery with unspecified angina pectoris
- Captures both atherosclerosis (etiology) and angina (manifestation)

Disease with Complication: Single codes including primary condition and associated complications.

Example:

- E11.40 Type 2 diabetes mellitus with diabetic neuropathy, unspecified
- Captures diabetes (primary) and neuropathy (complication)

Condition with Acuity/Severity: Single codes specifying both condition and current status.

Example:

- J44.1 Chronic obstructive pulmonary disease with acute exacerbation
- Captures COPD (condition) and acute worsening (status)

Complex Combination Code Scenarios

Scenario 1: Multiple Related Conditions

Documentation: "Hypertensive heart disease with congestive heart failure"

Incorrect Approach:

- I10 Essential hypertension
- I25.9 Chronic ischemic heart disease, unspecified
- I50.9 Heart failure, unspecified

Correct Approach:

- I11.0 Hypertensive heart disease with heart failure
- I50.9 Heart failure, unspecified (additional code per instruction)

Key Learning: Check for combination codes before assigning multiple separate codes for related conditions.

Scenario 2: Poisoning vs. Adverse Effect

Documentation: "Patient took too much prescribed warfarin, developed excessive bleeding"

Analysis:

- Prescribed medication taken as directed vs. overdose
- Determines whether poisoning or adverse effect coding applies
- Documentation indicates overdose ("too much")

Correct Coding:

- T45.511A Poisoning by anticoagulants, accidental (unintentional), initial encounter
- R58 Hemorrhage, not elsewhere classified

Alternative if taken as prescribed:

- T45.515A Adverse effect of anticoagulants, initial encounter
- R58 Hemorrhage, not elsewhere classified

Key Learning: Distinguish between poisoning (wrong dose/substance) and adverse effects (correct medication, unexpected reaction).

Manifestation Codes

Some conditions cannot be coded with combination codes and require dual coding: one code for the underlying etiology and another for the manifestation.

Identifying Manifestation Situations

Mandatory Dual Coding:

- Alphabetic index shows two codes separated by brackets
- Tabular list includes "Code first" or "Use additional code" instructions
- Underlying condition causes secondary condition

Example Structure:

Nephritis diabetic - see Diabetes, nephropathy

Following the cross-reference:

Diabetes, diabetic nephropathy E11.21

But in tabular list:

E11.21 Type 2 diabetes mellitus with diabetic nephropathy
Use additional code to identify stage of chronic kidney disease (N18.1-N18.6, N18.9)

Sequencing Rules for Manifestation Coding

"Code First" Instructions: When found in manifestation codes, sequence the underlying condition first.

Example:

G32.89 Other specified degenerative disorders of nervous system in diseases classified elsewhere
Code first underlying disease, such as:
amyloidosis (E85.-)
cerebral degeneration (G31.9)

Correct Sequencing:

1. E85.4 Organ-limited amyloidosis (underlying condition)
2. G32.89 Other specified degenerative disorders of nervous system (manifestation)

"Use Additional Code" Instructions: Found in etiology codes, indicating manifestation code should be added.

Example:

B37.1 Pulmonary candidiasis
Use additional code to identify manifestation, such as:
pneumonia (J17)

Advanced Manifestation Scenarios

Scenario 1: Diabetic Complications

Documentation: "Type 2 diabetes with diabetic retinopathy, proliferative, with macular edema, bilateral"

Coding Process:

1. **Start with diabetes:** E11.- Type 2 diabetes mellitus

2. **Add complication:** E11.35- with proliferative diabetic retinopathy with macular edema
3. **Add laterality:** E11.353 bilateral

Result: E11.353 (single combination code captures all elements)

Key Learning: Modern ICD-10-CM often provides detailed combination codes that eliminate need for separate manifestation codes.

Scenario 2: Infectious Disease with Neurological Manifestation

Documentation: "Cryptococcal meningitis in AIDS patient"

Coding Process:

1. **Underlying condition:** B20 Human immunodeficiency virus [HIV] disease
2. **Infectious agent:** B45.1 Cerebral cryptococcosis
3. **Manifestation:** Code first instruction in B45.1 indicates HIV disease should be sequenced first

Correct Sequencing:

1. B20 Human immunodeficiency virus [HIV] disease
2. B45.1 Cerebral cryptococcosis

Key Learning: Some conditions require specific sequencing even when combination codes don't exist.

Late Effects and Sequela

Late effects (sequela) represent residual conditions that remain after acute phase of illness or injury has resolved. These scenarios require understanding of time relationships and causation.

Defining Sequela

Time Factor:

- No specific time limit between original condition and late effect
- Can occur immediately or years later
- Original condition may or may not still be present

Causation:

- Clear relationship between original condition and current problem
- Documented by provider as related
- Not coincidental occurrence

Sequela Coding Structure

Seventh Character "S": Many injury codes use 7th character "S" to indicate sequela.

Example:

- S72.001A Fracture of unspecified part of neck of right femur, initial encounter
- S72.001S Fracture of unspecified part of neck of right femur, sequela

Dedicated Sequela Codes: Some conditions have specific sequela codes in appropriate chapters.

Example:

- B94.1 Sequelae of viral encephalitis
- I69.- Sequelae of cerebrovascular disease

Sequencing Rules for Sequela

General Rule:

1. Code describing residual condition (sequela) first
2. Sequela code or injury code with "S" 7th character second

Exception: When sequela code describes both residual and cause, use only the sequela code.

Complex Sequela Scenarios

Scenario 1: Stroke with Residual Effects

Documentation: "Right-sided hemiplegia due to old cerebral infarction 6 months ago"

Coding Process:

1. **Residual condition:** G81.91 Hemiplegia, unspecified affecting right dominant side
2. **Sequela cause:** I69.351 Hemiplegia and hemiparesis following cerebral infarction affecting right dominant side

Wait—there's a specific sequela code!

Correct Coding: I69.351 only (this sequela code describes both the residual and the cause)

Key Learning: Check for specific sequela codes before using general residual + cause coding.

Scenario 2: Late Effect of Injury

Documentation: "Chronic pain in left shoulder due to old fracture of humeral head 2 years ago"

Coding Process:

1. **Residual condition:** M25.512 Pain in left shoulder
2. **Sequela cause:** S42.292S Fracture of other part of upper end of left humerus, sequela

Correct Sequencing:

1. M25.512 Pain in left shoulder
2. S42.292S Fracture of other part of upper end of left humerus, sequela

Key Learning: When no specific sequela code exists, use residual condition first, then injury code with "S" 7th character.

Burns and Corrosions

Burn coding requires understanding of anatomical site, degree, extent, and external cause. Multiple coding is often required for complete documentation.

Burn Degree Classification

First Degree (Erythema):

- Redness, no blistering
- Involves epidermis only
- Generally not coded unless specifically documented

Second Degree (Partial Thickness):

- Blistering present
- Involves epidermis and dermis
- Most common burn requiring medical treatment

Third Degree (Full Thickness):

- Destruction through all skin layers
- May involve subcutaneous tissue
- Requires specialized treatment

Fourth Degree:

- Extends into muscle, tendon, or bone
- Most severe classification
- Life-threatening injuries

Burn Coding Structure

Site-Specific Codes: T20-T25 burns organized by body region with 4th character for specific sites and 5th character for degree.

Example: T22.012A Burn of first degree of left forearm, initial encounter

Rule of Nines for Extent: T31.- codes indicate percentage of body surface burned, important for severity assessment and treatment planning.

Complex Burn Scenarios

Scenario 1: Multiple Burn Sites and Degrees

Documentation: "Patient sustained burns in house fire: 3rd degree burns to chest (8% body surface), 2nd degree burns to both arms (9% body surface)"

Coding Process:

1. **Most severe burn first:** T21.31XA Burn of third degree of chest wall, initial encounter
2. **Additional burns:** T22.20XA Burn of second degree of shoulder and upper limb, except wrist and hand, unspecified site
3. **Total body surface:** T31.11 Burns involving 10-19% of body surface
4. **External cause:** X00.0XXA Exposure to flames in uncontrolled fire in building or structure, initial encounter
5. **Place of occurrence:** Y92.009 Unspecified place in unspecified non-institutional residence

Key Learning: Burn coding requires multiple codes for complete documentation: site/degree, extent, external cause, and place of occurrence.

Scenario 2: Chemical Burns (Corrosions)

Documentation: "Chemical burn from sulfuric acid to right hand, second degree"

Coding Process:

1. **Corrosion code:** T23.601A Corrosion of second degree of right hand, unspecified site, initial encounter
2. **Chemical agent:** T54.2X1A Toxic effect of corrosive acids and acid-like substances, accidental (unintentional), initial encounter
3. **External cause:** X47.XXXA Accidental poisoning by and exposure to other gases and vapors, initial encounter

Key Learning: Corrosions (chemical burns) require different codes than thermal burns and include specific chemical identification.

Fractures

Fracture coding involves complex decisions about type, displacement, encounter timing, and healing status. Understanding orthopedic terminology and healing processes is essential.

Fracture Classification Systems

By Bone Continuity:

- **Complete:** Bone completely broken through
- **Incomplete:** Bone partially broken (greenstick, torus, buckle)

By Displacement:

- **Displaced:** Bone fragments separated or angulated
- **Nondisplaced:** Bone fragments remain in anatomical alignment

By Skin Integrity:

- **Closed:** Skin remains intact
- **Open:** Bone fragments penetrate skin or external wound communicates with fracture

Gustilo Classification for Open Fractures:

- **Type I:** Clean wound <1cm
- **Type II:** Clean wound >1cm without extensive soft tissue damage
- **Type IIIA:** Extensive soft tissue damage, adequate coverage
- **Type IIIB:** Extensive soft tissue damage, inadequate coverage
- **Type IIIC:** Vascular injury requiring repair

Seventh Character Usage for Fractures

Initial Encounter (A, B, C):

- **A:** Closed fracture, initial encounter
- **B:** Open fracture type I or II, initial encounter
- **C:** Open fracture type IIIA, IIIB, or IIIC, initial encounter

Subsequent Encounter (D, E, F, G, H, J, K, M, N, P, Q, R):

- **D:** Closed fracture with routine healing
- **E:** Open fracture type I or II with routine healing
- **F:** Open fracture type IIIA, IIIB, or IIIC with routine healing
- **G:** Closed fracture with delayed healing
- **H:** Open fracture type I or II with delayed healing
- **J:** Open fracture type IIIA, IIIB, or IIIC with delayed healing
- **K:** Closed fracture with nonunion
- **M:** Open fracture type I or II with nonunion
- **N:** Open fracture type IIIA, IIIB, or IIIC with nonunion
- **P:** Closed fracture with malunion
- **Q:** Open fracture type I or II with malunion
- **R:** Open fracture type IIIA, IIIB, or IIIC with malunion

Sequela (S):

- Conditions resulting from fracture after healing is complete

Complex Fracture Scenarios

Scenario 1: Multiple Fractures, Same Bone

Documentation: "Comminuted fracture of mid-shaft and distal third of left femur"

Coding Decision:

- Multiple fracture sites on same bone
- Assign separate codes for each site when different anatomical locations

Correct Coding:

1. S72.352A Displaced comminuted fracture of shaft of left femur, initial encounter
2. S72.402A Unspecified fracture of lower end of left femur, initial encounter

Key Learning: Code each fracture site separately when involving different anatomical locations, even on the same bone.

Scenario 2: Pathological vs. Traumatic Fracture

Documentation: "Spontaneous vertebral compression fracture L1 in patient with osteoporosis"

Analysis:

- No trauma documented
- Underlying disease (osteoporosis) present
- Indicates pathological fracture

Correct Coding:

1. M80.08XA Age-related osteoporosis with current pathological fracture, vertebrae, initial encounter

Alternative if traumatic: S32.010A Wedge compression fracture of first lumbar vertebra, initial encounter

Key Learning: Distinguish between traumatic fractures (S-codes) and pathological fractures (M-codes) based on documentation and clinical context.

Scenario 3: Fracture Healing Complications

Documentation: "Patient returns 12 weeks post-fracture. X-ray shows femur fracture is not healing properly, nonunion present."

Coding Process:

1. **Determine original fracture type:** Was it open or closed?
2. **Identify complication:** Nonunion (delayed healing vs. complete failure)

3. **Select appropriate 7th character:** K, M, or N for nonunion

If closed fracture: S72.301K Unspecified fracture of shaft of right femur, subsequent encounter for closed fracture with nonunion

Key Learning: Subsequent encounter coding requires understanding of healing progress and complications.

Poisoning and Adverse Effects

Drug-related coding distinguishes between intentional and unintentional poisoning, adverse effects of properly administered medications, and underdosing scenarios.

Classification Framework

Poisoning:

- Wrong substance taken
- Correct substance taken incorrectly (overdose, wrong route, etc.)
- Substance taken by wrong person

Adverse Effect:

- Correct substance, correct dose, correct route, correct person
- Unexpected or undesired reaction occurs

Underdosing:

- Taking less medication than prescribed or instructed
- Can be intentional (patient choice) or unintentional (error)

Table of Drugs and Chemicals Navigation

Column Structure:

1. **Poisoning, Accidental (unintentional)**
2. **Poisoning, Intentional self-harm**
3. **Poisoning, Assault**
4. **Poisoning, Undetermined**
5. **Adverse Effect**
6. **Underdosing**

Sequencing Rules:

For Poisoning:

1. Poisoning code first
2. Manifestation codes (symptoms/conditions caused)

For Adverse Effects:

1. Condition/symptom caused by drug first
2. Adverse effect code second

Complex Poisoning/Adverse Effect Scenarios

Scenario 1: Medication Error by Healthcare Provider

Documentation: "Patient received 10mg morphine instead of prescribed 2mg, developed respiratory depression"

Analysis:

- Healthcare provider error = accidental poisoning
- Not adverse effect (wrong dose given)
- Respiratory depression is manifestation

Correct Coding:

1. T40.2X1A Poisoning by other opioids, accidental (unintentional), initial encounter
2. J96.90 Respiratory failure, unspecified, unspecified with hypoxia or hypercapnia

Scenario 2: Properly Administered Medication Reaction

Documentation: "Patient developed severe allergic reaction to penicillin given as prescribed"

Analysis:

- Correct medication, correct dose, prescribed route
- Unexpected reaction = adverse effect
- Allergic reaction is primary condition

Correct Coding:

1. T78.07XA Anaphylactic reaction due to other drug, initial encounter
2. T36.0X5A Adverse effect of penicillins, initial encounter

Key Learning: Sequencing differs between poisoning (poison code first) and adverse effects (reaction first).

Scenario 3: Patient Non-Compliance

Documentation: "Patient with diabetes stopped taking insulin, admitted in diabetic ketoacidosis"

Analysis:

- Patient choice to stop medication
- Underdosing scenario
- DKA is consequence of underdosing

Correct Coding:

1. E10.10 Type 1 diabetes mellitus with ketoacidosis without coma
2. T38.3X6A Underdosing of insulin and oral hypoglycemic [antidiabetic] drugs, initial encounter

Key Learning: Underdosing codes capture intentional or unintentional insufficient medication use.

Advanced Practice Scenarios

Test your mastery with complex, multi-system scenarios that mirror CPC exam difficulty.

Practice Scenario 1: Complex Medical Case

Documentation: "85-year-old female with history of hypertension and diabetes presents with altered mental status. Workup reveals sepsis due to E. coli UTI. Patient develops acute kidney injury secondary to sepsis. Blood cultures positive for E. coli. Patient is on chronic medications including lisinopril for hypertension and metformin for diabetes."

Coding Challenge: Identify all appropriate codes and sequencing.

Analysis Steps:

1. **Primary reason for encounter:** Sepsis (most severe, life-threatening)
2. **Organism identification:** E. coli specified
3. **Source of sepsis:** UTI
4. **Complications:** Acute kidney injury
5. **Chronic conditions:** Hypertension, diabetes (if being managed)

Correct Coding:

1. **A41.51** Sepsis due to Escherichia coli [E. coli]
2. **N39.0** Urinary tract infection, site not specified
3. **N17.9** Acute kidney failure, unspecified
4. **I10** Essential (primary) hypertension

5. **E11.9** Type 2 diabetes mellitus without complications

Key Learning Points:

- Sepsis sequenced first as most serious condition
- UTI coded separately as source (not integral to sepsis code)
- Acute kidney injury coded as complication
- Chronic conditions coded if being managed during encounter

Practice Scenario 2: Surgical Complication

Documentation: "Patient underwent laparoscopic cholecystectomy 5 days ago. Now presents with fever, abdominal pain, and leukocytosis. CT scan shows intra-abdominal abscess. Taken to OR for drainage of post-operative abscess."

Coding Challenge: Distinguish between complication and new condition.

Analysis Steps:

1. **Temporal relationship:** 5 days post-surgery
2. **Clinical connection:** Abscess in surgical area
3. **Provider documentation:** "Post-operative abscess"
4. **Current encounter focus:** Treatment of complication

Correct Coding:

1. **T81.4XXA** Infection following a procedure, initial encounter
2. **K68.11** Postprocedural retroperitoneal abscess

Alternative consideration: If provider doesn't establish causal relationship, might code as:

1. **K68.19** Other retroperitoneal abscess

Key Learning Points:

- Complication codes require provider documentation of relationship
- When relationship established, use complication codes
- Focus on reason for current encounter for sequencing

Practice Scenario 3: Pregnancy with Complications

Documentation: "28-year-old female at 32 weeks gestation presents with severe preeclampsia. Patient has gestational diabetes that has been well controlled with diet. No prior history of hypertension or diabetes."

Coding Challenge: Pregnancy-related conditions require O-codes.

Analysis Steps:

1. **Pregnancy status:** 32 weeks = third trimester
2. **Primary condition:** Severe preeclampsia
3. **Secondary condition:** Gestational diabetes
4. **Encounter focus:** Treatment of preeclampsia

Correct Coding:

1. **O14.13** Severe pre-eclampsia, third trimester
2. **O24.410** Gestational diabetes mellitus in pregnancy, diet controlled
3. **Z3A.32** 32 weeks gestation of pregnancy

Key Learning Points:

- Pregnancy conditions use O-codes, not general medical codes
- Gestational age coded when documented
- Pregnancy complications take precedence in sequencing

Chapter 8 Practice Questions

Test your complex scenario coding skills:

Question 1: A patient presents with acute exacerbation of COPD due to pneumonia. How should this be coded?

A) J44.1 only (COPD with acute exacerbation) B) J18.9 only (pneumonia) C) J44.1 first, then J18.9 D) J18.9 first, then J44.1

Answer: C Explanation: Code the exacerbated chronic condition first (J44.1), then the precipitating cause (J18.9). Both conditions should be coded when documented as the cause of exacerbation.

Question 2: For a patient with "metastatic lung cancer" with no other details, the correct interpretation is:

A) Primary lung cancer only B) Secondary lung cancer only C) Primary lung cancer with unspecified metastases D) Cannot determine without additional information

Answer: C Explanation: "Metastatic lung cancer" indicates primary lung cancer that has spread. Code C78.00 (primary lung) and C79.9 (secondary site unspecified) unless specific metastatic sites are documented.

Question 3: A burn described as "third-degree burn of chest, 8% of body surface" requires which codes?

A) T21.31XA only B) T21.31XA and T31.0 C) T21.31XA, T31.0, and external cause code D) T31.0 and external cause code only

Answer: C Explanation: Burn coding requires the specific site/degree code (T21.31XA), extent code (T31.0 for <10% body surface), and external cause code for complete documentation.

Question 4: For "Type 2 diabetes with diabetic nephropathy, patient uses insulin," the correct coding is:

A) E11.21 only B) E11.21 and Z79.4 C) E10.21 and Z79.4 D) E11.9 and Z79.4

Answer: B Explanation: Code the diabetes with specific complication (E11.21) and add Z79.4 for long-term insulin use. Type 2 diabetes doesn't change to Type 1 just because insulin is used.

Question 5: A patient has a nonunion of a previously closed femur fracture. The correct 7th character is:

A) A (initial encounter) B) D (routine healing) C) G (delayed healing) D) K (nonunion)

Answer: D Explanation: Nonunion represents complete failure of bone healing. For a closed fracture with nonunion, use 7th character "K" (closed fracture with nonunion).

Question 6: Patient took too much prescribed warfarin and developed bleeding. This should be coded as:

A) Adverse effect (T45.515A) B) Poisoning, accidental (T45.511A) C) Poisoning, intentional (T45.512A)
D) Underdosing (T45.516A)

Answer: B Explanation: Taking too much of a prescribed medication constitutes accidental poisoning, not an adverse effect. Adverse effects occur with correct dosing.

Question 7: For sequela of old stroke with current right-sided weakness, use:

A) I63.9 and G81.91 B) I69.351 only C) G81.91 and I63.9S D) G81.91 only

Answer: B Explanation: I69.351 (Hemiplegia following cerebral infarction affecting right dominant side) is a specific sequela code that captures both the residual condition and its cause.

Question 8: A patient develops anaphylactic shock from correctly administered penicillin. Sequence:

A) T36.0X5A first, then T78.2XXA B) T78.2XXA first, then T36.0X5A C) T36.0X5A only D) T78.2XXA only

Answer: B Explanation: For adverse effects, sequence the condition caused by the drug first (T78.2XXA - anaphylactic shock), then the adverse effect code (T36.0X5A - penicillin adverse effect).

Question 9: Combination codes should be used when:

A) Multiple conditions are present B) A single code describes multiple related conditions C) Documentation is unclear D) Provider requests specific coding

Answer: B Explanation: Use combination codes when a single code accurately describes multiple related conditions. Check for combination codes before assigning separate codes for related conditions.

Question 10: For diabetes with multiple complications, you should:

A) Use only the most severe complication code B) Code each complication separately with multiple diabetes codes C) Use the most specific combination code available D) Code diabetes once and list all complications separately

Answer: C Explanation: Use the most specific combination code available that captures all documented complications. ICD-10-CM often provides detailed combination codes for diabetes with multiple complications.

Chapter 8 Summary: Mastering Complex Coding

You've now conquered the most challenging aspects of ICD-10-CM coding. Your achievements include:

Advanced Decision-Making: You can navigate ambiguous documentation and make appropriate coding decisions using available evidence.

Complex Sequencing: You understand sophisticated sequencing rules for multiple conditions, complications, and manifestations.

Specialized Scenarios: You can handle burns, fractures, poisoning, adverse effects, and other complex coding situations that require specialized knowledge.

System Integration: You see how multiple body systems interact and affect coding decisions in real-world scenarios.

Professional Judgment: You've developed the clinical understanding necessary for accurate coding in complex situations.

Remember: Complex coding scenarios test not just your knowledge of codes, but your understanding of medicine, documentation, and the relationships between conditions. The patterns you've mastered here separate expert coders from those who simply look up codes.

You're now ready to apply this diagnostic coding expertise to the procedural side of medical coding. Your next challenge: mastering CPT® procedure coding, where precision meets medical procedures in ways that directly impact healthcare delivery and reimbursement.

The journey continues with even greater rewards ahead. Every complex scenario you've mastered builds confidence for both the CPC exam and your future career as a coding professional.

Final Chapter 8 Practice Questions

Test your mastery of complex ICD-10-CM scenarios:

Question 11: A pregnant woman at 28 weeks with gestational hypertension should be coded with:

A) I10 Essential hypertension B) O13.3 Gestational hypertension, third trimester C) O16.3 Unspecified maternal hypertension, third trimester D) O10.13 Pre-existing essential hypertension complicating pregnancy, third trimester

Answer: B Explanation: Gestational hypertension (hypertension that develops during pregnancy) is coded with O13.3 for third trimester. This is different from pre-existing hypertension complicating pregnancy.

Question 12: For late effects of poliomyelitis with current muscle weakness, code:

A) A80.9 and M62.81 B) B91 only C) B91 and M62.81 D) A80.9 only

Answer: C Explanation: Code the residual condition first (M62.81 muscle weakness), then the sequela code (B91 sequelae of poliomyelitis). Both are needed to completely describe the situation.

Question 13: A patient with breast cancer receives chemotherapy. The encounter is primarily for chemotherapy. Sequence:

A) C50.911 first, then Z51.11 B) Z51.11 first, then C50.911 C) Z51.11 only D) C50.911 only

Answer: B Explanation: When encounter is primarily for chemotherapy, sequence Z51.11 (chemotherapy encounter) first, followed by the neoplasm code. The primary reason for encounter drives sequencing.

Question 14: Multiple trauma with fractures of right femur and left tibia requires:

A) One code for multiple trauma B) Two separate fracture codes C) S06.9XXA Multiple injuries, unspecified D) T07 Unspecified multiple injuries

Answer: B Explanation: Each fracture should be coded separately when involving different bones. Multiple injury codes are used only when specific injuries cannot be identified.

Question 15: Patient admitted for rule-out myocardial infarction. Final diagnosis: chest pain, MI ruled out. Code:

A) I21.9 Acute myocardial infarction B) R06.02 Shortness of breath C) R06.00 Dyspnea, unspecified D) R07.9 Chest pain, unspecified

Answer: D Explanation: In outpatient settings, don't code rule-out diagnoses. Code the documented signs and symptoms. Chest pain is the documented finding after MI was ruled out.

Congratulations! You've completed Part III: ICD-10-CM Diagnosis Coding. You now possess the comprehensive knowledge and practical skills needed to handle any diagnosis coding scenario with confidence and accuracy.

Your diagnostic coding foundation is complete. Next, you'll build upon this expertise as you master CPT® procedure coding, where your understanding of anatomy, medical terminology, and clinical relationships becomes even more critical for success.

PART IV: CPT® PROCEDURE CODING

"Success is not final, failure is not fatal: it is the courage to continue that counts." - Winston Churchill

Welcome to the heart of medical coding where precision meets medicine. CPT® procedure coding transforms complex medical procedures into standardized codes that enable healthcare communication, billing, and quality measurement worldwide. This isn't just about memorizing numbers—you're learning to speak the universal language of healthcare procedures.

Your diagnostic coding foundation now supports everything you'll learn here. The anatomy knowledge, medical terminology, and systematic thinking you've developed will help you master CPT® coding with confidence and accuracy.

Every procedure performed in healthcare requires accurate CPT® coding. From routine office visits to complex surgeries, your coding decisions directly impact patient care, provider reimbursement, and healthcare statistics. The responsibility is significant, but so are the rewards for those who master these skills.

You're about to join the ranks of coding professionals who ensure healthcare runs smoothly behind the scenes. Let's begin this journey together.

Chapter 9: CPT® Coding Fundamentals

"Excellence is not a skill, it's an attitude." - Ralph Marston

CPT® coding success starts with understanding the systematic approach that transforms medical procedures into standardized codes. This chapter builds your foundation for confident, accurate procedure coding that will serve you throughout your career.

You'll discover how CPT® organizes over 10,000 procedure codes, learn the conventions that govern code selection, and master the modifier system that adds precision to your coding. Most importantly, you'll develop the analytical thinking that separates expert coders from those who simply look up codes.

CPT® Structure and Organization

CPT® follows a logical structure designed to organize medical procedures systematically. Understanding this organization helps you locate codes efficiently and ensures you're using the most appropriate codes available.

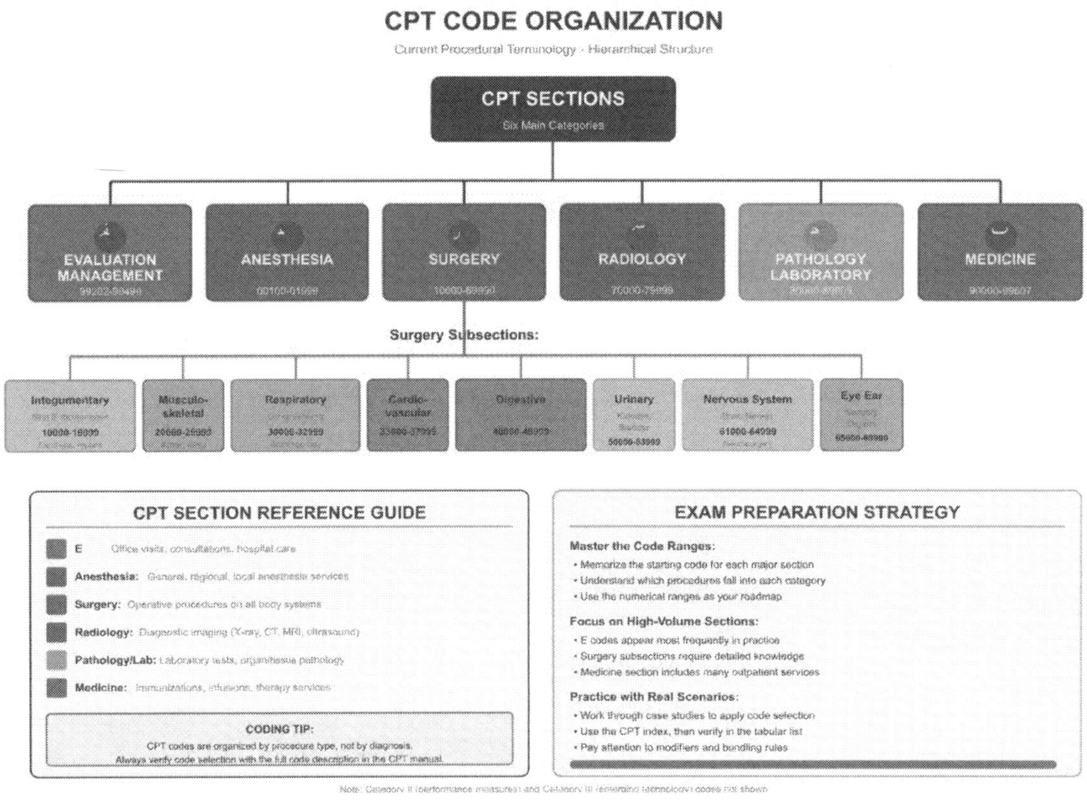

The Six Main Sections

Evaluation and Management (99202-99499):

- Office visits, consultations, hospital care
- Most frequently used codes in medical practices
- Foundation for all other coding decisions

Anesthesia (00100-01999):

- Anesthesia services for surgical procedures
- Organized by anatomical site
- Uses unique base unit + time unit methodology

Surgery (10000-69990):

- All surgical procedures organized by body system
- Largest section with most complex guidelines
- Includes both major and minor surgical procedures

Radiology (70010-79999):

- Diagnostic imaging and radiation therapy
- Organized by anatomical area and procedure type
- Includes supervision and interpretation services

Pathology and Laboratory (80047-89398):

- Laboratory tests and pathological examinations
- Organized by test type and complexity
- Includes both automated and manual testing procedures

Medicine (90281-99607):

- Non-surgical procedures and services
- Immunizations, injections, therapeutic procedures
- Includes various specialized services

Understanding Code Structure

Five-Digit Format: All CPT® codes follow a consistent five-digit structure:

- No decimal points or alpha characters in standard codes
- Consistent length makes codes easy to recognize and process

Category I Codes (10000-99999):

- Permanent codes for established procedures
- Annually updated by the AMA
- Most commonly used codes in medical practice

Category II Codes (0001F-9999F):

- Performance measurement codes (optional)
- End with "F" to distinguish from Category I
- Used for quality reporting and improvement

Category III Codes (0001T-0999T):

- Temporary codes for emerging technologies
- End with "T" to distinguish from Category I
- May become permanent Category I codes over time

Code Range Organization

Each section organizes codes by anatomical site or procedure type:

Surgery Section Example:

- 10000-10999: Integumentary System
- 20000-20999: Musculoskeletal System
- 30000-30999: Respiratory System
- 40000-40999: Digestive System

This organization helps you quickly locate the appropriate code range for any procedure.

Understanding CPT® Guidelines

Guidelines provide the rules that govern proper code usage. These aren't suggestions—they're binding requirements that determine correct code assignment.

Types of Guidelines

Section Guidelines:

- Apply to entire sections (e.g., all Surgery codes)
- Most comprehensive and authoritative
- Override general coding principles when conflicts exist

Subsection Guidelines:

- Apply to anatomical systems within sections
- More specific than section guidelines
- Address common coding scenarios within specialties

Subheading Guidelines:

- Apply to specific groups of related procedures
- Most detailed and specific guidelines
- Essential for complex procedure coding

Category Guidelines:

- Apply to individual code families
- Provide specific instructions for related procedures
- Critical for accurate code selection

Essential Guideline Concepts

Global Surgical Package: Understanding what's included in surgical codes prevents unbundling:

Preoperative Care:

- Related E/M services day before or day of surgery
- Immediate preoperative services
- Local infiltration anesthesia

Intraoperative Services:

- The surgical procedure itself
- Normal, uncomplicated postoperative care
- Writing orders and dictating operative reports

Postoperative Care:

- Follow-up visits during global period
- Postoperative pain management
- Suture removal and wound care

- Return to operating room for complications

Global Period Lengths:

- 0 days: Minor procedures (endoscopies, injections)
- 10 days: Minor surgical procedures
- 90 days: Major surgical procedures

Separate Procedure Concept: Procedures commonly performed alone but may be part of larger procedures:

Code Separately When:

- Performed alone
- Unrelated to other procedures performed
- Performed on different anatomical sites

Don't Code Separately When:

- Part of a larger, more comprehensive procedure
- Performed through same incision
- Considered incidental to main procedure

Professional vs. Technical Components:

Professional Component:

- Physician's interpretation and report
- Uses modifier -26 when billing separately

Technical Component:

- Equipment, technician, supplies
- Uses modifier -TC when billing separately

Global Service:

- Both professional and technical components
- No modifier needed

Modifiers: Purpose and Proper Usage

Modifiers provide additional information about how, where, or under what circumstances procedures were performed. Correct modifier usage prevents claim denials and ensures appropriate reimbursement.

Essential CPT® Modifiers

Modifier -22 (Increased Procedural Services): Use when procedure required significantly more work than typically required.

Requirements:

- Procedure must be substantially more difficult
- Documentation must support increased complexity
- Usually requires special reports

Example: Appendectomy complicated by extensive adhesions requiring 3 hours instead of typical 45 minutes

Modifier -24 (Unrelated E/M Service During Postoperative Period): Use when E/M service during global period is unrelated to original surgery.

Requirements:

- Service must be unrelated to surgical procedure
- Different diagnosis typically required
- Documentation must clearly show relationship

Example: Post-operative patient seen for unrelated diabetes management

Modifier -25 (Significant, Separately Identifiable E/M Service): Use when E/M service and procedure performed same day are both significant.

Requirements:

- E/M service must be significant and separately identifiable
- Different diagnosis or separate problem preferred
- Documentation must support both services

Example: Patient seen for routine physical exam, skin lesion discovered and removed same day

Modifier -26 (Professional Component): Use when billing only interpretation portion of procedure that has both professional and technical components.

Example: Radiologist interpreting X-ray taken at different facility

Modifier -50 (Bilateral Procedure): Use when identical procedure performed on both sides of body.

Requirements:

- Procedure must be capable of being performed bilaterally
- Must be performed during same operative session
- Code description doesn't already specify bilateral

Example: Bilateral carpal tunnel release

Modifier -51 (Multiple Procedures): Use when multiple procedures performed during same session.

Guidelines:

- List primary procedure first (highest RVU)
- Add -51 to secondary procedures
- Some codes exempt from -51 (marked with ⊕)

Modifier -52 (Reduced Services): Use when procedure partially reduced or eliminated at physician discretion.

Example: Planned colonoscopy stopped due to patient condition, only partial examination completed

Modifier -53 (Discontinued Procedure): Use when procedure discontinued due to extenuating circumstances after anesthesia administration.

Modifier -58 (Staged or Related Procedure): Use when procedure performed during postoperative period was planned or related to original procedure.

Requirements:

- Procedure must be planned, staged, or more extensive than original
- Performed during global period
- Related to original procedure

Modifier -59 (Distinct Procedural Service): Use to identify procedures/services that are not normally reported together but are appropriate under circumstances.

Requirements:

- Different session or patient encounter
- Different procedure or surgery
- Different site or organ system
- Separate incision/excision
- Separate lesion
- Separate injury

Anatomical Modifiers

Digital Modifiers:

- F1: Left hand, second digit
- F2: Left hand, third digit
- F3: Left hand, fourth digit
- F4: Left hand, fifth digit
- F5: Right hand, thumb
- F6: Right hand, second digit
- F7: Right hand, third digit
- F8: Right hand, fourth digit
- F9: Right hand, fifth digit
- FA: Left hand, thumb

Eyelid Modifiers:

- E1: Upper left, eyelid
- E2: Lower left, eyelid
- E3: Upper right, eyelid
- E4: Lower right, eyelid

Coronary Artery Modifiers:

- LC: Left circumflex coronary artery
- LD: Left anterior descending coronary artery
- LM: Left main coronary artery
- RC: Right coronary artery
- RI: Ramus intermedius coronary artery

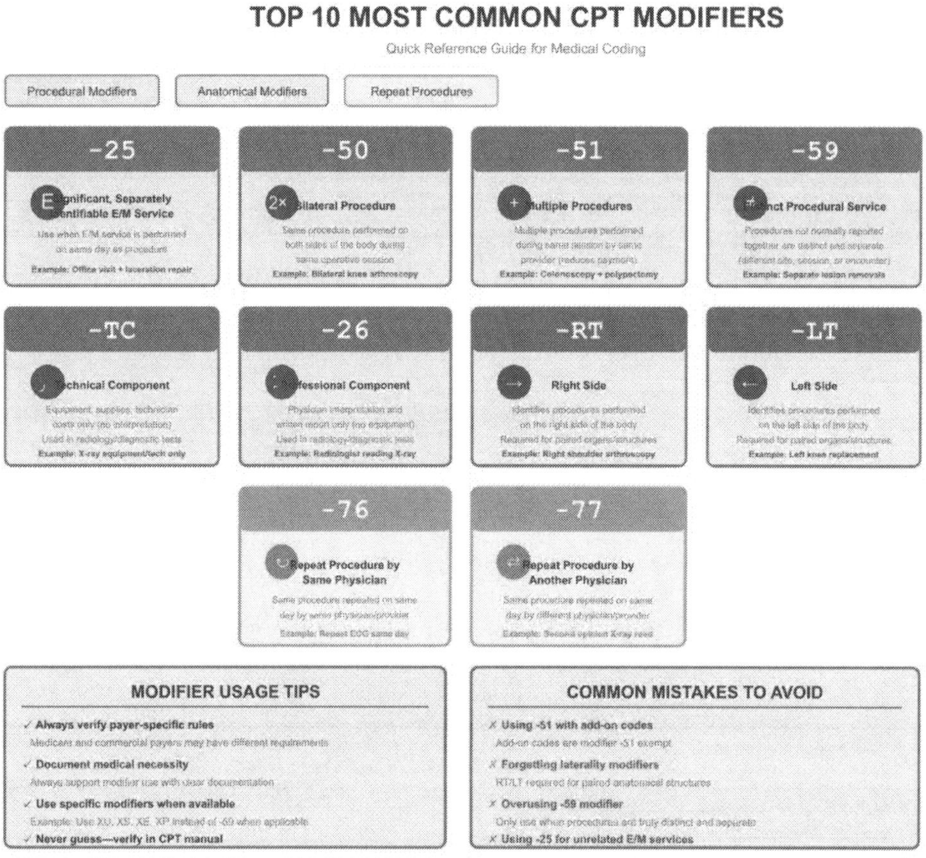

Unlisted Procedures and Category III Codes

When established CPT® codes don't exist for procedures, alternative coding options ensure all services can be reported.

Unlisted Procedure Codes

Purpose: Report procedures/services for which no specific CPT® code exists.

Characteristics:

- End in -99 (e.g., 19499, 27599, 64999)
- Exist in every CPT® section and subsection
- Require special reports explaining procedure
- Often require manual review by payers

Documentation Requirements:

- Detailed procedure description
- Medical necessity justification
- Comparison to similar established procedures
- Operative report when applicable

Example Unlisted Codes:

- 17999: Unlisted procedure, skin, mucous membrane and subcutaneous tissue
- 27599: Unlisted procedure, femur or knee
- 43499: Unlisted procedure, esophagus
- 64999: Unlisted procedure, nervous system

When to Use Unlisted Codes:

- New surgical techniques not yet in CPT®
- Significant modifications of existing procedures
- Combination procedures not covered by existing codes
- Investigational procedures

Category III Codes (Emerging Technology)

Purpose: Temporary codes for new and emerging technologies, services, and procedures.

Identification:

- Four digits followed by "T" (e.g., 0001T, 0123T)
- Updated twice yearly (July 1 and January 1)
- May be archived if not widely adopted

Advantages Over Unlisted Codes:

- More specific than unlisted procedures
- Easier claims processing
- Better data collection for new technologies
- May transition to permanent Category I codes

Tracking and Updates:

- Monitor AMA updates for new Category III codes
- Watch for transitions to Category I status
- Archive codes are deleted from active use

Example Category III Codes:

- 0001T: Endovascular repair of infrarenal aortic aneurysm
- 0071T: Focused ultrasound ablation of uterine leiomyomata
- 0085T: Breath test for heart transplant rejection

Add-on Codes and Exempt Codes

Some procedures require special handling for multiple procedure scenarios and global surgery rules.

Add-on Codes (+)

Identification:

- Marked with "+" symbol in CPT® book
- Cannot be reported alone
- Always used with primary procedure code
- Represent additional work beyond base procedure

Characteristics:

- Never use modifier -51 with add-on codes

- No reduction in reimbursement for multiple add-ons
- May be reported multiple times when appropriate
- Always list after primary procedure

Examples:

- +11001: Each additional 10 sq cm of skin repair (with 11000)
- +22614: Each additional vertebral segment (with 22612)
- +93320: Doppler echocardiography (with 93318)
- +99354: Prolonged physician service (with E/M codes)

Proper Usage:

Example: Excision of three skin lesions, 2.5 cm, 1.8 cm, and 1.2 cm

Correct Coding:
11403 (lesion 2.1-3.0 cm) - primary code
+11402 (lesion 1.1-2.0 cm) - add-on
+11402 (lesion 1.1-2.0 cm) - add-on

Incorrect: Using modifier -51 with add-on codes

Modifier -51 Exempt Codes (⊕)

Identification:

- Marked with ⊕ symbol in CPT® book
- Exempt from multiple procedure payment reduction
- Don't use modifier -51 with these codes

Types of Exempt Codes:

- Add-on codes (already covered above)
- Some radiology codes
- Some pathology codes
- Some E/M codes

Examples:

- 93320: Doppler echocardiography, complete
- 88305: Tissue examination by pathologist
- 93000: Electrocardiogram, complete

Chapter 9 Practice Questions

Test your understanding of CPT® fundamentals:

Question 1: Which CPT® section contains the most codes?

A) Evaluation and Management B) Surgery C) Radiology D) Medicine

Answer: B Explanation: The Surgery section (10000-69990) contains the most CPT® codes, covering all surgical procedures organized by body system. This section includes both major and minor surgical procedures across all medical specialties.

Question 2: Category III codes are identified by:

A) Ending in -99 B) Ending with the letter "F" C) Ending with the letter "T" D) Having six digits instead of five

Answer: C Explanation: Category III codes end with the letter "T" and represent temporary codes for emerging technologies and procedures. They consist of four digits followed by "T" (e.g., 0001T).

Question 3: The global surgical package includes all of the following EXCEPT:

A) Related E/M services the day before surgery B) The surgical procedure itself C) Complications requiring return to OR D) Normal postoperative follow-up visits

Answer: C Explanation: Complications requiring return to the operating room are NOT included in the global surgical package and should be coded separately. The global package includes routine, uncomplicated care only.

Question 4: Modifier -25 should be used when:

A) A procedure is performed bilaterally B) An E/M service and procedure are both significant and performed the same day C) A procedure is discontinued due to patient condition D) Multiple procedures are performed during the same session

Answer: B Explanation: Modifier -25 indicates a significant, separately identifiable E/M service performed on the same day as a procedure. Both services must be significant and separately identifiable.

Question 5: Add-on codes are identified in the CPT® book by:

A) The ⊕ symbol B) The "+" symbol
C) The letter "T" after the code D) Ending in -99

Answer: B Explanation: Add-on codes are identified by the "+" symbol in the CPT® book. These codes cannot be reported alone and must be used with a primary procedure code.

Question 6: When should you use an unlisted procedure code?

A) When you can't find the exact code quickly B) When no specific CPT® code exists for the procedure C) When the procedure is performed bilaterally D) When multiple procedures are performed

Answer: B Explanation: Unlisted procedure codes (ending in -99) should only be used when no specific CPT® code exists for the procedure performed. They require special documentation and often manual review.

Question 7: The professional component modifier is:

A) -22 B) -24 C) -26 D) -50

Answer: C Explanation: Modifier -26 indicates the professional component of a procedure that has both professional and technical components. It's used when billing only the interpretation portion of a service.

Question 8: Which modifier indicates a bilateral procedure?

A) -25 B) -50 C) -51 D) -59

Answer: B Explanation: Modifier -50 indicates that identical procedures were performed on both sides of the body during the same operative session. The procedure must be capable of being performed bilaterally.

Question 9: Modifier -51 (Multiple Procedures) should NOT be used with:

A) The primary procedure code B) Add-on codes marked with "+" C) Bilateral procedures D) Reduced services

Answer: B Explanation: Modifier -51 should not be used with add-on codes (marked with "+") because these codes are already designed to be used in addition to primary procedures and are exempt from multiple procedure payment reductions.

Question 10: The global period for major surgical procedures is typically:

A) 0 days B) 10 days
C) 30 days D) 90 days

Answer: D Explanation: Major surgical procedures typically have a 90-day global period, during which routine postoperative care is included in the surgical code. Minor procedures may have 0-day or 10-day global periods.

Chapter 9 Summary: Building Your CPT® Foundation

You've established the fundamental knowledge necessary for successful CPT® procedure coding. Your achievements include:

Structural Understanding: You know how CPT® organizes over 10,000 codes into logical sections and subsections, making code location systematic rather than random.

Guideline Mastery: You understand the hierarchy of guidelines and can apply section, subsection, and category-specific rules to ensure accurate coding.

Modifier Expertise: You can select and apply the most commonly used modifiers to provide additional information about procedures and prevent claim denials.

Special Situations: You know when to use unlisted codes, Category III codes, add-on codes, and exempt codes for unusual coding scenarios.

Professional Foundation: You've developed the analytical thinking and systematic approach that underlies all expert coding decisions.

This foundation supports everything that follows. As you progress through evaluation and management coding, surgery coding, and other specialized areas, these fundamental concepts will guide your decision-making and ensure your coding accuracy.

Remember: CPT® coding isn't about memorizing thousands of codes—it's about understanding the system and applying consistent principles. The foundation you've built here will serve you throughout your coding career.

Next, you'll apply these fundamentals to master Evaluation and Management coding, the most frequently used codes in medical practice and a critical component of CPC exam success.

Additional Chapter 9 Practice Questions

Continue building your CPT® fundamentals:

Question 11: Which statement about Category II codes is correct?

A) They are mandatory for all procedures B) They end with the letter "F" C) They replace Category I codes D) They are used for experimental procedures

Answer: B Explanation: Category II codes end with the letter "F" and are optional performance measurement codes used for quality reporting. They supplement, but do not replace, Category I codes.

Question 12: The "separate procedure" designation means:

A) The procedure must always be coded separately B) The procedure cannot be performed with other procedures C) The procedure is commonly part of another procedure D) The procedure requires a separate operative session

Answer: C Explanation: "Separate procedure" indicates that the procedure is commonly performed as part of a larger procedure. It should only be coded separately when performed alone or unrelated to other procedures.

Question 13: Modifier -52 (Reduced Services) is used when:

A) A procedure is performed bilaterally B) A procedure is partially reduced at physician discretion C) A procedure is discontinued due to complications D) A procedure requires increased work

Answer: B Explanation: Modifier -52 is used when a procedure is partially reduced or eliminated at the physician's discretion, indicating that less work was performed than typically required for that procedure code.

Question 14: Global surgical package components include:

A) Only the surgical procedure itself B) All services from decision for surgery through complete recovery C) Preoperative, intraoperative, and normal postoperative care D) Any complications that occur during the global period

Answer: C Explanation: The global surgical package includes preoperative care (day before/day of surgery), the intraoperative procedure, and normal uncomplicated postoperative care during the global period.

Question 15: When multiple procedures are performed, they should be sequenced:

A) Alphabetically by procedure name B) By anatomical location C) By the highest RVU (relative value unit) first D) In the order they were performed

Answer: C Explanation: When multiple procedures are performed during the same session, sequence them with the highest RVU procedure first, followed by additional procedures with modifier -51 (unless exempt).

Chapter 10: Evaluation and Management (E/M) Coding

"The expert in anything was once a beginner who refused to give up." - Helen Hayes

Evaluation and Management coding represents the foundation of medical practice—every patient encounter involves some level of evaluation and management. These codes capture the cognitive work physicians perform: thinking, analyzing, deciding, and managing patient care.

E/M coding has evolved significantly with recent revisions that emphasize medical decision-making and time-based coding. Understanding these changes and mastering both traditional and current guidelines will make you a more versatile and valuable coder.

This chapter transforms complex E/M guidelines into practical, applicable knowledge. You'll learn to analyze documentation systematically, select appropriate codes confidently, and handle the most challenging E/M scenarios that appear on the CPC exam.

By the end of this chapter, you'll think like the physicians who perform these services, understanding not just what codes to assign, but why those codes accurately reflect the work performed.

E/M Guidelines and Documentation Requirements

E/M coding success depends on understanding what work these codes represent and how documentation supports code selection. The 2021 and 2023 E/M guideline changes modernized these requirements while maintaining the precision needed for accurate coding.

The Three Key Components (Historical Foundation)

While newer guidelines emphasize different elements, understanding the traditional three key components remains important for many E/M categories:

1. History

- Chief Complaint (CC): Always required
- History of Present Illness (HPI): 1-3 elements = brief, 4+ elements = extended
- Review of Systems (ROS): Constitutional and affected system = problem pertinent, 2-9 systems = extended, 10+ systems = complete
- Past, Family, Social History (PFSH): 1 area = pertinent, 2+ areas = complete

2. Examination

- Problem Focused: Limited to affected body area
- Expanded Problem Focused: Limited body area plus related systems
- Detailed: Extended examination of affected area and related systems
- Comprehensive: General multi-system or complete single system examination

3. Medical Decision Making (MDM)

- Straightforward: Minimal diagnosis/management options, minimal data, minimal risk
- Low Complexity: Limited options/data, low risk
- Moderate Complexity: Multiple options/data, moderate risk
- High Complexity: Extensive options/data, high risk

EVALUATION MANAGEMENT (E/M) TIME-BASED CODING

Office Visit Code Selection Based on Total Time (2023 Guidelines)

CPT CODE	TIME RANGE	COMPLEXITY LEVEL	MEDICAL DECISION MAKING
NEW PATIENT OFFICE VISITS		(99202-99205)	
99202	15-29 minutes	**STRAIGHTFORWARD** Minimal complexity	Self-limited/minor problem
99203	30-44 minutes	**LOW COMPLEXITY** Limited examination	2+ self-limited problems or 1 stable chronic illness
99204	45-59 minutes	**MODERATE COMPLEXITY** Detailed examination	1+ chronic illness with exacerbation or progression
99205	60-74 minutes	**HIGH COMPLEXITY** Comprehensive examination	Severe exacerbation or threat to life/function
ESTABLISHED PATIENT OFFICE VISITS		(99212-99215)	
99212	10-19 minutes	**STRAIGHTFORWARD** Minimal complexity	Self-limited/minor problem
99213	20-29 minutes	**LOW COMPLEXITY** Limited examination	2+ self-limited problems or 1 stable chronic illness
99214	30-39 minutes	**MODERATE COMPLEXITY** Detailed examination	1+ chronic illness with

Current E/M Guidelines (2021/2023 Changes)

Office/Outpatient E/M (99202-99215):

- Level selection based on MDM OR time
- History and examination performed as clinically appropriate
- No longer required to meet specific documentation thresholds

Medical Decision Making Framework: Three elements determine MDM level:

1. **Number and complexity of problems addressed**
2. **Amount and/or complexity of data reviewed and analyzed**
3. **Risk of complications and/or morbidity or mortality of patient management**

Time-Based Coding:

- Total time on date of encounter
- Includes face-to-face and non-face-to-face time
- Specific time thresholds for each level

Understanding Medical Decision Making

Element 1: Problems Addressed

Minimal (1 problem):

- Self-limited or minor problem

Low (2 problems):

- Self-limited or minor problems
- Stable chronic illness
- Acute uncomplicated illness or injury

Moderate (1-2 problems):

- Chronic illness with exacerbation, progression, or side effects
- Undiagnosed new problem with uncertain prognosis
- Acute illness with systemic symptoms
- Acute complicated injury

High (3+ problems OR 1 chronic illness with severe exacerbation):

- Chronic illness with severe exacerbation, progression, or side effects
- Acute or chronic illness/injury that poses threat to life or bodily function

Element 2: Data Reviewed and Analyzed

Categories and Points:

- Tests ordered, reviewed, or interpreted: 1 point each category
- Independent interpretation of tests: 2 points each category
- Discussion with external physician/qualified healthcare professional: 1 point
- Discussion with patient/family/caregiver: 1 point

Complexity Levels:

- **Minimal:** No data or minimal data (1 point)

- **Low:** Limited data (2 points)
- **Moderate:** Moderate data (3 points)
- **High:** Extensive data (4+ points)

Element 3: Risk of Management

Risk Levels:

- **Minimal:** Minimal risk of morbidity from additional testing/treatment
- **Low:** Low risk of morbidity from additional testing/treatment
- **Moderate:** Moderate risk of morbidity from additional testing/treatment
- **High:** High risk of morbidity from additional testing/treatment

Risk Examples:

- **Low:** Rest, superficial dressings, over-the-counter drugs
- **Moderate:** Minor surgery with no identified risk factors, prescription drug management
- **High:** Major surgery, drug therapy requiring intensive monitoring, emergency major surgery

Office and Other Outpatient Services (99202-99215)

These codes represent the most frequently used E/M codes in medical practice. Mastering these codes is essential for CPC exam success and professional practice.

New Patient Codes (99202-99205)

99202 - Office/outpatient visit, new patient, low level:

- **MDM:** Straightforward medical decision making
- **Time:** 15-29 minutes
- **Typical patients:** Minor acute illness, routine preventive care

Documentation Example: "24-year-old presents with 2-day history of sore throat. Physical exam reveals mild erythema, no exudate. Diagnosis: viral pharyngitis. Plan: supportive care, return if worsens."

99203 - Office/outpatient visit, new patient, moderate level:

- **MDM:** Low complexity medical decision making
- **Time:** 30-44 minutes
- **Typical patients:** Acute uncomplicated illness, stable chronic condition

Documentation Example: "45-year-old with new-onset chest pain, exercise-related. EKG normal, chest X-ray normal. Diagnosis: atypical chest pain, rule out cardiac etiology. Plan: stress test, follow up in 1 week."

99204 - Office/outpatient visit, new patient, high level:

- **MDM:** Moderate complexity medical decision making

- **Time:** 45-59 minutes
- **Typical patients:** Chronic illness with exacerbation, acute complicated illness

Documentation Example: "58-year-old diabetic with worsening control, HbA1c 9.2%, new peripheral neuropathy symptoms. Multiple medication adjustments needed, diabetic education provided. Comprehensive plan developed."

99205 - Office/outpatient visit, new patient, comprehensive:

- **MDM:** High complexity medical decision making
- **Time:** 60-74 minutes
- **Typical patients:** Multiple chronic conditions, severe acute illness

Documentation Example: "72-year-old with congestive heart failure exacerbation, diabetes, hypertension, and COPD. Multiple medication adjustments, hospital vs. home management decision, extensive counseling provided."

Established Patient Codes (99211-99215)

99211 - Office/outpatient visit, established patient, minimal:

- **MDM:** Minimal medical decision making
- **Time:** No time requirement
- **Typical services:** Blood pressure check, simple dressing change
- **May be performed by clinical staff under physician supervision**

99212 - Office/outpatient visit, established patient, low level:

- **MDM:** Straightforward medical decision making
- **Time:** 10-19 minutes
- **Typical patients:** Minor acute illness, stable chronic condition monitoring

99213 - Office/outpatient visit, established patient, moderate level:

- **MDM:** Low complexity medical decision making
- **Time:** 20-29 minutes
- **Typical patients:** Acute uncomplicated illness, routine chronic disease management

99214 - Office/outpatient visit, established patient, high level:

- **MDM:** Moderate complexity medical decision making
- **Time:** 30-39 minutes
- **Typical patients:** Chronic illness with changes, acute complicated illness

99215 - Office/outpatient visit, established patient, comprehensive:

- **MDM:** High complexity medical decision making
- **Time:** 40-54 minutes
- **Typical patients:** Multiple complex conditions, severe exacerbations

Key Coding Considerations

New vs. Established Patient:

- **New:** No professional services within past 3 years from same physician/group, same specialty
- **Established:** Professional services within past 3 years from same physician/group, same specialty

Time Counting Rules:

- **Includes:** Face-to-face time, non-face-to-face time on date of service
- **Examples:** Reviewing records, interpreting tests, communicating with other providers, documentation
- **Excludes:** Travel time, teaching time for trainees

MDM vs. Time Selection:

- Use whichever method (MDM or time) supports the higher level of service
- Cannot combine elements from both methods
- Document the method used for level selection

Hospital Observation Services (99217-99226)

Observation services bridge the gap between emergency department care and inpatient admission, requiring understanding of Medicare guidelines and appropriate utilization.

Observation Care Delivery Codes

99217 - Observation care discharge:

- All levels of discharge services
- Includes final examination, discharge instructions, preparation of discharge records
- Used regardless of length of observation stay

99218 - Initial observation care, low level:

- **History:** Detailed or comprehensive
- **Examination:** Detailed or comprehensive
- **MDM:** Straightforward or low complexity
- **Time:** Usually 30 minutes

99219 - Initial observation care, moderate level:

- **History:** Comprehensive
- **Examination:** Comprehensive
- **MDM:** Moderate complexity
- **Time:** Usually 50 minutes

99220 - Initial observation care, high level:

- **History:** Comprehensive

- **Examination:** Comprehensive
- **MDM:** High complexity
- **Time:** Usually 70 minutes

Subsequent observation care follows same patterns as subsequent hospital care (99231-99233).

Observation Coding Guidelines

Same Day Admission and Discharge:

- Use 99234-99236 (same day observation codes)
- Represents continuous care from admission through discharge
- More appropriate than separate admission and discharge codes

Observation vs. Inpatient Status:

- Observation: Patient status determination by physician order
- Inpatient: Medical necessity for inpatient level of care
- Status affects code selection and reimbursement

Medicare Requirements:

- Must meet Medicare medical necessity criteria
- Physician must order observation status
- Usually requires minimum 8-hour stay for separate billing

Hospital Inpatient Services (99221-99239)

Inpatient E/M coding requires understanding of complex medical conditions, care coordination, and the higher intensity of inpatient management.

Initial Hospital Care (99221-99223)

99221 - Initial hospital care, low level:

- **History:** Detailed or comprehensive
- **Examination:** Detailed or comprehensive
- **MDM:** Straightforward or low complexity
- **Time:** Usually 30 minutes

99222 - Initial hospital care, moderate level:

- **History:** Comprehensive
- **Examination:** Comprehensive
- **MDM:** Moderate complexity
- **Time:** Usually 50 minutes

99223 - Initial hospital care, high level:

- **History:** Comprehensive
- **Examination:** Comprehensive
- **MDM:** High complexity
- **Time:** Usually 70 minutes

Subsequent Hospital Care (99231-99233)

99231 - Subsequent hospital care, low level:

- **History:** Problem focused interval history
- **Examination:** Problem focused
- **MDM:** Straightforward or low complexity
- **Time:** Usually 15 minutes

99232 - Subsequent hospital care, moderate level:

- **History:** Expanded problem focused interval history
- **Examination:** Expanded problem focused
- **MDM:** Moderate complexity
- **Time:** Usually 25 minutes

99233 - Subsequent hospital care, high level:

- **History:** Detailed interval history
- **Examination:** Detailed
- **MDM:** High complexity
- **Time:** Usually 35 minutes

Hospital Discharge Services (99238-99239)

99238 - Hospital discharge, 30 minutes or less:

- Final examination of patient
- Discussion of hospital stay
- Instructions for continuing care
- Preparation of discharge records
- Prescriptions and referrals

99239 - Hospital discharge, more than 30 minutes:

- Same services as 99238 but requiring more than 30 minutes
- Often involves complex patients with multiple conditions
- May include family conferences and extensive planning

Inpatient Coding Considerations

Admission Date Services:

- Only one physician can bill initial hospital care per admission
- Other physicians use consultation codes or subsequent care codes
- Admitting physician relationship determines code selection

Care Plan Oversight:

- Inpatient E/M includes routine care plan oversight
- Separate care plan oversight codes exist for complex cases
- Time thresholds determine when separate billing appropriate

Consultations (99241-99255)

Consultation coding requires understanding of the referral relationship and the specific requirements that distinguish consultations from other E/M services.

Consultation Requirements (The 3 R's)

1. Request:

- Written or verbal request from another physician or appropriate source

- Request must be documented in medical record
- Self-referrals don't qualify for consultation codes

2. Render:

- Consultant must render an opinion or advice
- May include initiation of treatment
- Must provide expertise beyond referring physician's scope

3. Report:

- Written report of findings and recommendations
- Must be communicated back to requesting physician
- Documentation in medical record satisfies requirement

Office/Outpatient Consultations (99241-99245)

99241 - Office consultation, low level:

- **History:** Problem focused
- **Examination:** Problem focused
- **MDM:** Straightforward
- **Time:** Usually 15 minutes

99242 - Office consultation, moderate-low level:

- **History:** Expanded problem focused
- **Examination:** Expanded problem focused
- **MDM:** Straightforward
- **Time:** Usually 30 minutes

99243 - Office consultation, moderate level:

- **History:** Detailed
- **Examination:** Detailed
- **MDM:** Low complexity
- **Time:** Usually 40 minutes

99244 - Office consultation, moderate-high level:

- **History:** Comprehensive
- **Examination:** Comprehensive
- **MDM:** Moderate complexity
- **Time:** Usually 60 minutes

99245 - Office consultation, high level:

- **History:** Comprehensive
- **Examination:** Comprehensive
- **MDM:** High complexity
- **Time:** Usually 80 minutes

Inpatient Consultations (99251-99255)

Follow same level structure as office consultations but represent inpatient setting services with typically higher complexity due to hospitalized patient status.

Medicare Consultation Policy:

- Medicare no longer recognizes consultation codes
- Use appropriate new or established patient codes instead
- Private payers may still accept consultation codes
- Verify payer-specific policies before coding

Consultation vs. Referral:

Consultation Characteristics:

- Temporary relationship
- Report back to requesting physician
- May or may not initiate treatment
- Requesting physician maintains primary responsibility

Referral Characteristics:

- Transfer of care responsibility
- Ongoing treatment relationship
- Use new/established patient codes

- Referred-to physician assumes primary care

Emergency Department Services (99281-99288)

ED coding reflects the unique environment where physicians must be prepared to handle any condition at any time, often with limited patient history and high-acuity situations.

ED Service Levels (99281-99285)

99281 - ED visit, low level:

- **History:** Problem focused
- **Examination:** Problem focused
- **MDM:** Straightforward
- **Time:** Usually 10 minutes
- **Typical cases:** Minor injuries, simple acute illnesses

99282 - ED visit, moderate-low level:

- **History:** Expanded problem focused
- **Examination:** Expanded problem focused
- **MDM:** Low complexity
- **Time:** Usually 20 minutes
- **Typical cases:** Moderate injuries, uncomplicated acute illnesses

99283 - ED visit, moderate level:

- **History:** Expanded problem focused
- **Examination:** Expanded problem focused
- **MDM:** Moderate complexity
- **Time:** Usually 30 minutes
- **Typical cases:** Moderately severe injuries, acute illnesses requiring multiple interventions

99284 - ED visit, high level:

- **History:** Detailed
- **Examination:** Detailed
- **MDM:** Moderate complexity
- **Time:** Usually 45 minutes
- **Typical cases:** Severe injuries, acute illnesses with systemic symptoms

99285 - ED visit, comprehensive:

- **History:** Comprehensive
- **Examination:** Comprehensive
- **MDM:** High complexity
- **Time:** Usually 60 minutes
- **Typical cases:** Life-threatening conditions, multiple trauma, cardiac arrest

ED Coding Considerations

No New vs. Established Patient Distinction:

- All ED patients coded with same codes regardless of prior relationship
- Emergency nature supersedes established patient criteria

Critical Care Integration:

- If critical care provided, use critical care codes (99291-99292)
- Cannot bill both ED and critical care codes for same time period
- Document critical care time separately from ED time

Observation from ED:

- May bill both ED code and observation admission
- Must meet criteria for both services
- Observation must be separate decision from ED care

Critical Care Services (99291-99292)

Critical care represents the highest level of E/M services, requiring intensive monitoring and frequent physician intervention for patients with life-threatening conditions.

Critical Care Criteria

Patient Condition Requirements:

- High probability of imminent or life-threatening deterioration
- Requires constant physician availability
- Requires frequent vital sign monitoring
- Often involves multiple organ system failure

Physician Work Requirements:

- Direct personal management by physician
- Frequent reassessment and intervention
- Complex medical decision making
- Immediate availability for patient needs

Location Requirements:

- Usually ICU, CCU, ED, or similar setting
- Location less important than patient acuity and physician work
- Can be provided in any location meeting care criteria

Critical Care Codes

99291 - Critical care, first 30-74 minutes:

- Minimum 30 minutes required for billing
- Maximum 74 minutes covered by this code
- Includes all critical care services during this time

99292 - Critical care, each additional 30 minutes:

- Used for time beyond initial 74 minutes
- Report in addition to 99291
- May be reported multiple times per day

Time Reporting Examples:

- 45 minutes: 99291 only
- 90 minutes: 99291 + 99292
- 150 minutes: 99291 + 99292 + 99292

Services Included in Critical Care:

- Interpretation of cardiac output measurements
- Chest X-rays (professional component)
- Blood gases and pH
- Gastric intubation
- Temporary transvenous pacing
- Ventilator management
- Vascular access procedures

Services NOT Included (Bill Separately):

- Procedures with their own CPT® codes

- Services performed by other physicians
- Transport services

- Separate billable procedures performed during critical care

Nursing Facility Services (99304-99318)

Nursing facility coding addresses the unique needs of patients requiring skilled nursing care, with emphasis on care plan development and interdisciplinary coordination.

Initial Nursing Facility Care (99304-99306)

99304 - Initial nursing facility care, low level:

- **History:** Detailed or comprehensive
- **Examination:** Detailed or comprehensive
- **MDM:** Straightforward or low complexity

99305 - Initial nursing facility care, moderate level:

- **History:** Comprehensive
- **Examination:** Comprehensive
- **MDM:** Moderate complexity

99306 - Initial nursing facility care, high level:

- **History:** Comprehensive
- **Examination:** Comprehensive
- **MDM:** High complexity

Subsequent Nursing Facility Care (99307-99310)

99307 - Subsequent nursing facility care, low level:

- **History:** Problem focused interval history
- **Examination:** Problem focused
- **MDM:** Straightforward

99308 - Subsequent nursing facility care, moderate level:

- **History:** Expanded problem focused
- **Examination:** Expanded problem focused
- **MDM:** Low complexity

99309 - Subsequent nursing facility care, moderate-high level:

- **History:** Detailed interval history
- **Examination:** Detailed
- **MDM:** Moderate complexity

99310 - Subsequent nursing facility care, high level:

- **History:** Comprehensive interval history
- **Examination:** Comprehensive
- **MDM:** High complexity

Annual Assessments and Discharges

99318 - Annual nursing facility assessment:

- Comprehensive assessment required by regulations
- Medical appropriateness of placement
- Health status evaluation
- Care plan review and revision

99315-99316 - Nursing facility discharge services:

- Similar to hospital discharge services
- Time-based coding (30 minutes or less vs. more than 30 minutes)

- Includes final examination and care transition planning

Domiciliary, Rest Home Services (99324-99337)

These codes address care provided in residential facilities that don't meet nursing facility criteria but house patients needing medical supervision.

Service Categories:

- New patient codes (99324-99328)
- Established patient codes (99334-99337)
- Similar level structure to office visits
- Emphasize care coordination and patient/family counseling

Coding Considerations:

- Facility type determines code selection
- Patient's primary residence vs. temporary stay
- Level of medical supervision available
- Integration with community care resources

Prolonged Services and Other E/M Services

Prolonged Services (99354-99359)

99354 - Prolonged physician service, first hour:

- Used with office/outpatient E/M codes
- Requires face-to-face time beyond highest E/M level
- Minimum 30 minutes beyond typical time

99355 - Prolonged physician service, each additional 30 minutes:

- Add-on code for use with 99354
- Extends prolonged service reporting

99356-99357 - Prolonged services without direct patient contact:

- Pre-service and post-service work
- Chart review, test interpretation, communication with other providers
- Must exceed typical pre/post work for E/M level

Other E/M Services

Preventive Medicine Services (99381-99397):

- Age-based coding structure
- New vs. established patient categories
- Focus on health maintenance and disease prevention
- Separate from problem-oriented E/M codes

Case Management Services (99490-99491):

- Complex chronic care management
- Transitional care management
- Behavioral health integration services
- Time-based and complexity-based coding

E/M Practice Questions

Test your understanding of E/M coding principles:

Question 1: A new patient is seen for 45 minutes with moderate complexity medical decision making. The correct code is:

A) 99203 (30-44 minutes, low complexity MDM) B) 99204 (45-59 minutes, moderate complexity MDM) C) 99205 (60-74 minutes, high complexity MDM) D) Either 99203 or 99204 depending on documentation

Answer: B Explanation: For new patients, 99204 covers 45-59 minutes OR moderate complexity MDM. Since both criteria are met (45 minutes AND moderate MDM), 99204 is correct. Use whichever method (time or MDM) supports the appropriate level.

Question 2: An established patient is seen for routine blood pressure monitoring by a nurse under physician supervision. The appropriate code is:

A) 99211 B) 99212 C) 99213 D) No E/M code appropriate

Answer: A Explanation: 99211 is the only E/M code that can be performed by clinical staff under physician supervision. It represents minimal physician work and is appropriate for routine monitoring visits.

Question 3: A consultation requires all of the following EXCEPT:

A) Written request from another physician B) Written report back to requesting physician C) Transfer of care to the consulting physician D) Rendering of an opinion or advice

Answer: C Explanation: Consultations do NOT require transfer of care. The requesting physician maintains primary responsibility while the consultant provides opinion/advice and reports back. Transfer of care would make it a referral, not a consultation.

Question 4: Critical care services require a minimum of how many minutes?

A) 15 minutes B) 20 minutes C) 30 minutes D) 45 minutes

Answer: C Explanation: Critical care services (99291) require a minimum of 30 minutes to be billable. Less than 30 minutes should be coded with appropriate E/M codes based on level of service provided.

Question 5: For Medicare patients, consultation codes should be:

A) Used as normal for all consultations B) Replaced with new/established patient codes C) Used only for office consultations D) Used only for inpatient consultations

Answer: B Explanation: Medicare no longer recognizes consultation codes. For Medicare patients, use appropriate new patient or established patient E/M codes based on the patient's relationship with the physician.

Question 6: An established patient is seen for 25 minutes with low complexity medical decision making. The correct code is:

A) 99212 (10-19 minutes, straightforward MDM) B) 99213 (20-29 minutes, low complexity MDM) C) 99214 (30-39 minutes, moderate complexity MDM) D) Either 99212 or 99213

Answer: B Explanation: 99213 is correct because it covers 20-29 minutes OR low complexity MDM. Since both the time (25 minutes) and MDM (low complexity) criteria are met, 99213 is the appropriate level.

Question 7: Hospital discharge services are reported with:

A) The same code regardless of time spent B) 99238 for 30 minutes or less, 99239 for more than 30 minutes C) The final subsequent hospital care code D) No separate code—included in final hospital day

Answer: B Explanation: Hospital discharge services are time-based: 99238 for 30 minutes or less, and 99239 for more than 30 minutes. These are separate from subsequent hospital care codes.

Question 8: Emergency department coding differs from office coding because:

A) It uses different code ranges B) It has no new vs. established patient distinction C) It requires different documentation D) All of the above

Answer: D Explanation: ED coding uses different code ranges (99281-99285), makes no distinction between new and established patients, and often involves different documentation patterns due to the emergency nature of care.

Question 9: Time-based E/M coding includes:

A) Only face-to-face time with the patient B) Only time spent in the examination room C) Total time on the date of encounter including non-face-to-face activities D) Only time spent documenting the encounter

Answer: C Explanation: Current E/M time-based coding includes total time on the date of encounter, including both face-to-face time and non-face-to-face time related to the encounter (reviewing records, arranging care, etc.).

Question 10: Prolonged services codes (99354-99355) are used when:

A) Any E/M service takes longer than expected B) Face-to-face time significantly exceeds the typical time for the highest level E/M code C) Documentation takes longer than usual D) The patient requires extensive counseling

Answer: B Explanation: Prolonged service codes are used when face-to-face time significantly exceeds the typical time associated with the highest level E/M service that can be reported for that encounter type.

Chapter 10 Summary: E/M Coding Mastery

You've now mastered the most complex and frequently used codes in medical practice. Your achievements include:

Guideline Expertise: You understand both historical and current E/M guidelines, enabling you to work with various documentation styles and requirements.

Code Selection Accuracy: You can analyze documentation and select appropriate E/M levels using either medical decision making or time-based criteria.

Setting-Specific Knowledge: You know the unique requirements for office, hospital, ED, nursing facility, and other E/M services.

Special Situations: You can handle consultations, critical care, prolonged services, and other complex E/M scenarios.

Professional Application: You understand the clinical context behind E/M codes and can make appropriate coding decisions in ambiguous situations.

Remember: E/M coding represents the cognitive work physicians perform—the thinking, analyzing, and decision-making that drives all medical care. Your expertise in these codes reflects your understanding of the medical decision-making process itself.

This foundation now supports your journey into procedural coding, where you'll learn to code the hands-on procedures and interventions that E/M services often lead to. The analytical skills you've developed here will serve you well as you master surgery coding and other procedural areas.

Next, you'll tackle surgery coding by body system, where anatomical knowledge and procedural understanding combine to create the most detailed and specific codes in all of medicine.

Additional Chapter 10 Practice Questions

Continue refining your E/M coding expertise:

Question 11: An established patient presents with multiple chronic conditions requiring extensive review of outside records and consultation with specialists. The physician spends 50 minutes total time on the encounter. The correct code is:

A) 99213 (20-29 minutes) B) 99214 (30-39 minutes) C) 99215 (40-54 minutes) D) 99215 + 99354 (prolonged services)

Answer: C Explanation: 99215 covers 40-54 minutes, which includes the 50 minutes spent. Prolonged services are only used when time significantly exceeds the highest level E/M service (beyond 54 minutes for established patients).

Question 12: A physician provides 45 minutes of critical care to an unstable patient in the ICU. The correct coding is:

A) 99291 only B) 99232 (subsequent hospital care) C) 99291 + 99292 D) Cannot bill less than 60 minutes of critical care

Answer: A Explanation: 99291 covers 30-74 minutes of critical care, so 45 minutes is appropriately coded with 99291 only. The minimum is 30 minutes, not 60 minutes.

Question 13: For nursing facility services, the annual assessment is coded with:

A) The highest level subsequent nursing facility code B) 99318 (annual nursing facility assessment) C) A preventive medicine code D) The initial nursing facility care code

Answer: B Explanation: 99318 is specifically designated for the annual nursing facility assessment required by regulations. It's distinct from routine subsequent care codes.

Question 14: A patient is seen in the ED for chest pain. After evaluation, the physician admits the patient to observation. The correct coding approach is:

A) ED code only B) Observation admission code only C) Both ED code and observation admission code D) Initial hospital care code

Answer: C Explanation: When a patient receives distinct services in the ED followed by a separate decision for observation admission, both services can typically be coded if they represent separate physician work and meet respective criteria.

Question 15: Medical decision making complexity is determined by which three elements?

A) History, examination, and time B) Problems addressed, data reviewed, and risk of management C) Chief complaint, assessment, and plan D) Diagnosis complexity, treatment options, and patient compliance

Answer: B Explanation: Current E/M guidelines base medical decision making complexity on three elements: (1) number and complexity of problems addressed, (2) amount and/or complexity of data reviewed and analyzed, and (3) risk of complications and/or morbidity or mortality of patient management.

Chapter 11: Surgery Coding by Body System

"Precision is not just a goal—it's the only acceptable standard." - Anonymous Surgeon

Surgery coding represents the pinnacle of medical coding complexity and precision. Every surgical procedure tells a story of anatomical knowledge, technical skill, and life-changing intervention. Your role as a surgical coder is to translate these complex procedures into accurate codes that ensure proper reimbursement and maintain detailed healthcare records.

This chapter transforms your anatomical knowledge into practical coding expertise across all surgical specialties. You'll master the systematic approach that makes complex surgical coding manageable, learn the specialty-specific guidelines that govern accurate code selection, and develop the confidence to handle even the most challenging surgical scenarios.

Surgery coding isn't just about finding the right code—it's about understanding the procedure well enough to select the most appropriate and specific code available. By the end of this chapter, you'll think like a surgical coder who truly understands the medicine behind the codes.

Your anatomy foundation, medical terminology mastery, and E/M coding skills now combine to support this advanced surgical coding knowledge. You're ready to tackle the most detailed and challenging codes in all of healthcare.

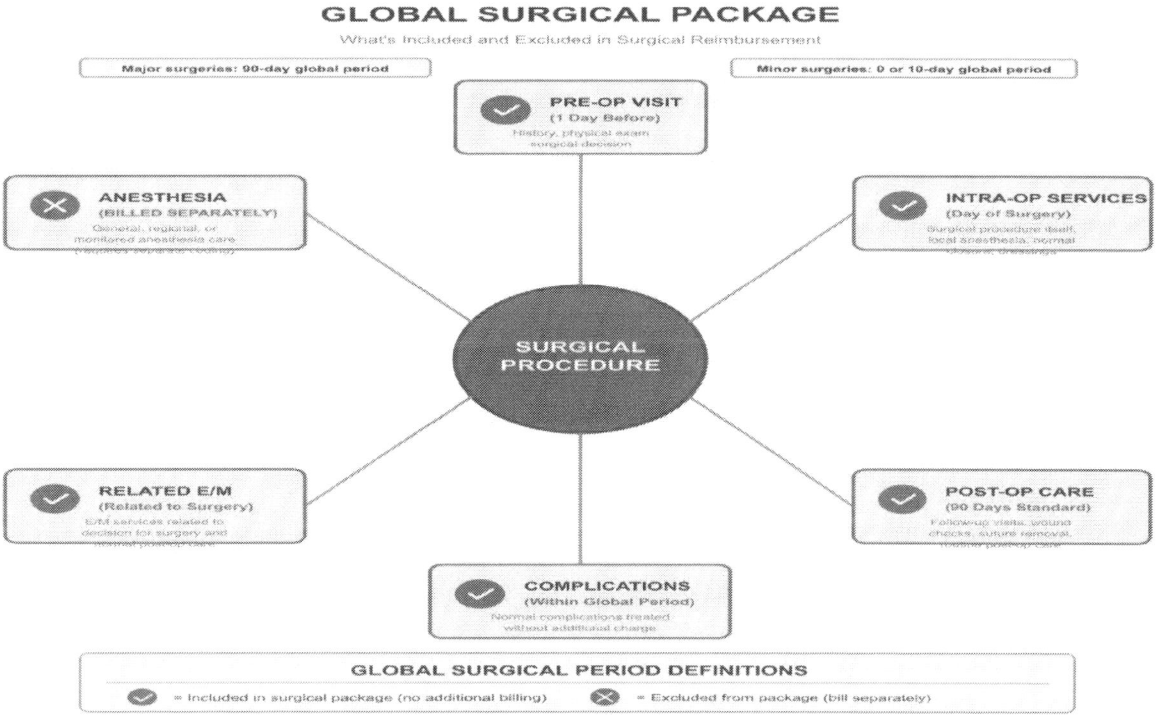

Integumentary System (10000-19999)

The integumentary system generates high coding volume in medical practices, from simple skin repairs to complex reconstructive procedures. Understanding skin anatomy, wound classification, and repair techniques is essential for accurate coding.

Skin, Subcutaneous and Accessory Structures

Understanding Wound Classifications

Simple Repair (12001-12021):

- Superficial wounds involving epidermis, dermis, and subcutaneous tissue
- Single-layer closure
- Minimal undermining
- No significant contamination or tissue loss

Coding Structure: Organized by anatomical location and wound length:

- 12001-12007: Scalp, neck, axilla, external genitalia, trunk, extremities
- 12011-12018: Face, ears, eyelids, nose, lips, mucous membranes
- 12020-12021: Scalp, arms, legs (complex simple repairs)

Length Calculations: Add all wounds in same classification and location:

- Example: 2.5 cm + 1.8 cm + 3.2 cm = 7.5 cm total
- Use total length to select appropriate code
- Don't add lengths from different anatomical groups

Intermediate Repair (12031-12057):

- Layered closure of deeper wounds
- Extensive cleaning or removal of particulate matter
- Layered closure of subcutaneous tissue and superficial fascia
- Single-layer closure of heavily contaminated wounds

Complex Repair (13100-13160):

- More than layered closure
- Extensive undermining, stents, or retention sutures
- Creation of defect for repair or revision
- Debridement of complicated lacerations
- Repair of avulsion wounds

Surgical Wound Scenarios

Scenario 1: Multiple Simple Repairs

Documentation: "Patient sustained lacerations in motor vehicle accident: 4 cm laceration to forehead, 2 cm laceration to cheek, 3 cm laceration to chin. All repaired with simple sutures."

Analysis:

- All wounds on face (same anatomical group)
- All simple repairs (same classification)

- Total length: 4 + 2 + 3 = 9 cm

Correct Coding: 12014 Simple repair of superficial wounds of face, ears, eyelids, nose, lips, mucous membranes; 7.6 cm to 12.5 cm

Key Learning: Add lengths within same anatomical group and repair type.

Scenario 2: Different Repair Types

Documentation: "Complex laceration to scalp requiring layered closure and extensive undermining (6 cm). Simple laceration to arm repaired with single-layer closure (3 cm)."

Analysis:

- Two different repair types (complex vs. simple)
- Different anatomical locations
- Code each separately

Correct Coding:

1. 13120 Repair, complex, scalp, arms, and/or legs; 2.6 cm to 7.5 cm
2. 12002 Simple repair of superficial wounds of scalp, neck, axillae, external genitalia, trunk and/or extremities; 2.6 cm to 7.5 cm

Key Learning: Different repair types require separate coding, even if lengths could be combined.

Excision Procedures (11400-11471)

Excision of Benign Lesions: Organized by anatomical site and specimen diameter:

- Includes simple closure
- Measure greatest clinical diameter plus margin
- Document pathology findings for medical necessity

Excision of Malignant Lesions:

- Higher reimbursement than benign lesions
- Requires pathology confirmation for final coding
- More extensive margins typically required

Lesion Coding Decision Tree:

1. **Determine lesion type:** Benign vs. malignant (from pathology)
2. **Identify location:** Trunk/arms/legs, scalp/neck/hands/feet, face/ears/lips
3. **Measure total diameter:** Lesion + margins removed
4. **Select appropriate code range**
5. **Apply modifiers if needed** (multiple lesions, bilateral procedures)

Mohs Micrographic Surgery (17311-17315):

- Specialized technique for skin cancer removal
- Real-time microscopic examination
- Layer-by-layer removal until clear margins
- Separate coding for stages and repair

Breast Procedures

Breast procedures require understanding of anatomy, cancer staging, and reconstruction options.

Breast Anatomy Review:

- Four quadrants: upper outer, upper inner, lower outer, lower inner
- Central portion (subareolar region)
- Axillary tail (extension toward axilla)
- Lymphatic drainage patterns

Breast Biopsy Procedures

Needle Biopsy (19081-19086):

- Image-guided procedures
- Multiple sampling techniques
- Includes imaging guidance when performed
- Marker placement when performed

19081 - Biopsy, breast, with placement of breast localization device:

- Percutaneous needle core biopsy
- Placement of localization device
- Includes imaging guidance

Surgical Biopsy (19101-19103):

- Open surgical approach
- When needle biopsy not feasible or adequate
- May be incisional or excisional

Mastectomy Procedures (19300-19307)

19300 - Mastectomy for gynecomastia:

- Male breast tissue removal
- Benign condition
- May be unilateral or bilateral

19301 - Partial mastectomy, lumpectomy:

- Breast-conserving surgery
- Removal of tumor with surrounding tissue
- Preserves breast contour

19302 - Simple mastectomy:

- Complete removal of breast tissue
- Nipple-areolar complex removed
- Pectoral fascia may be removed

19303 - Mastectomy, radical:

- Breast, pectoral muscles, lymph nodes
- Most extensive mastectomy procedure
- Rarely performed today

Reconstruction Procedures

Immediate vs. Delayed Reconstruction:

- Timing affects code selection
- Different techniques available
- May require multiple stages

Common Reconstruction Methods:

- Implant-based reconstruction
- Autologous tissue reconstruction (TRAM, DIEP flaps)
- Combined approaches
- Nipple-areolar reconstruction

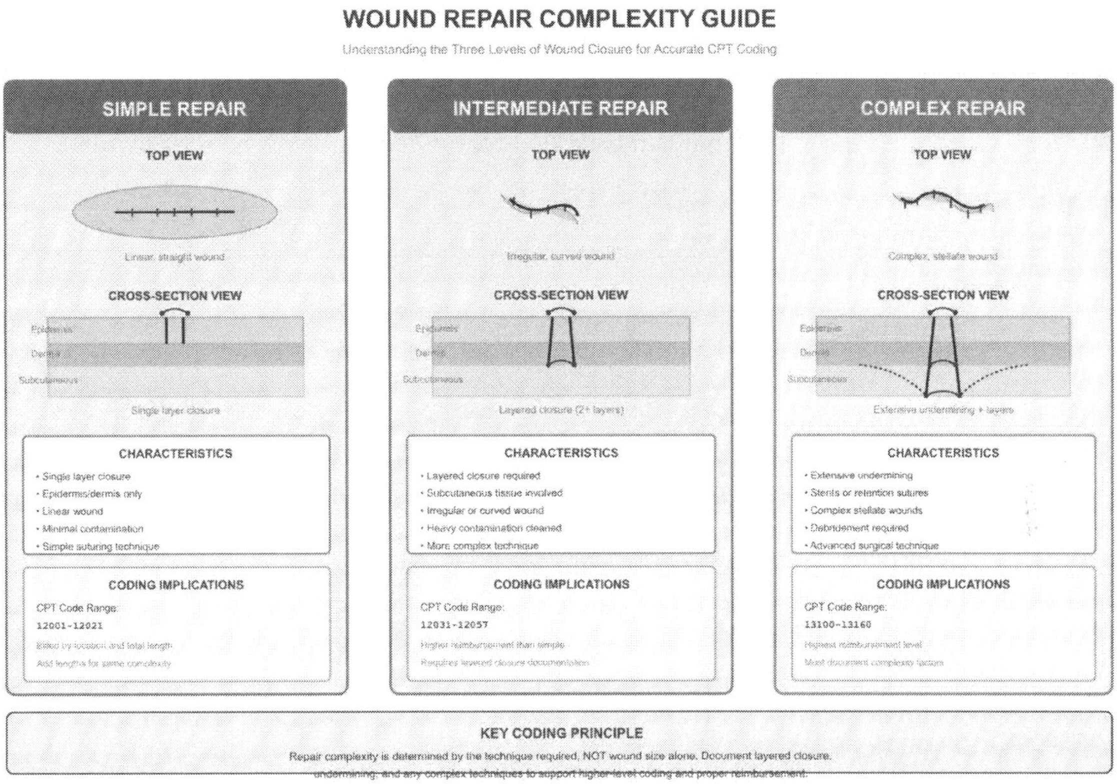

Practice Questions - Integumentary System

Test your understanding of skin and breast coding:

Question 1: A patient has three lacerations repaired: 3 cm on forehead (simple), 2 cm on cheek (simple), and 4 cm on scalp (intermediate). How should this be coded?

A) 12014 only (9 cm total, face) B) 12013 (5 cm face) + 12032 (4 cm scalp) C) 12014 (face) + 12032 (scalp) D) Three separate codes for each laceration

Answer: B Explanation: Simple repairs on face total 5 cm (12013), intermediate repair on scalp is 4 cm (12032). Different anatomical groups and repair types require separate coding.

Question 2: Excision of a 1.5 cm malignant lesion from the back with 0.5 cm margins should be coded as:

A) 11402 (1.1 to 2.0 cm, benign) B) 11603 (1.1 to 2.0 cm, malignant) C) 11604 (2.1 to 3.0 cm, malignant) D) Cannot code until pathology results available

Answer: C Explanation: Total diameter is lesion (1.5 cm) + margins (0.5 cm × 2) = 2.5 cm. Malignant lesion on trunk codes to 11604 for 2.1-3.0 cm range.

Question 3: A partial mastectomy with sentinel lymph node biopsy should be coded as:

A) 19301 only B) 19301 + 38500 C) 19302 + 38525 D) 38525 only

Answer: B Explanation: Partial mastectomy (19301) and sentinel lymph node biopsy (38500) are separate procedures that can be coded together when both are performed.

Musculoskeletal System (20000-29999)

Musculoskeletal coding requires precise anatomical knowledge and understanding of surgical approaches, fixation methods, and bone healing processes.

General Procedures (20005-20999)

Incision and Drainage (20005):

- Deep abscess or hematoma
- Soft tissue of pelvis and/or hip
- Requires deep dissection

Arthrocentesis and Injection Procedures (20600-20615):

- Joint aspiration and/or injection
- Organized by joint size
- May include imaging guidance

20600 - Small joints: Fingers, toes **20605 - Intermediate joints:** Wrist, elbow, ankle **20610 - Major joints:** Shoulder, hip, knee

Bone and Joint Infections (20240-20245):

- Bone biopsy procedures
- Drainage of bone abscess
- Treatment of osteomyelitis

Fracture Care Principles

Understanding fracture treatment methods is essential for accurate orthopedic coding.

Treatment Types:

Closed Treatment:

- No surgical exposure of fracture site
- With or without manipulation
- External stabilization methods

Open Treatment:

- Surgical exposure of fracture site
- Internal fixation typically used
- Direct visualization of fracture

Percutaneous Skeletal Fixation:

- Fixation placed through skin without open exposure
- Image guidance typically used
- Intermediate between closed and open treatment

Fracture Coding Components:

1. **Anatomical site:** Specific bone and location
2. **Treatment method:** Closed, open, or percutaneous
3. **Manipulation:** With or without reduction
4. **Fixation type:** Internal, external, or none

Application of Casts and Strapping (29000-29799):

- Separate procedure when not part of fracture treatment
- Included in fracture care when performed by same physician
- Removal and replacement may be separately billable

Spine and Pelvis Procedures

Spinal procedures require understanding of vertebral anatomy, approach methods, and fusion techniques.

Spinal Anatomy Review:

- 7 cervical vertebrae (C1-C7)
- 12 thoracic vertebrae (T1-T12)
- 5 lumbar vertebrae (L1-L5)
- Sacrum (S1-S5 fused)
- Coccyx

Vertebral Levels and Coding:

- Single level: One vertebral segment
- Additional levels: Add-on codes available
- Approach affects code selection

Common Spinal Procedures:

Laminectomy (63030-63091):

- Removal of lamina
- Decompression of neural elements
- May include discectomy
- Organized by spinal region and levels

Spinal Fusion (22558-22819):

- Arthrodesis procedures
- Multiple approach options
- Graft materials separately coded
- Instrumentation separately coded

Discectomy (63020-63078):

- Removal of intervertebral disc

- May be part of larger procedure
- Different approaches available

Upper and Lower Extremities

Extremity procedures require understanding of anatomical relationships and functional restoration goals.

Shoulder Procedures (23000-23929):

- Complex ball-and-socket joint
- High mobility requires stability compromise
- Common procedures include rotator cuff repairs, shoulder replacements

Elbow Procedures (24000-24999):

- Hinge joint with complex articulations
- Tennis elbow, fracture repairs common
- Ulnar nerve procedures included

Wrist and Hand Procedures (25000-26989):

- High-precision functional requirements
- Carpal tunnel syndrome very common
- Tendon and nerve repairs frequent

Hip Procedures (27000-27299):

- Weight-bearing ball-and-socket joint
- Hip replacements increasingly common
- Fracture repairs in elderly patients

Knee Procedures (27300-27599):

- Complex hinge joint with menisci
- Arthroscopic procedures very common
- Ligament reconstructions in athletes

Ankle and Foot Procedures (27600-28899):

- Weight-bearing and balance functions
- Bunion corrections common
- Fracture repairs frequent

Arthroscopy

Arthroscopic procedures use small incisions and cameras for joint visualization and treatment.

Arthroscopy Advantages:

- Minimal invasive approach
- Reduced recovery time
- Lower infection risk
- Better cosmetic results

Common Arthroscopic Procedures:

Knee Arthroscopy (29870-29887):

- Diagnostic arthroscopy
- Meniscal repair/removal
- Ligament reconstruction
- Cartilage procedures

Shoulder Arthroscopy (29805-29828):

- Rotator cuff repairs
- Labral repairs
- Subacromial decompression
- Capsular releases

Arthroscopy Coding Principles:

- Multiple procedures common in single session
- Some procedures include diagnostic arthroscopy
- Bilateral procedures require modifier -50
- Surgical approach affects code selection

Practice Questions - Musculoskeletal System

Question 4: Closed treatment of a displaced femur fracture with manipulation should be coded as:

A) 27500 (closed treatment without manipulation) B) 27502 (closed treatment with manipulation) C) 27506 (open treatment) D) 27509 (percutaneous skeletal fixation)

Answer: B Explanation: Closed treatment with manipulation (27502) is correct when fracture fragments are realigned without surgical exposure. The manipulation component increases the work performed.

Question 5: Arthroscopic partial meniscectomy of the knee should be coded as:

A) 29870 (arthroscopy, diagnostic) B) 29880 (arthroscopy with meniscectomy) C) 29881 (arthroscopy with meniscectomy including repair) D) 27332 (open meniscectomy)

Answer: B Explanation: 29880 represents arthroscopic meniscectomy (partial or total removal). Diagnostic arthroscopy is included when performed during the same session as the surgical procedure.

Question 6: Application of a short arm cast for a fracture treated by the same physician should be:

A) Coded separately with 29075 B) Included in the fracture treatment code C) Coded only if applied later D) Never coded separately

Answer: B Explanation: Cast application is included in fracture treatment when performed by the same physician. Separate coding is appropriate when applied by different physician or as replacement/adjustment.

Respiratory System (30000-39999)

Respiratory system coding requires understanding of airway anatomy, breathing physiology, and the relationship between upper and lower respiratory tract procedures.

Nose and Sinuses (30000-30999)

Nasal Anatomy Review:

- External nose: Cartilaginous and bony framework
- Nasal cavity: Divided by septum into right and left sides
- Turbinates: Superior, middle, inferior - increase surface area
- Sinuses: Frontal, ethmoid, sphenoid, maxillary

Common Nasal Procedures:

30000 - Drainage of nasal abscess or hematoma:

- Simple incision and drainage
- External approach

30020 - Drainage of nasal septal abscess:

- Internal approach
- More complex than simple nasal drainage

Rhinoplasty Procedures (30400-30630):

- Cosmetic vs. functional procedures
- Medical necessity documentation important
- Primary vs. secondary procedures

30400 - Rhinoplasty, primary, lateral and alar cartilages:

- Cosmetic nose surgery
- Reshaping nasal tip and nostrils

30410 - Rhinoplasty, primary, complete:

- Comprehensive nasal reshaping
- Both cosmetic and functional components

Sinus Surgery (31000-31299): Endoscopic sinus surgery has largely replaced open approaches:

31231 - Nasal endoscopy, diagnostic:

- Includes inspection of nasal cavity and sinuses
- Often part of more extensive procedures

31237 - Nasal/sinus endoscopy, surgical, with biopsy:

- Tissue sampling for diagnosis
- May be multiple sites

31254 - Ethmoidectomy, partial:

- Removal of ethmoid air cells
- Unilateral procedure

31255 - Ethmoidectomy, total:

- Complete removal of ethmoid air cells
- More extensive than partial

31256 - Maxillary antrostomy:

- Opening of maxillary sinus
- Drainage and ventilation

Larynx and Trachea (31300-31899)

Laryngeal Anatomy:

- Supraglottis: Above vocal cords
- Glottis: Vocal cords and immediate area
- Subglottis: Below vocal cords

Laryngoscopy Procedures:

31575 - Laryngoscopy, flexible fiberoptic, diagnostic:

- Office-based procedure
- Evaluation of vocal cord function
- Assessment of airway abnormalities

31579 - Laryngoscopy, flexible or rigid telescopic, with stroboscopy:

- Advanced vocal cord assessment
- Evaluation of vocal cord vibration patterns

Vocal Cord Procedures:

31540 - Laryngoscopy, direct, with excision of tumor:

- Removal of laryngeal masses
- Direct visualization approach

31541 - Laryngoscopy, direct, with excision of tumor, requiring tracheostomy:

- More extensive tumor removal
- Temporary or permanent airway needed

Tracheostomy (31600-31614):

- Surgical opening in trachea
- Emergency vs. planned procedures
- Temporary vs. permanent airways

31603 - Tracheostomy, emergency procedure:

- Life-threatening airway obstruction
- Performed under emergency conditions
- Higher complexity than planned procedure

31605 - Tracheostomy, planned procedure:

- Scheduled surgical airway
- More controlled conditions
- Extensive preoperative planning

Bronchi and Lungs (32000-32999)

Pulmonary Anatomy:

- Right lung: Upper, middle, lower lobes
- Left lung: Upper, lower lobes (lingula part of upper lobe)
- Bronchial tree: Main, lobar, segmental bronchi
- Pleural space: Potential space between visceral and parietal pleura

Bronchoscopy (31622-31654):

31622 - Bronchoscopy, diagnostic:

- Inspection of tracheobronchial tree
- Assessment of airways and secretions

31625 - Bronchoscopy with bronchial or endobronchial biopsy:

- Tissue sampling from airways
- Multiple samples common

31628 - Bronchoscopy with transbronchial lung biopsy:

- Sampling of lung parenchyma
- Through bronchial wall approach

Lung Biopsy Procedures:

32405 - Biopsy, lung or mediastinum, percutaneous needle:

- Image-guided needle sampling

- Less invasive than surgical biopsy
- CT or ultrasound guidance

32607 - Thoracoscopy, with diagnostic biopsy:

- Video-assisted thoracoscopic surgery (VATS)
- Direct visualization of pleural surfaces
- Multiple biopsy sites possible

Lung Resection (32440-32505):

32480 - Partial pulmonary decortication:

- Removal of fibrous tissue from lung surface
- Allows lung expansion

32482 - Bilobectomy:

- Removal of two lung lobes
- Usually right middle and lower lobes

32484 - Pneumonectomy:

- Complete lung removal
- Most extensive pulmonary resection

Pleural Procedures:

32554 - Thoracentesis, needle or catheter:

- Drainage of pleural fluid
- Diagnostic or therapeutic
- Image guidance when used

32560 - Pleural drainage, open:

- Surgical drainage approach
- More invasive than needle drainage

•

Practice Questions - Respiratory System

Question 7: A diagnostic nasal endoscopy followed by ethmoidectomy should be coded as:

A) 31231 + 31254 B) 31254 only C) 31231 only
D) 31255 only

Answer: B Explanation: Diagnostic endoscopy (31231) is included when performed as part of a more extensive endoscopic procedure like ethmoidectomy (31254). Only the surgical procedure should be coded.

Question 8: Flexible laryngoscopy performed in the office should be coded as:

A) 31575 (flexible laryngoscopy, diagnostic) B) 31576 (flexible laryngoscopy with biopsy) C) 31540 (direct laryngoscopy with excision) D) 31579 (laryngoscopy with stroboscopy)

Answer: A Explanation: 31575 is the appropriate code for diagnostic flexible fiberoptic laryngoscopy performed in the office setting without additional procedures.

Question 9: Thoracentesis with image guidance should be coded as:

A) 32554 only B) 32554 + imaging guidance code C) 32555 only D) 32560 only

Answer: A Explanation: Current thoracentesis codes (32554-32557) include imaging guidance when performed. Separate imaging codes should not be reported.

Digestive System (40000-49999)

Digestive system coding spans from lips to anus, requiring understanding of anatomy, physiology, and both endoscopic and open surgical approaches.

Lips through Anus Overview

Digestive Tract Organization:

- Lips and mouth (40490-40899)
- Tongue and floor of mouth (41000-41599)
- Dentoalveolar structures (41800-41899)
- Palate and uvula (42000-42299)
- Salivary glands (42300-42699)
- Pharynx, adenoids, tonsils (42700-42999)
- Esophagus (43020-43499)
- Stomach (43500-43999)
- Intestines (44005-44799)
- Meckel's diverticulum (44800-44899)
- Appendix (44900-44979)
- Colon and rectum (45000-45999)
- Anus (46020-46999)

Endoscopic Procedures

Endoscopy allows direct visualization and treatment of the GI tract with minimal invasion.

Upper Endoscopy (43235-43259):

43235 - Esophagogastroduodenoscopy (EGD), diagnostic:

- Examination of esophagus, stomach, duodenum
- Assessment of symptoms like dysphagia, pain, bleeding

43239 - EGD with biopsy:

- Tissue sampling during upper endoscopy
- Multiple sites commonly biopsied

43249 - EGD with balloon dilation:

- Treatment of strictures
- Gradual expansion of narrowed areas

43255 - EGD with control of bleeding:

- Therapeutic intervention for GI bleeding
- Various methods: injection, thermal, mechanical

Lower Endoscopy (45330-45398):

45330 - Sigmoidoscopy, diagnostic:

- Examination of rectum and sigmoid colon
- Limited scope compared to colonoscopy

45378 - Colonoscopy, diagnostic:

- Complete examination of colon
- From rectum to cecum visualization

45380 - Colonoscopy with biopsy:

- Tissue sampling during colonoscopy

- Screening and surveillance procedures

45385 - Colonoscopy with removal of tumor, polyp, or other lesion:

- Polypectomy procedures
- Various removal techniques

Endoscopy Coding Guidelines:

Incomplete Procedures:

- Use modifier -52 (reduced services) when procedure terminated early
- Modifier -53 (discontinued procedure) when stopped due to patient condition
- Document reason for incomplete examination

Multiple Procedures:

- Different techniques during same session may be coded separately
- Same technique at multiple sites typically included in single code
- Follow CCI edits for appropriate combinations

Hernia Repairs

Hernia procedures are among the most common surgical procedures, requiring understanding of anatomical locations and repair techniques.

Types of Hernias:

Inguinal Hernias (49495-49525):

- Most common type of hernia
- Direct vs. indirect classification
- Unilateral vs. bilateral occurrence

49505 - Inguinal hernia repair, age 5 years or older:

- Initial repair
- Unilateral procedure
- Various surgical techniques

49507 - Incarcerated or strangulated inguinal hernia repair:

- Emergency procedure
- Higher complexity due to complication
- Risk of bowel compromise

Ventral Hernias (49560-49568):

- Incisional hernias: Through previous surgical site
- Umbilical hernias: Through umbilical ring
- Epigastric hernias: Above umbilicus

49560 - Ventral hernia repair, initial:

- First-time repair
- Various sizes and locations

49565 - Ventral hernia repair, recurrent:

- Previous repair has failed
- More complex due to scar tissue
- Higher recurrence risk

Hernia Repair Methods:

Open Repair:

- Traditional surgical exposure
- Direct visualization and repair
- Various suture and mesh techniques

Laparoscopic Repair:

- Minimally invasive approach

- Mesh placement from inside abdomen
- Faster recovery, less pain

Mesh vs. Non-mesh Repairs:

- Mesh reduces recurrence rates
- Synthetic vs. biological materials
- Long-term considerations

Liver, Pancreas, and Abdomen

Hepatic Procedures (47000-47399):

47562 - Laparoscopic cholecystectomy:

- Most common approach for gallbladder removal
- Minimally invasive technique
- Standard treatment for gallbladder disease

47563 - Laparoscopic cholecystectomy with cholangiography:

- Includes intraoperative imaging
- Assessment of bile duct anatomy
- Detection of retained stones

Pancreatic Procedures (48000-48999):

48150 - Pancreatectomy, proximal subtotal:

- Whipple procedure
- Complex procedure for pancreatic head lesions
- High morbidity procedure

48160 - Pancreatectomy, total:

- Complete pancreas removal
- Requires lifelong diabetes management
- Reserved for extensive disease

Practice Questions - Digestive System

Question 10: A colonoscopy with biopsy and polyp removal should be coded as:

A) 45380 (colonoscopy with biopsy) only B) 45385 (colonoscopy with polyp removal) only C) 45380 + 45385 (both procedures) D) 45378 (diagnostic colonoscopy) + 45380 + 45385

Answer: B Explanation: When multiple endoscopic procedures are performed during the same session, code only the most extensive procedure. Polyp removal (45385) includes any biopsies performed and is more extensive than biopsy alone.

Question 11: Laparoscopic repair of recurrent ventral hernia should be coded as:

A) 49560 (ventral hernia repair, initial) B) 49565 (ventral hernia repair, recurrent) C) 49650 (laparoscopic hernia repair) D) 49651 (laparoscopic hernia repair, recurrent)

Answer: D Explanation: 49651 specifically addresses laparoscopic repair of recurrent ventral hernia. The approach (laparoscopic) and status (recurrent) both affect code selection.

Question 12: EGD with control of bleeding using injection therapy should be coded as:

A) 43235 (EGD, diagnostic) B) 43255 (EGD with control of bleeding) C) 43236 (EGD with injection)
D) 43239 (EGD with biopsy)

Answer: B Explanation: 43255 covers EGD with control of bleeding regardless of the method used (injection, thermal coagulation, etc.). The specific technique doesn't change the code selection.

Chapter 11 Summary: Surgery Coding Mastery by System

You've now mastered surgery coding across four major body systems, developing the systematic approach that makes complex surgical coding manageable. Your achievements include:

Anatomical Precision: You can identify specific anatomical structures and understand how surgical approach affects code selection.

Procedure Classification: You understand the difference between simple, intermediate, and complex procedures and can select appropriate codes based on documentation.

System-Specific Guidelines: You've mastered the unique coding rules that apply to each body system, from wound repair measurements to endoscopy bundling rules.

Clinical Understanding: You can connect surgical techniques to their clinical indications and understand why certain procedures are performed.

Coding Integration: You see how surgical procedures relate to the diagnostic codes and E/M services that support them.

Remember: Surgery coding requires understanding the medicine behind the codes. The anatomical knowledge, terminology mastery, and systematic thinking you've developed here will serve you throughout your coding career.

The patterns you've learned—understanding anatomy, classifying procedures, applying guidelines, and integrating clinical knowledge—apply to all remaining surgical specialties. You're now equipped with the foundation to tackle any surgical coding challenge.

Next, you'll apply these same principles to the remaining surgical systems, building comprehensive expertise across all surgical specialties tested on the CPC exam.

Continue building your surgical coding expertise:

Question 13: Simple repair of a 3.0 cm laceration on the face and a 2.5 cm laceration on the scalp should be coded as:

A) 12013 (face, 2.6-5.0 cm) + 12002 (scalp, 2.6-7.5 cm) B) 12014 (face, 7.6-12.5 cm) for combined length C) 12013 (face, 2.6-5.0 cm) only D) Two separate simple repair codes

Answer: A Explanation: Face and scalp are different anatomical groups in wound repair coding. Each location should be coded separately: face 3.0 cm (12013) and scalp 2.5 cm (12002).

Question 14: Arthroscopic meniscectomy with repair of anterior cruciate ligament should be coded as:

A) 29880 (meniscectomy) only B) 29888 (ACL reconstruction) only C) 29880 + 29888 (both procedures) D) 29870 (diagnostic arthroscopy) + 29880 + 29888

Answer: C Explanation: Arthroscopic meniscectomy (29880) and ACL reconstruction (29888) are separate, distinct procedures that can be performed during the same operative session and should be coded separately.

Question 15: Emergency tracheostomy for acute airway obstruction should be coded as:

A) 31600 (tracheostomy, planned) B) 31601 (tracheostomy, emergency) C) 31603 (tracheostomy, emergency procedure) D) 31605 (tracheostomy, planned procedure)

Answer: C Explanation: 31603 specifically identifies emergency tracheostomy procedures performed under emergency conditions for acute airway obstruction, which carries higher risk and complexity than planned procedures.

Your surgical coding foundation across these major body systems is now solid. You understand the fundamental principles that apply across all surgical specialties and can apply systematic approaches to complex coding scenarios.

Urinary System (50000-53899)

Urological procedures require understanding of complex anatomy, from kidney function to bladder dynamics, and the intricate relationships between urinary and reproductive systems.

Kidney and Ureter Procedures

Renal Anatomy Review:

- Kidneys: Retroperitoneal organs with cortex, medulla, and pelvis
- Ureters: Muscular tubes connecting kidneys to bladder
- Three natural constriction points: ureteropelvic junction, crossing iliac vessels, ureterovesical junction
- Blood supply: Renal arteries with multiple branches

Kidney Biopsy and Aspiration (50200-50290):

50200 - Renal biopsy, percutaneous needle:

- Image-guided tissue sampling
- Diagnosis of glomerular disease, transplant rejection
- Less invasive than surgical biopsy

50205 - Renal biopsy, by surgical exposure:

- Open surgical approach
- When needle biopsy insufficient or contraindicated
- Direct visualization of kidney

Nephrolithotomy Procedures (50060-50081):

50060 - Nephrolithotomy, removal of calculus:

- Open surgical stone removal
- Large or complex stones
- When less invasive methods unsuccessful

50065 - Nephrolithotomy, secondary surgical operation:

- Removal of residual or recurrent stones
- More complex due to prior surgery
- Higher risk of complications

Nephrectomy (50220-50365):

50220 - Nephrectomy, including partial ureterectomy:

- Complete kidney removal
- Includes portion of ureter
- Benign disease indications

50225 - Nephrectomy, complicated:

- Difficult technical circumstances
- Previous surgery, inflammation, large tumors
- Requires additional surgical skill

50230 - Nephrectomy, radical:

- Kidney, adrenal gland, surrounding fascia, lymph nodes
- Cancer treatment procedure
- Most extensive kidney removal

Partial Nephrectomy (50240-50290):

50240 - Nephrectomy, partial:

- Kidney-sparing procedure
- Removal of diseased portion only

- Preserves renal function

Ureteral Procedures (50600-50980):

50600 - Ureterotomy with exploration:

- Surgical opening of ureter
- Stone removal or stricture treatment
- Direct visualization approach

50650 - Ureterectomy, with bladder cuff:

- Complete ureter removal
- Includes portion of bladder
- Cancer treatment

Endoscopic Procedures (50551-50580):

50551 - Renal endoscopy through established nephrostomy:

- Flexible or rigid scope
- Stone removal, biopsy, treatment
- Through existing tract

50561 - Renal endoscopy through established nephrostomy, with removal of foreign body or calculus:

- Stone removal procedures
- Foreign body extraction
- Therapeutic intervention

Bladder and Urethra Procedures

Bladder Anatomy:

- Detrusor muscle: Main bladder muscle
- Trigone: Triangular area between ureteral orifices and urethra
- Bladder neck: Junction with urethra
- Internal and external sphincters: Continence mechanisms

Cystoscopy Procedures (52000-52010):

52000 - Cystourethroscopy:

- Diagnostic examination
- Bladder and urethra visualization
- Assessment of symptoms

52005 - Cystourethroscopy, with ureteral catheterization:

- Catheter placement into ureter
- Drainage or contrast injection
- Diagnostic or therapeutic

Cystoscopy with Biopsy (52204-52224):

52204 - Cystourethroscopy, with biopsy:

- Cold cup biopsy of bladder lesion
- Tissue sampling for diagnosis
- Multiple sites possible

52224 - Cystourethroscopy, with fulguration of minor lesions:

- Destruction of small bladder lesions
- Electrocautery treatment
- Benign lesions typically

Transurethral Procedures (52234-52318):

52234 - Cystourethroscopy, with fulguration and/or resection of small bladder tumors:

- Treatment of bladder cancer
- Complete tumor removal
- Staging information obtained

52235 - Cystourethroscopy, with fulguration and/or resection of medium bladder tumors:

- Larger tumor procedures
- More extensive resection
- Higher complexity

Prostate Procedures (52400-52700):

52450 - Transurethral incision of prostate:

- Treatment of benign prostatic hyperplasia
- Less extensive than TURP
- Outpatient procedure typically

52601 - Transurethral electrosurgical resection of prostate:

- TURP procedure
- Gold standard for BPH treatment
- Significant symptom improvement

Urethral Procedures (53000-53899):

53000 - Urethrotomy, external:

- Treatment of urethral stricture
- External incision approach
- Stricture division

53040 - Drainage of deep periurethral abscess:

- Treatment of infection
- Deep tissue involvement
- May require extensive dissection

Practice Questions - Urinary System

Question 16: Cystoscopy with biopsy of bladder tumor and fulguration of small lesion should be coded as:

A) 52000 (cystoscopy, diagnostic) B) 52204 (cystoscopy with biopsy) + 52224 (fulguration) C) 52234 (cystoscopy with fulguration/resection of small tumor) D) 52204 (cystoscopy with biopsy) only

Answer: C Explanation: When multiple cystoscopic procedures are performed during the same session, code the most extensive procedure. Fulguration/resection (52234) includes any biopsy performed and represents the most comprehensive service.

Question 17: Radical nephrectomy for renal cell carcinoma should be coded as:

A) 50220 (nephrectomy, including partial ureterectomy) B) 50225 (nephrectomy, complicated) C) 50230 (nephrectomy, radical) D) 50240 (nephrectomy, partial)

Answer: C Explanation: Radical nephrectomy (50230) is the appropriate code for cancer treatment, which includes removal of kidney, adrenal gland, surrounding fascia, and lymph nodes. This is more extensive than simple nephrectomy.

Question 18: TURP (transurethral resection of prostate) should be coded as:

A) 52450 (transurethral incision of prostate) B) 52500 (transurethral balloon dilation of prostate) C) 52601 (transurethral electrosurgical resection of prostate) D) 52700 (drainage of prostatic abscess)

Answer: C Explanation: 52601 specifically represents TURP (transurethral electrosurgical resection of prostate), which is the complete removal of prostatic tissue through the urethra using electrocautery.

Male/Female Genital Systems (54000-58999)

Reproductive system coding requires understanding of complex anatomy, hormonal relationships, and procedures that may significantly impact patients' quality of life and reproductive capacity.

Male Reproductive System (54000-55899)

Male Genital Anatomy:

- Penis: Corpora cavernosa, corpus spongiosum, glans
- Scrotum: Contains testes and epididymides
- Testes: Sperm and hormone production
- Epididymis: Sperm maturation and storage
- Vas deferens: Sperm transport
- Prostate: Alkaline fluid production
- Seminal vesicles: Fructose-rich secretions

Penile Procedures (54000-54450):

54000 - Slitting of prepuce, dorsal or lateral:

- Treatment of phimosis or paraphimosis
- Emergency or elective procedure
- Preserves foreskin

54001 - Slitting of prepuce, dorsal or lateral, newborn:

- Age-specific procedure
- Different anatomy and considerations
- Often emergency procedure

54150 - Circumcision, using clamp or other device:

- Newborn circumcision
- Religious or medical indications
- Standard technique with device

54161 - Circumcision, surgical excision other than clamp:

- More complex technique
- May be required for anatomical variations
- Higher physician work

Testicular Procedures (54500-54699):

54500 - Biopsy of testis, needle:

- Fertility evaluation
- Sperm retrieval procedures
- Less invasive than open biopsy

54505 - Biopsy of testis, incisional:

- Open surgical approach
- When needle biopsy insufficient
- Direct visualization

54520 - Orchiectomy, simple:

- Testis removal
- Benign conditions

- Standard surgical approach

54535 - Orchiectomy, radical, for tumor:

- Cancer treatment
- Includes spermatic cord removal
- More extensive procedure

54560 - Orchiopexy, inguinal approach:

- Treatment of cryptorchidism
- Brings undescended testis to scrotum
- Preserves fertility potential

Vas Deferens Procedures (55250-55450):

55250 - Vasectomy, unilateral or bilateral:

- Male sterilization procedure
- Elective contraceptive surgery
- Outpatient procedure

55400 - Vasovasostomy, vasoepididymostomy:

- Vasectomy reversal
- Microsurgical technique
- Fertility restoration attempt

Female Reproductive System (56405-58999)

Female Genital Anatomy:

- Vulva: External genital structures
- Vagina: Muscular canal
- Cervix: Lower portion of uterus
- Uterus: Fundus, body, cervix
- Fallopian tubes: Egg transport
- Ovaries: Egg and hormone production

Vulvar and Vaginal Procedures (56405-57426):

56405 - Incision and drainage of vulvar or perineal abscess:

- Treatment of localized infection
- External genital area
- Simple drainage procedure

56420 - Incision and drainage of Bartholin's gland abscess:

- Specific gland involvement
- Common gynecologic procedure
- May require marsupialization

57454 - Biopsy of cervix, single or multiple:

- Evaluation of abnormal Pap smear
- Colposcopy-directed typically
- Rule out cervical cancer

57456 - Endocervical curettage:

- Sampling of cervical canal
- Often combined with colposcopy
- Cancer screening procedure

Cervical Procedures (57500-57800):

57500 - Biopsy of cervix, single or multiple:

- Punch biopsy technique
- Outpatient procedure
- Diagnostic evaluation

57522 - Conization of cervix, with or without fulguration:

- Cone-shaped tissue removal
- Treatment and diagnosis
- Preserves fertility potential

57530 - Trachelectomy, radical:

- Cervix removal with preservation of uterus
- Fertility-sparing cancer treatment
- Complex procedure

Hysterectomy Procedures (58150-58294):

58150 - Total abdominal hysterectomy:

- Removal of uterus and cervix
- Abdominal approach
- Ovaries may be preserved

58152 - Total abdominal hysterectomy with bilateral salpingo-oophorectomy:

- Includes fallopian tubes and ovaries
- More extensive procedure
- Complete reproductive organ removal

58260 - Vaginal hysterectomy:

- Vaginal approach
- Faster recovery than abdominal
- Limited to appropriate anatomy

58570 - Laparoscopy, surgical, with total hysterectomy:

- Minimally invasive approach
- Combines laparoscopic and vaginal techniques
- Reduced recovery time

Ovarian and Tubal Procedures (58600-58770):

58661 - Laparoscopy, surgical, with removal of adnexal structures:

- Ovary and/or fallopian tube removal
- Minimally invasive approach
- Benign or malignant indications

58700 - Salpingectomy, complete or partial, unilateral or bilateral:

- Fallopian tube removal
- Open surgical approach
- Various indications

In Vitro Fertilization Procedures (58970-58976):

58970 - Follicle puncture for oocyte retrieval:

- Egg harvest procedure
- Transvaginal ultrasound guidance
- Part of IVF cycle

58974 - Embryo transfer, intrauterine:

- Placement of embryos in uterus
- Transcervical approach
- Final step of IVF cycle

Practice Questions - Reproductive Systems

Question 19: Bilateral orchiectomy for prostate cancer treatment should be coded as:

A) 54520 (orchiectomy, simple) × 2 B) 54520 with modifier -50 (bilateral) C) 54522 (orchiectomy, partial bilateral) D) 54535 (orchiectomy, radical)

Answer: B Explanation: Simple bilateral orchiectomy for hormone ablation in prostate cancer treatment should be coded as 54520 with modifier -50 (bilateral procedure) rather than coding the procedure twice.

Question 20: Laparoscopic total hysterectomy with bilateral salpingo-oophorectomy should be coded as:

A) 58570 (laparoscopic total hysterectomy) + 58661 (removal of adnexal structures) B) 58571 (laparoscopic total hysterectomy with removal of tubes and ovaries) C) 58150 (total abdominal hysterectomy) + 58720 (salpingo-oophorectomy) D) 58260 (vaginal hysterectomy) + 58661

Answer: B Explanation: 58571 specifically describes laparoscopic total hysterectomy with removal of fallopian tubes and ovaries in a single code, which is more appropriate than multiple separate codes.

Question 21: Vasectomy reversal (vasovasostomy) should be coded as:

A) 55250 (vasectomy) B) 55400 (vasovasostomy, vasoepididymostomy) C) 55450 (ligation of vas deferens) D) 54900 (epididymectomy)

Answer: B Explanation: 55400 covers both vasovasostomy (vas deferens reconnection) and vasoepididymostomy (vas deferens to epididymis connection), both of which are vasectomy reversal procedures.

Nervous System (61000-64999)

Neurological procedures require precise anatomical knowledge and understanding of complex relationships between brain, spinal cord, and peripheral nerves.

Skull, Brain, and Spine Procedures

Neuroanatomy Review:

- Central Nervous System: Brain and spinal cord
- Peripheral Nervous System: Cranial nerves, spinal nerves, autonomic nerves
- Meninges: Dura mater, arachnoid mater, pia mater
- Cerebrospinal fluid: Cushioning and nutrition

Skull Procedures (61000-61253):

61000 - Subdural tap through fontanelle:

- Pediatric procedure
- CSF sampling or pressure relief
- Through soft spot in skull

61020 - Ventricular puncture through previous burr hole:

- CSF sampling
- Pressure monitoring
- Through existing skull opening

61105 - Craniotomy for excision of brain tumor:

- Open surgical approach
- Direct tumor visualization
- Various tumor types and locations

Brain Procedures (61304-61576):

61304 - Craniectomy or craniotomy for exploration or decompression:

- Relief of intracranial pressure

- Exploration of brain injury
- Emergency or planned procedure

61312 - Craniectomy or craniotomy for evacuation of hematoma, supratentorial:

- Blood clot removal
- Above tentorium cerebelli
- Often emergency procedure

61510 - Craniectomy, trephination, bone flap craniotomy for excision of brain tumor:

- Tumor removal procedure
- Various surgical approaches
- Depends on tumor location

Spinal Procedures (62263-63746):

63005 - Laminectomy with exploration and/or decompression of spinal cord:

- Spinal stenosis treatment
- Pressure relief on spinal cord
- Single level procedure

63030 - Laminectomy with exploration and/or decompression of spinal cord, lumbar:

- Lower back procedures
- Common for spinal stenosis
- May include multiple levels

63650 - Percutaneous implantation of spinal neurostimulator electrode array:

- Pain management procedure
- Minimally invasive approach
- Trial before permanent implant

Nerves and Neurostimulation

Peripheral Nerve Procedures (64400-64999):

64400 - Injection, anesthetic agent, trigeminal nerve:

- Facial pain treatment
- Diagnostic or therapeutic
- Various injection sites

64483 - Injection, anesthetic agent and/or steroid, transforaminal epidural:

- Back and leg pain treatment
- Image-guided procedure
- Single level

64721 - Neuroplasty and/or transposition, median nerve at carpal tunnel:

- Carpal tunnel syndrome treatment
- Nerve decompression
- Outpatient procedure

64831 - Suture of digital nerve:

- Finger nerve repair
- Trauma or surgical injury
- Microsurgical technique often required

Question 22: Carpal tunnel release should be coded as:

A) 64721 (neuroplasty of median nerve at carpal tunnel) B) 25000 (incision, extensor tendon sheath, wrist) C) 64831 (suture of digital nerve) D) 20526 (injection, carpal tunnel)

Answer: A Explanation: 64721 specifically describes neuroplasty (nerve decompression) and/or transposition of the median nerve at the carpal tunnel, which is the standard carpal tunnel release procedure.

Question 23: Epidural steroid injection at L5-S1 level should be coded as:

A) 64483 (transforaminal epidural injection, single level) B) 64484 (transforaminal epidural injection, each additional level) C) 62311 (lumbar epidural injection) D) 20610 (arthrocentesis, major joint)

Answer: A Explanation: 64483 represents transforaminal epidural injection of anesthetic and/or steroid at a single level. This is the appropriate code for L5-S1 epidural injection.

Question 24: Laminectomy for spinal stenosis at L4-L5 and L5-S1 should be coded as:

A) 63030 (laminectomy, lumbar) × 2 B) 63030 + 63035 (each additional segment) C) 63047 + 63048 (each additional segment) D) 22630 (spinal fusion)

Answer: B Explanation: Laminectomy procedures use primary codes for the first level and add-on codes for each additional level. 63030 covers the first level, and 63035 is the add-on code for each additional segment.

Chapter 11 Surgery Summary: Complete Mastery

You have now achieved comprehensive mastery of surgery coding across all major body systems. Your expertise encompasses:

Anatomical Precision: Deep understanding of surgical anatomy across all body systems and how anatomical variations affect code selection.

Procedural Classification: Ability to distinguish between different types of procedures and select the most specific codes available.

Approach Recognition: Understanding how surgical approach (open, laparoscopic, endoscopic, percutaneous) affects code assignment.

Complexity Assessment: Skills to evaluate procedure complexity and apply appropriate modifiers and add-on codes.

System Integration: Knowledge of how different body systems interact and affect surgical coding decisions.

Clinical Context: Understanding of medical indications, surgical techniques, and expected outcomes that support accurate coding.

Professional Application: Ability to handle complex scenarios, incomplete documentation, and ambiguous situations with confidence.

Key Coding Principles Mastered:

Systematic Approach:

1. Identify anatomical location
2. Determine procedure type and extent
3. Consider surgical approach
4. Apply appropriate guidelines
5. Select most specific code available

Documentation Analysis:

- Extract key procedural elements from operative reports
- Identify when additional codes or modifiers are needed
- Recognize when procedures are bundled vs. separately reportable

Guideline Application:

- Apply global surgical package rules
- Use modifier system correctly
- Follow CCI edits and bundling rules
- Handle multiple procedures appropriately

Quality Assurance:

- Verify anatomical accuracy
- Ensure procedural specificity
- Confirm appropriate code relationships
- Validate clinical appropriateness

Preparing for Advanced Coding:

Your surgical coding mastery now supports progression to other CPT® sections:

Anesthesia Coding: Understanding of surgical procedures enhances anesthesia code selection **Radiology Coding:** Knowledge of anatomical locations supports imaging procedure coding
Pathology Coding: Surgical specimens and biopsy procedures connect to laboratory testing
Medicine Coding: Non-surgical procedures often relate to surgical diagnoses and treatments

Professional Development:

This comprehensive surgical coding expertise positions you for:

CPC Exam Success: Surgery coding represents the largest portion of procedure coding questions **Career Advancement:** Surgical coding specialists are highly valued in healthcare organizations **Specialty Opportunities:** Foundation for subspecialty coding in orthopedics, neurosurgery, cardiovascular surgery **Consulting Potential:** Advanced surgical coding knowledge enables teaching and consulting opportunities

Remember: Surgery coding excellence comes from understanding the intersection of anatomy, physiology, and surgical technique. You've mastered not just codes, but the medical knowledge that makes accurate coding possible.

Chapter 12: Anesthesia Coding (00100-01999)

"The best preparation for tomorrow is doing your best today." - H. Jackson Brown Jr.

Anesthesia coding stands apart from every other section of CPT® as the only area that requires mathematical calculations to determine the final billable units. While other specialties focus on selecting the right code, anesthesia coding demands that you master a systematic formula that combines base units, time units, and qualifying circumstances to arrive at the total reportable units.

Understanding anesthesia coding opens the door to one of the most specialized and well-compensated areas of medical coding. Anesthesia providers depend on accurate coding not just for proper reimbursement, but for demonstrating the complexity and risk management inherent in their services. Your expertise in this area directly impacts their financial success and professional recognition.

This chapter transforms what many consider the most intimidating aspect of medical coding into a manageable, step-by-step process. You'll develop confidence in the mathematical calculations, master the clinical concepts that drive anesthesia decision-making, and learn to handle complex scenarios that separate expert anesthesia coders from those who simply follow formulas.

Your surgical coding knowledge now becomes invaluable. Understanding which procedures require anesthesia, how surgical complexity affects anesthesia management, and why certain patients need more intensive monitoring will make you a more thoughtful and accurate anesthesia coder.

By the end of this chapter, you'll approach anesthesia coding with the same confidence you have in any other specialty, knowing that your systematic approach ensures accuracy every time.

Understanding Anesthesia as a Medical Specialty

Before diving into coding calculations, it's essential to understand what anesthesiologists actually do and why their services are coded differently from other medical specialties. This clinical foundation makes the coding rules more logical and helps you make better decisions in ambiguous situations.

The Anesthesiologist's Role

Anesthesiologists are physicians who specialize in perioperative medicine, pain management, and critical care. Their responsibilities extend far beyond simply "putting patients to sleep" and encompass comprehensive patient care before, during, and after surgical procedures.

Preoperative Assessment and Planning: Every surgical patient requires careful evaluation to determine the safest anesthetic approach. The anesthesiologist reviews medical history, current medications, allergies, and previous anesthetic experiences. They assess cardiovascular status, respiratory function, kidney and liver health, and neurological condition. This evaluation leads to an individualized anesthetic plan that balances surgical requirements with patient safety.

For example, a healthy 25-year-old having an appendectomy requires vastly different preparation than a 75-year-old with diabetes, heart disease, and kidney impairment having the same procedure. The older patient might need specialized monitoring, medication adjustments, and extended recovery planning. This difference in complexity is reflected in physical status modifiers that directly affect anesthesia billing.

Intraoperative Management: During surgery, anesthesiologists provide continuous patient monitoring and physiologic support. They manage blood pressure, heart rate, breathing, body temperature, and fluid balance while maintaining appropriate levels of unconsciousness, pain relief, and muscle relaxation. Modern anesthetic management involves sophisticated monitoring equipment, multiple medications, and split-second decision-making.

Consider a cardiac surgery patient whose blood pressure drops suddenly during the procedure. The anesthesiologist must immediately assess potential causes—blood loss, medication effects, heart rhythm problems, or equipment malfunction—while implementing corrective measures. This level of intensity and expertise justifies the time-based component of anesthesia billing.

Postoperative Care: Anesthesia services continue through the immediate recovery period, ensuring patients wake up safely and comfortably. This includes pain management, nausea prevention, and monitoring for complications. The anesthesiologist must ensure patients meet specific criteria before transferring care to recovery room nurses.

Why Anesthesia Coding Is Different

The unique nature of anesthesia services explains why they're coded differently from other medical specialties. Understanding these differences helps you apply anesthesia coding rules more effectively.

Continuous, Time-Based Services: Unlike surgeons who perform discrete procedures, anesthesiologists provide continuous care throughout the entire surgical experience. A surgeon might spend 20 minutes removing an appendix, but the anesthesiologist is actively involved from the patient's arrival in the operating room until they're safely recovered. This continuous responsibility justifies time-based billing that's unique to anesthesia services.

Variable Complexity Within Same Procedure: The same surgical procedure can require vastly different anesthesia management depending on patient condition. A healthy patient having gallbladder surgery might need routine monitoring, while a critically ill patient having the same surgery might require invasive monitoring, multiple medications, and specialized techniques. The base unit system recognizes this inherent complexity, while physical status modifiers adjust for individual patient factors.

Risk and Liability Considerations: Anesthesiologists accept significant liability for patient safety during vulnerable periods of unconsciousness and altered physiology. They must be prepared to manage life-threatening emergencies at any moment, from allergic reactions to cardiac arrest. This level of responsibility and required expertise supports the professional fee structure reflected in anesthesia coding.

Anesthesia Code Structure and Organization

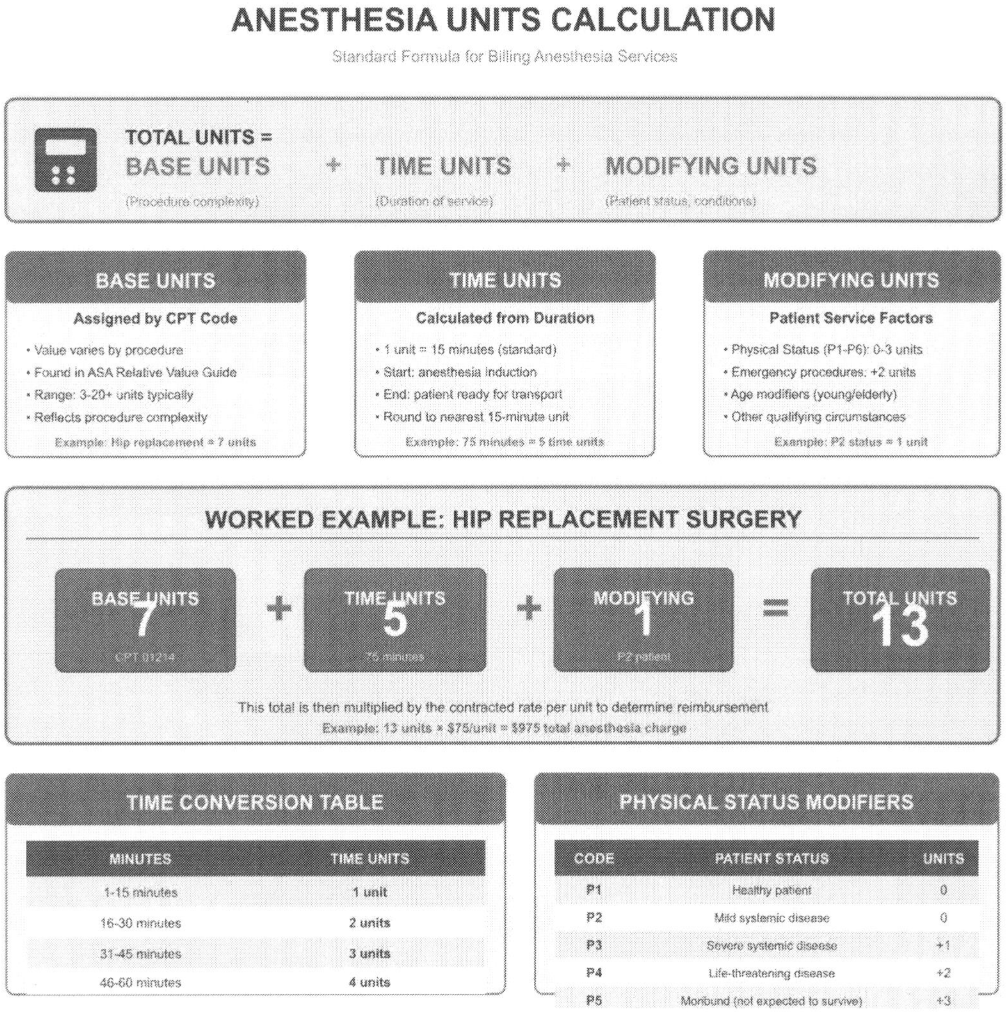

Anesthesia codes follow a systematic organization that reflects anatomical regions and surgical complexity. Understanding this structure helps you locate codes quickly and ensures you're using the most appropriate code for each situation.

Anatomical Organization Principles

CPT® organizes anesthesia codes by the anatomical region where surgery is performed, not by the type of anesthesia provided. This organization recognizes that the surgical site primarily determines anesthesia complexity, regardless of whether general, regional, or local anesthesia is used.

Head and Neck Procedures (00100-00222): This section covers anesthesia for procedures involving the scalp, face, nose, mouth, and neck. These procedures often involve airway management challenges due to shared anatomy between surgical and anesthetic access routes. For example, nasal surgery might require oral intubation with careful positioning to avoid interfering with the surgical field.

Code 00100 (anesthesia for procedures on salivary glands) carries 4 base units, reflecting moderate complexity. The surgical site near critical nerves and blood vessels requires careful monitoring, but the procedure typically doesn't involve major physiologic stress. Compare this to code 00190 (anesthesia for procedures on facial bones or skull), which carries 6 base units due to increased complexity from potential blood loss and longer operative times.

Intrathoracic Procedures (00500-00580): Chest procedures present unique anesthesia challenges due to effects on breathing and circulation. Many require single-lung ventilation, where the anesthesiologist selectively ventilates one lung while the surgeon operates on the other. This technique requires specialized equipment and expertise.

Code 00560 (anesthesia for procedures on heart, pericardial sac, and great vessels) carries 15 base units—among the highest in the anesthesia section. This reflects the extreme complexity of cardiac anesthesia, which requires advanced monitoring, specialized medications, and management of cardiopulmonary bypass machines. Patients undergoing cardiac surgery often have multiple medical problems that further complicate anesthetic management.

Intra-abdominal Procedures (00700-00882): Abdominal surgery anesthesia involves managing the physiologic effects of pneumoperitoneum (gas insufflation), patient positioning, and potential for significant fluid shifts. Laparoscopic procedures create unique challenges as gas pressure affects breathing and circulation.

Code 00840 (anesthesia for intraperitoneal procedures in lower abdomen) carries 6 base units, representing moderate complexity. However, the same surgical procedure might require different anesthesia management depending on patient position, surgical approach, and expected duration. This variability is captured through time units and qualifying circumstances rather than different base codes.

Base Unit Assignment Logic

Understanding how base units are assigned helps you appreciate the relative complexity different procedures represent and makes anesthesia coding more intuitive.

Factors Influencing Base Unit Values:

Surgical Stress and Physiologic Impact: Procedures that create significant physiologic stress receive higher base unit values. For example, cardiac surgery (15 base units) creates massive physiologic disruption requiring intensive monitoring and intervention. In contrast, cataract surgery (3 base units) creates minimal physiologic stress and requires mainly ensuring patient comfort and stillness.

Anesthetic Complexity and Risk: Some procedures require specialized anesthetic techniques that increase complexity and risk. Neurosurgical procedures often require precise blood pressure control, specialized positioning, and monitoring of brain function. These factors are reflected in higher base unit assignments.

Monitoring Requirements: Procedures requiring extensive monitoring receive higher base units. Cardiac surgery requires arterial lines, central venous catheters, transesophageal echocardiography, and specialized laboratory monitoring. This intensive monitoring reflects the high base unit assignment and acknowledges the anesthesiologist's expanded responsibilities.

Duration and Intensity: While time is separately captured in time units, the typical intensity of anesthetic management influences base unit assignment. Procedures requiring constant adjustment and intervention receive higher base units than those allowing more routine management.

Understanding Code Ranges and Their Clinical Significance

Each anesthesia code range reflects specific clinical challenges and management considerations that affect both coding and patient care.

Spine and Spinal Cord Procedures (00600-00670): Spinal surgery anesthesia requires careful attention to patient positioning, potential for significant blood loss, and neurological monitoring. Many procedures use neurophysiologic monitoring to detect nerve damage in real-time, requiring anesthetic techniques that don't interfere with these signals.

Prone positioning (face-down) creates unique challenges for airway management and circulation. The anesthesiologist must ensure adequate padding to prevent nerve damage and maintain careful blood pressure control to ensure spinal cord perfusion. These complexities justify moderate to high base unit assignments in this section.

Upper and Lower Extremity Procedures (01200-01782): Extremity surgery often allows regional anesthesia techniques like nerve blocks, which can provide excellent surgical conditions while reducing systemic medication requirements. However, these techniques require specialized skills and monitoring for complications like local anesthetic toxicity.

The base unit assignments in this section generally reflect lower complexity than major body cavity procedures, but certain factors can increase requirements. For example, tourniquets used to create bloodless surgical fields can cause significant physiologic stress when deflated, requiring careful anesthetic management.

Radiological Procedures (01810-01860): Anesthesia for radiological procedures often involves unique challenges like restricted access to the patient during imaging, radiation safety considerations, and the need for absolute stillness during scans. MRI anesthesia requires non-magnetic equipment and monitoring devices, adding complexity and expense.

These procedures typically involve healthy patients requiring anesthesia for comfort rather than medical necessity, but the unique environmental constraints justify specific coding recognition.

The Mathematics of Anesthesia Billing

Anesthesia billing calculations follow a specific formula that combines several components to determine total billable units. Mastering this calculation is essential for accurate anesthesia coding and forms the foundation for handling complex scenarios.

The Basic Formula Explained

Total Anesthesia Units = Base Units + Time Units + Qualifying Circumstances + Physical Status Modifiers

Each component of this formula serves a specific purpose in capturing the work performed by the anesthesiologist:

Base Units: Reflect the inherent complexity of providing anesthesia for the specific surgical procedure **Time Units:** Capture the duration of anesthesia services provided **Qualifying Circumstances:** Account for unusual conditions that significantly complicate anesthesia management **Physical Status Modifiers:** Adjust for patient condition complexity (note: not all payers recognize physical status modifiers for reimbursement)

Time Unit Calculations in Detail

Time units represent one of the most critical components of anesthesia billing, as they often constitute the largest portion of total billable units. Understanding proper time calculation ensures accurate billing and appropriate recognition of anesthesiologist services.

Defining Anesthesia Time: Anesthesia time begins when the anesthesiologist starts preparing the patient for anesthesia induction and ends when the patient is safely placed under post-anesthesia care supervision. This definition captures the anesthesiologist's responsibility for patient safety throughout the entire perioperative period.

Start Time Determination: The start time is recorded when the anesthesiologist begins preparing the patient for anesthetic induction. This might include placing monitoring devices, starting intravenous lines, or beginning premedication. It does not include time spent reviewing charts or discussing the case with surgeons before patient contact.

For example, if an anesthesiologist enters the operating room at 8:00 AM to review equipment but doesn't begin patient preparation until 8:15 AM, the billable anesthesia time starts at 8:15 AM. However, if the anesthesiologist begins placing monitors immediately upon entering at 8:00 AM, that becomes the start time.

End Time Determination: The end time is recorded when the anesthesiologist transfers responsibility for patient monitoring to post-anesthesia care unit (PACU) staff or other qualified personnel. This typically occurs when the patient meets specific criteria for safe transfer, including stable vital signs, adequate breathing, and appropriate level of consciousness.

The end time is not when surgery finishes, when the patient leaves the operating room, or when the anesthesiologist stops administering anesthetic medications. It's specifically when responsibility for patient monitoring transfers to recovery room staff.

Time Calculation Examples:

Example 1: Standard Calculation

- Start time: 9:30 AM
- End time: 11:45 AM
- Total time: 2 hours 15 minutes = 135 minutes
- Time units: 135 ÷ 15 = 9 time units

Example 2: Rounding Scenarios

- 67 minutes: 67 ÷ 15 = 4.47 → rounds to 4 time units
- 68 minutes: 68 ÷ 15 = 4.53 → rounds to 5 time units
- 75 minutes: 75 ÷ 15 = 5.00 → exactly 5 time units

The rounding rule follows standard mathematical principles: 0.5 and above rounds up, below 0.5 rounds down.

Time Documentation Requirements: Accurate time documentation requires clear records of start and end times, including any interruptions or transfers of care. Many anesthesia providers use automated record-keeping systems that timestamp key events, reducing documentation errors and supporting billing accuracy.

Physical Status Modifiers in Practice

Physical status modifiers describe the patient's overall health condition and its impact on anesthesia risk. While these modifiers affect billing calculations, their primary purpose is communicating patient acuity and justifying the level of anesthesia care provided.

P1 - Normal Healthy Patient: These patients have no organic, physiologic, or psychiatric disturbances beyond the surgical condition requiring treatment. They represent the baseline risk for anesthetic management and require routine monitoring and care.

Clinical Example: A 28-year-old athlete having arthroscopic knee surgery for a sports injury. No medical history, takes no medications, excellent functional capacity. The anesthetic plan can be straightforward with standard monitoring.

P2 - Patient with Mild Systemic Disease: These patients have controlled medical conditions that don't significantly limit functional capacity. The conditions are stable and well-managed, creating only minor increases in anesthetic risk.

Clinical Example: A 45-year-old office worker having gallbladder surgery. Medical history includes well-controlled hypertension on one medication, BMI of 28, and seasonal allergies. The hypertension requires blood pressure monitoring and possible medication adjustments, but doesn't significantly complicate anesthetic management.

P3 - Patient with Severe Systemic Disease: These patients have medical conditions that create functional limitations but aren't immediately life-threatening. Multiple conditions or poorly controlled single conditions may place patients in this category.

Clinical Example: A 65-year-old having colon surgery. Medical history includes diabetes with peripheral neuropathy (HbA1c 8.5%), moderate COPD requiring inhaler use, and osteoarthritis limiting mobility. The diabetes requires careful glucose monitoring, COPD affects ventilation planning, and multiple medications create interaction risks.

P4 - Patient with Severe Systemic Disease Constituting Constant Threat to Life: These patients have poorly controlled or end-stage medical conditions that create significant anesthetic risk. They require intensive monitoring and may need specialized care.

Clinical Example: A 72-year-old having emergency bowel surgery. Medical history includes severe heart failure (ejection fraction 25%), recent myocardial infarction, kidney failure requiring dialysis, and insulin-dependent diabetes. Every aspect of anesthetic management requires careful planning and monitoring.

P5 - Moribund Patient Not Expected to Survive Without Operation: These patients are critically ill with little chance of survival regardless of surgical intervention. Anesthetic management focuses on maintaining minimal physiologic function long enough to complete necessary surgery.

Clinical Example: A patient with ruptured aortic aneurysm, massive blood loss, and cardiovascular collapse requiring emergency surgical repair. The anesthetic management involves aggressive resuscitation while preparing for surgery that represents the only chance for survival.

P6 - Declared Brain-Dead Patient for Organ Donation: These patients present unique challenges as the goal is maintaining organ viability rather than patient survival. Anesthetic management focuses on optimizing organ function for transplantation.

Qualifying Circumstances: When Standard Care Isn't Enough

Qualifying circumstances recognize situations where anesthesia management becomes significantly more complex than typical for the procedure being performed. These circumstances justify additional reimbursement by acknowledging the extra work and risk involved.

+99100 - Anesthesia for Patient of Extreme Age

Age significantly affects anesthetic management due to physiologic changes and increased medical complexity common in very young and very old patients.

Patients Under One Year: Infants present unique challenges that make anesthesia management significantly more complex than adult cases. Their cardiovascular and respiratory systems are immature, creating different responses to medications and increased sensitivity to physiologic changes.

Physiologic Differences: Infants have higher heart rates, different blood pressure norms, and proportionally larger heads that affect airway management. Their higher metabolic rates increase oxygen consumption and carbon dioxide production, requiring careful ventilation management.

Medication Considerations: Drug dosing in infants requires weight-based calculations with careful attention to organ maturity. Liver and kidney function differences affect medication metabolism and elimination, requiring modified drug choices and dosing intervals.

Temperature Regulation: Infants lose heat rapidly due to high surface area to body weight ratios and immature temperature regulation mechanisms. Maintaining normal body temperature requires special warming devices and careful monitoring.

Fluid Management: Infant fluid requirements differ significantly from adults, with higher baseline needs and increased sensitivity to both dehydration and fluid overload. Careful calculation and monitoring prevent serious complications.

Patients Over 70 Years: Elderly patients typically have multiple medical conditions, take multiple medications, and have physiologic changes that complicate anesthetic management.

Cardiovascular Changes: Aging affects heart function, blood vessel elasticity, and blood pressure regulation. These changes require modified medication choices and careful hemodynamic monitoring.

Respiratory Changes: Lung function decreases with age, affecting oxygen exchange and ventilation requirements. Elderly patients may need longer recovery times and more intensive respiratory support.

Medication Interactions: Elderly patients often take multiple medications that can interact with anesthetic agents. Careful review and planning prevent dangerous drug interactions and adverse effects.

Cognitive Considerations: Some elderly patients have cognitive impairment that affects cooperation and recovery. Anesthetic plans must account for these factors while maintaining patient dignity and comfort.

+99116 - Anesthesia Complicated by Utilization of Total Body Hypothermia

Deliberate cooling of patients below normal body temperature creates significant anesthetic challenges that require specialized monitoring and management techniques.

Cardiac Surgery Applications: Many cardiac surgeries use hypothermia to protect organs during periods when blood circulation is stopped or reduced. The anesthesiologist must carefully manage the cooling and rewarming process while monitoring for complications.

Cooling Process Management: Gradual temperature reduction requires coordination between anesthesiologist and surgeon. Too rapid cooling can cause dangerous heart rhythm changes, while inadequate cooling doesn't provide organ protection.

Physiologic Effects: Hypothermia affects all organ systems, changing heart function, blood clotting, kidney function, and medication metabolism. The anesthesiologist must adjust medications and monitoring throughout the temperature changes.

Rewarming Challenges: Bringing patients back to normal temperature creates unique risks including heart rhythm disturbances, blood pressure changes, and increased bleeding tendency. Careful management prevents serious complications.

Monitoring Requirements: Hypothermia requires specialized temperature monitoring at multiple body sites, modified blood gas analysis for temperature effects, and careful assessment of blood clotting function.

+99135 - Anesthesia Complicated by Utilization of Controlled Hypotension

Deliberately lowering blood pressure below normal levels reduces surgical bleeding and improves visualization in certain procedures, but creates significant anesthetic challenges.

Surgical Benefits: Controlled hypotension dramatically reduces bleeding during certain procedures, allowing surgeons better visualization of anatomical structures and reducing need for blood transfusions. This technique is particularly valuable in spine surgery, plastic surgery, and certain neurosurgical procedures.

Anesthetic Challenges: Maintaining safe blood pressure reduction requires specialized medications, continuous monitoring, and careful assessment of organ perfusion. The anesthesiologist must balance surgical benefits against risks of inadequate organ blood flow.

Medication Management: Achieving controlled hypotension requires precise titration of specialized medications that lower blood pressure while maintaining heart function. These medications require careful monitoring and adjustment throughout the procedure.

Organ Perfusion Monitoring: While blood pressure is deliberately lowered, the anesthesiologist must ensure adequate blood flow to vital organs including brain, heart, kidneys, and spinal cord. This requires sophisticated monitoring and clinical assessment.

Patient Selection: Not all patients are candidates for controlled hypotension. Those with cardiovascular disease, cerebrovascular disease, or other conditions affecting blood flow may not tolerate blood pressure reduction safely.

+99140 - Anesthesia Complicated by Emergency Conditions

Emergency surgery creates unique anesthetic challenges due to limited preparation time, patient instability, and increased risk of complications.

Time Pressure Challenges: Emergency procedures don't allow the usual preoperative optimization that improves anesthetic safety. Patients may not be fasting appropriately, increasing aspiration risk. Medical conditions may not be optimally controlled, creating additional management challenges.

Patient Instability: Emergency patients often present with hemodynamic instability, blood loss, or other physiologic derangements that complicate anesthetic management. The anesthesiologist must simultaneously address these problems while providing appropriate anesthesia for surgery.

Limited Information: Emergency situations may not allow complete medical history gathering or diagnostic testing. The anesthesiologist must make management decisions with incomplete information while preparing for potential complications.

Increased Aspiration Risk: Emergency patients often haven't fasted appropriately, creating significant risk of vomiting and aspiration during anesthesia induction. Special techniques and equipment may be required to manage this risk safely.

Resource Limitations: Emergency procedures may occur during off-hours when specialized personnel or equipment isn't immediately available. The anesthesiologist may need to modify techniques based on available resources while maintaining patient safety.

Comprehensive Anesthesia Coding Examples

Real-world anesthesia coding requires integrating all components of the billing formula while considering clinical factors that affect each element. These comprehensive examples demonstrate the thought process expert anesthesia coders use.

Complex Case Study 1: Emergency Surgery in High-Risk Patient

Clinical Scenario: Mrs. Johnson, an 82-year-old woman, presents to the emergency department with severe abdominal pain. CT scan reveals a perforated colon requiring emergency surgery. Her medical history includes severe heart failure, diabetes with kidney complications, and chronic lung disease. She takes 12 different medications and uses supplemental oxygen at home.

Anesthetic Challenges: This case presents multiple factors that significantly complicate anesthetic management:

Age Factor: At 82 years old, Mrs. Johnson qualifies for the extreme age qualifying circumstance (+99100).

Emergency Nature: The perforated colon requires immediate surgery without time for medical optimization, qualifying for emergency conditions (+99140).

Medical Complexity: Severe heart failure with kidney complications and chronic lung disease places her in P4 category (severe systemic disease constituting constant threat to life).

Surgery Duration: The surgery takes 3 hours and 45 minutes (225 minutes) due to extensive infection and difficult anatomy.

Coding Calculation:

- **Anesthesia Code:** 00840 (Anesthesia for intraperitoneal procedures in lower abdomen)
- **Base Units:** 6 units
- **Time Units:** 225 minutes ÷ 15 = 15 time units
- **Physical Status:** P4 (severe systemic disease, constant threat to life)
- **Qualifying Circumstances:** +99100 (extreme age, 1 unit) + +99140 (emergency conditions, 1 unit)

Total Calculation: 6 + 15 + 0 + 1 + 1 = 23 total anesthesia units

Clinical Justification: This high unit total reflects the extraordinary complexity of providing anesthesia for an elderly, critically ill patient requiring emergency surgery. The anesthesiologist must manage multiple medical conditions, coordinate with surgical and nursing teams, and maintain patient stability throughout a prolonged procedure under emergency conditions.

Complex Case Study 2: Cardiac Surgery with Complications

Clinical Scenario: Mr. Rodriguez, a 65-year-old man, undergoes cardiac bypass surgery for severe coronary artery disease. During the procedure, complications require additional surgical time and specialized management including controlled hypotension and careful temperature management.

Anesthetic Challenges: Cardiac surgery represents one of the most complex anesthetic managements in medicine:

Procedure Complexity: Cardiac bypass surgery requires specialized monitoring, blood management, and coordination with cardiopulmonary bypass team.

Temperature Management: The procedure requires careful cooling and rewarming as part of cardiac protection strategy.

Blood Pressure Control: Certain phases of the procedure require controlled hypotension to improve surgical conditions and reduce bleeding.

Extended Duration: The surgery takes 6 hours and 30 minutes (390 minutes) due to complex anatomy and surgical complications.

Patient Condition: Severe coronary disease with moderate heart function places him in P3 category.

Coding Calculation:

- **Anesthesia Code:** 00560 (Anesthesia for procedures on heart, pericardial sac, and great vessels)
- **Base Units:** 15 units (highest complexity)
- **Time Units:** 390 minutes ÷ 15 = 26 time units
- **Physical Status:** P3 (severe systemic disease with functional limitation)
- **Qualifying Circumstances:** +99116 (total body hypothermia, 1 unit) + +99135 (controlled hypotension, 1 unit)

Total Calculation: 15 + 26 + 0 + 1 + 1 = 43 total anesthesia units

Clinical Justification: This extremely high unit total reflects the maximum complexity of anesthetic management. Cardiac surgery with complications requires specialized expertise, intensive monitoring, and management of multiple physiologic systems throughout an extended procedure.

Advanced Anesthesia Coding Scenarios

Multiple Procedures and Concurrent Care

Scenario: Sequential Procedures A patient undergoes arthroscopic knee surgery followed immediately by manipulation under anesthesia of the same knee.

Coding Approach: When multiple procedures are performed during continuous anesthesia care, use the code with the highest base unit value. Time units reflect the total anesthesia time for all procedures combined.

Calculation:

- Primary code: Higher base unit procedure
- Time units: Total time for all procedures
- Qualifying circumstances: Apply if relevant to any part of care

Scenario: Concurrent Anesthesiologist Supervision One anesthesiologist supervises multiple CRNAs providing anesthesia for different cases simultaneously.

Coding Considerations:

- Each case coded separately
- Qualifying circumstances apply to individual cases
- Medical direction rules may affect billing
- Documentation must support level of supervision provided

Anesthesia Billing Practice Questions

Test your mastery of anesthesia coding calculations and principles:

Question 1: Anesthesia for appendectomy (00840, 6 base units) in a healthy 25-year-old patient lasting 90 minutes. Calculate total units:

A) 12 units (6 base + 6 time + 0 qualifying circumstances) B) 13 units (6 base + 6 time + 1 physical status) C) 14 units (6 base + 7 time + 1 qualifying circumstances) D) 11 units (6 base + 5 time + 0 qualifying circumstances)

Answer: A Explanation: Base units (6) + Time units (90 ÷ 15 = 6) + P1 physical status (0 additional units) = 12 total units. Healthy 25-year-old doesn't qualify for age-related qualifying circumstances.

Question 2: An 85-year-old patient with severe heart disease undergoes emergency gallbladder surgery lasting 120 minutes (00790, 7 base units). Calculate total units:

A) 15 units (7 base + 8 time + 0 modifiers) B) 17 units (7 base + 8 time + 1 age + 1 emergency) C) 18 units (7 base + 8 time + 1 age + 1 emergency + 1 P4) D) 16 units (7 base + 8 time + 1 emergency)

Answer: B Explanation: Base units (7) + Time units (120 ÷ 15 = 8) + Age >70 (+99100, 1 unit) + Emergency (+99140, 1 unit) = 17 total units. Physical status modifiers don't add units in most billing systems.

Question 3: Which qualifying circumstance applies to a 6-month-old infant having hernia repair?

A) +99100 (extreme age) B) +99116 (controlled hypotension) C) +99135 (total body hypothermia) D) +99140 (emergency conditions)

Answer: A Explanation: +99100 applies to patients under 1 year of age or over 70 years old. A 6-month-old infant qualifies due to extreme young age.

Question 4: Anesthesia time starts when:

A) The patient enters the operating room B) Surgery begins C) The anesthesiologist begins preparing the patient for anesthesia D) The patient is unconscious

Answer: C Explanation: Anesthesia time begins when the anesthesiologist starts preparing the patient for anesthetic induction, which may include placing monitors, starting IVs, or beginning premedication.

Question 5: A patient with well-controlled diabetes and mild hypertension should be assigned which physical status modifier?

A) P1 (normal healthy patient) B) P2 (mild systemic disease) C) P3 (severe systemic disease) D) P4 (severe systemic disease, constant threat to life)

Answer: B Explanation: Well-controlled diabetes and mild hypertension represent mild systemic diseases without functional limitations, qualifying for P2 physical status modifier.

Chapter 12 Summary: Mastering Anesthesia Coding

You have now mastered the most mathematically complex section of CPT® coding. Your achievements include:

Formula Mastery: You can accurately calculate total anesthesia units using base units, time units, and qualifying circumstances with confidence in any scenario.

Clinical Understanding: You understand the medical complexity that drives anesthesia coding rules and can make appropriate decisions when documentation is incomplete.

Component Recognition: You can identify when physical status modifiers and qualifying circumstances apply and understand their clinical significance.

Complex Scenario Management: You can handle multiple procedures, emergency situations, and high-risk patients while maintaining coding accuracy.

Professional Application: You understand how anesthesia coding affects provider reimbursement and can communicate effectively with anesthesia providers about coding requirements.

The systematic approach you've developed here—understanding the clinical context, identifying all relevant components, applying the mathematical formula, and verifying the result—serves as a model for handling complex coding in any specialty.

Your anesthesia coding expertise now positions you as a valuable specialist in one of healthcare's most technically demanding coding areas. This knowledge opens opportunities in anesthesia practices, surgery centers, and hospitals where accurate anesthesia coding directly impacts financial performance.

Next, you'll apply similar analytical skills to radiology coding, where understanding imaging techniques and anatomical visualization becomes key to accurate code selection. The foundation you've built in systematic analysis and clinical understanding will serve you well as you master the remaining CPT® sections.

Remember: Anesthesia coding excellence comes from understanding both the mathematics and the medicine. You've mastered both, making you a complete anesthesia coding professional.

Chapter 13: Radiology Coding (70010-79999)

"A picture is worth a thousand words, but accurate radiology coding is worth proper reimbursement and quality patient care." - Anonymous Radiologist

Radiology coding opens a fascinating window into modern medicine's most sophisticated diagnostic tools. Every X-ray, CT scan, MRI, and ultrasound tells a story—not just about what's happening inside the patient's body, but about the complex intersection of medical technology, clinical expertise, and healthcare economics.

Understanding radiology coding means understanding how physicians see inside the human body without making a single incision. You'll learn to translate the sophisticated world of medical imaging into accurate codes that ensure radiologists are properly compensated for their expertise while maintaining the detailed records that drive quality patient care.

This chapter transforms the complex world of radiology services into manageable, logical coding concepts. You'll master the critical distinction between technical and professional components, understand how different imaging modalities answer different clinical questions, and develop the confidence to handle even the most challenging radiology scenarios that appear on the CPC exam.

Your anatomy knowledge becomes absolutely critical here. Understanding what structures different imaging techniques can visualize, why specific views are obtained, and how contrast materials enhance diagnostic capability will make you a more insightful and accurate radiology coder.

By the end of this chapter, you'll think like a radiologist who understands not just what codes to assign, but why those codes accurately reflect the sophisticated medical services provided. You'll appreciate the technology behind modern medical imaging and the expertise required to interpret these studies accurately.

Understanding Radiology as a Medical Specialty

Before diving into specific coding rules, it's essential to understand what radiologists do and why their services are structured differently from other medical specialties. This clinical foundation makes the coding rules more logical and helps you make better decisions when documentation is incomplete or ambiguous.

The Radiologist's Dual Role

Radiologists function as both technical experts and clinical consultants, requiring them to master sophisticated imaging technology while maintaining deep knowledge of anatomy, pathology, and clinical medicine. This dual expertise explains why radiology coding recognizes both technical and professional components of imaging services.

Technical Expertise and Equipment Management: Modern medical imaging requires some of the most sophisticated and expensive equipment in healthcare. A single MRI machine can cost several million dollars and requires specialized facilities with magnetic shielding, cryogenic cooling systems, and precise environmental controls. CT scanners use complex X-ray systems that can create thousands of cross-sectional images in seconds, requiring computer processing power that was unimaginable just decades ago.

Radiologists must understand how each imaging modality works, what factors affect image quality, and how to optimize scanning parameters for different clinical situations. They make real-time decisions about contrast administration, scanning protocols, and image reconstruction techniques. This technical expertise represents a significant component of radiology services and justifies the technical component billing structure.

Clinical Interpretation and Consultation: Beyond operating sophisticated equipment, radiologists serve as expert consultants who translate images into clinically meaningful information. They identify subtle abnormalities that might be missed by others, distinguish between normal variants and pathology, and provide clinical recommendations that directly impact patient care.

A chest X-ray that appears normal to most healthcare providers might reveal early pneumonia, a small pneumothorax, or the first signs of heart failure to a trained radiologist. This interpretive expertise requires years of specialized training and continuous education to stay current with evolving imaging techniques and disease patterns.

Communication and Clinical Correlation: Radiologists don't work in isolation—they serve as consultants to referring physicians who need imaging expertise to answer specific clinical questions. A good radiologist considers the clinical history, physical examination findings, and laboratory results when interpreting images, providing context that makes their interpretations more valuable and accurate.

This consultative role explains why radiologists often communicate directly with referring physicians about urgent findings, recommend additional imaging studies, or suggest alternative diagnostic approaches. These communications represent significant professional work that goes beyond simply reading images.

How Radiology Services Are Structured

Understanding the business and operational structure of radiology services helps explain why coding rules exist and how they affect different practice settings.

Hospital-Based Radiology: Most hospitals employ or contract with radiologists to provide imaging services. In this model, the hospital typically owns the expensive imaging equipment and employs technologists who operate the machines. Radiologists provide professional interpretation services, either as employees or independent contractors.

This arrangement creates a natural split between technical and professional components. The hospital bills for equipment, technologist services, and supplies (technical component), while radiologists bill for interpretation and consultation services (professional component). Understanding this split is crucial for accurate component coding.

Private Practice Radiology: Some radiologists operate private practices where they own imaging equipment and employ their own technologists. In this model, the practice provides both technical and professional components of imaging services, justifying global billing without component modifiers.

Private practice radiologists often specialize in particular imaging modalities or body systems, developing expertise that justifies premium fees for complex interpretations. They may also provide services to multiple hospitals or imaging centers, creating complex billing scenarios that require careful attention to component coding.

Imaging Centers and Outpatient Facilities: Freestanding imaging centers represent a growing segment of radiology services, often providing high-quality imaging in more convenient, less expensive settings than hospitals. These facilities typically own their equipment and employ technologists, but may contract with radiologists for professional interpretations.

Understanding these different practice models helps you apply component coding rules correctly and appreciate why certain billing patterns exist in radiology.

Diagnostic Radiology Guidelines: The Foundation of Accurate Coding

Radiology coding success begins with mastering the fundamental principles that govern how imaging services are coded, billed, and reimbursed. These guidelines form the foundation for everything else you'll learn in this chapter.

The Four Components of Radiology Services

Every radiology procedure potentially consists of four distinct components, though not all procedures include all components. Understanding these components is essential for accurate coding and appropriate use of modifiers.

1. Technical Component (TC) - The Technology and Support Infrastructure: The technical component encompasses all the resources required to produce diagnostic images: sophisticated equipment worth millions of dollars, skilled technologists who position patients and operate machines, specialized supplies including contrast materials and protective devices, and the physical facilities that house imaging equipment.

Consider a CT scan of the abdomen: The technical component includes the CT scanner itself with its complex X-ray systems and computer processing capabilities, the technologist who positions the patient and monitors the scan, the contrast material injected to enhance visualization, and the specialized room with radiation shielding and emergency equipment. The technical component also includes quality assurance testing, equipment maintenance, and regulatory compliance activities that ensure safe, accurate imaging.

The technical component represents the largest financial investment in radiology services and typically accounts for the majority of total reimbursement for most imaging procedures. This component is usually billed by hospitals, imaging centers, or other facilities that own the equipment.

2. Professional Component (PC) - The Medical Expertise and Interpretation: The professional component represents the radiologist's medical expertise in interpreting images and providing clinical recommendations. This includes reviewing images systematically, identifying normal and abnormal findings, correlating imaging findings with clinical history and other diagnostic information, generating written reports that communicate findings clearly to referring physicians, and providing consultation services when physicians have questions about imaging results.

The professional component requires extensive medical training, including four years of medical school, one year of internship, and four years of radiology residency. Many radiologists complete additional fellowship training in subspecialties like neuroradiology, body imaging, or interventional radiology.

A radiologist interpreting that same abdominal CT scan must systematically evaluate multiple organ systems, identify subtle abnormalities that might be missed by others, distinguish between normal variants and pathology, consider the clinical context provided by the referring physician, and generate a comprehensive report that guides further patient management. This expertise represents years of specialized training and justifies separate professional component billing.

3. Supervision Component - Real-Time Guidance and Quality Control: Some imaging procedures require direct physician supervision during image acquisition. This supervision involves real-time guidance of technologists, adjustment of imaging parameters based on initial findings, monitoring of patient safety during procedures, and immediate decision-making about additional imaging needs.

Supervision is particularly important for complex procedures like interventional radiology, where radiologists guide catheters and needles using real-time imaging, or specialized studies where imaging parameters must be adjusted based on preliminary findings. The supervision component ensures optimal image quality and patient safety.

4. Global Service - Complete Imaging Service: When the same provider or entity performs both technical and professional components, the service is billed globally without component modifiers. Global billing is appropriate when a single practice owns the equipment, employs the technologists, and provides the professional interpretation.

Global services are common in private radiology practices and some imaging centers where radiologists have ownership interests in the facilities. Understanding when global billing is appropriate prevents incorrect use of component modifiers.

Component Coding Rules and Modifier Usage

Proper component coding requires understanding when and how to use modifiers -26 (professional component) and -TC (technical component). These modifiers ensure accurate billing and prevent payment errors that can affect both providers and patients.

When to Use Modifier -26 (Professional Component): Use modifier -26 when billing only the professional interpretation of an imaging study. This situation occurs when the radiologist interprets images obtained at a different facility, when a radiologist provides interpretation services as an independent contractor, or when hospital-employed radiologists bill separately from the hospital's technical component charges.

Real-World Example: Dr. Smith, a radiologist in private practice, contracts with Regional Hospital to provide evening and weekend coverage for emergency radiology interpretations. When Dr. Smith interprets a chest X-ray performed at Regional Hospital, he bills 71045-26 (Radiologic examination, chest; single view, professional component). Regional Hospital bills 71045-TC for the technical component.

This arrangement allows the hospital to provide 24-hour radiology coverage without employing full-time radiologists for all shifts, while ensuring radiologists are compensated appropriately for their expertise regardless of when they provide services.

When to Use Modifier -TC (Technical Component): Use modifier -TC when billing only the technical portion of an imaging service. This occurs when facilities provide equipment, technologist services, and supplies but arrange for professional interpretation elsewhere.

Real-World Example: Community Imaging Center performs MRI studies using their equipment and technologists, but contracts with Metropolitan Radiology Group for all professional interpretations. When a patient has a knee MRI, Community Imaging Center bills 73721-TC (Magnetic resonance imaging, any joint of lower extremity; without contrast material, technical component). Metropolitan Radiology Group bills 73721-26 for the professional component.

This arrangement allows imaging centers to focus on operational efficiency and patient service while ensuring professional interpretations are provided by radiologists with appropriate subspecialty expertise.

When to Bill Globally (No Modifier): Bill globally when the same provider or entity performs both technical and professional components. This typically occurs in private radiology practices that own their equipment or when radiologists are employed by facilities that want to bill globally for imaging services.

Billing Scenarios to Avoid: Never bill both -26 and -TC modifiers for the same patient encounter from the same provider. This would represent double billing for the same service.

Similarly, don't bill globally and also bill component services—this also represents inappropriate duplicate billing.

Understanding Supervision and Interpretation

Many radiology codes include "supervision and interpretation" in their descriptions, indicating that the procedure includes both performance of the imaging study and professional interpretation of the results. Understanding this concept prevents coding errors and ensures appropriate billing.

Procedures That Include Supervision and Interpretation: Most diagnostic imaging procedures include supervision and interpretation as part of the global service. For example, 74170 (Computed tomography, abdomen; without contrast material, followed by contrast material and further sections) includes both performing the CT scan and providing professional interpretation.

When supervision and interpretation are included in the procedure description, you cannot bill separately for these services. The global code encompasses all components of the imaging service.

Procedures Requiring Separate Supervision Coding: Some interventional radiology procedures require separate coding for imaging supervision. These procedures typically involve using imaging guidance to perform therapeutic interventions, where the imaging guidance represents additional work beyond the basic procedure.

For example, percutaneous drainage of an abdominal fluid collection might require separate coding for the drainage procedure and the imaging guidance used to place the drainage catheter safely. Understanding which procedures include guidance and which require separate coding prevents both undercoding and inappropriate unbundling.

Documentation Requirements for Component Billing: Proper component billing requires clear documentation of which services were provided and by whom. This documentation should include identification of the interpreting radiologist, the facility where images were obtained, the type and extent of professional services provided, and any unusual circumstances that affected service provision.

Without proper documentation, component billing disputes can arise that affect payment and create compliance issues. Clear documentation protects both providers and patients while ensuring accurate billing.

Diagnostic Ultrasound: Sound Waves as Medical Tools

Ultrasound represents one of medicine's most versatile and patient-friendly imaging modalities. Using high-frequency sound waves instead of ionizing radiation, ultrasound provides real-time imaging that's safe for pregnant patients, children, and patients requiring multiple follow-up studies.

Understanding ultrasound coding requires appreciating both the technology's capabilities and limitations, the skill required for proper technique, and the wide range of clinical applications that make ultrasound essential in modern medical practice.

The Science and Art of Ultrasound Imaging

How Ultrasound Technology Works: Ultrasound imaging uses sound waves at frequencies above human hearing range (typically 2-15 MHz) that penetrate body tissues and reflect back to create images. Different tissues reflect sound waves differently—fluid appears black (anechoic), soft tissues appear gray, and dense structures like bone appear bright white (hyperechoic).

The ultrasound machine processes these reflected sound waves to create real-time images that show both structure and movement. This real-time capability makes ultrasound invaluable for evaluating fetal development, heart function, blood flow, and organ movement during breathing or other activities.

Operator Dependency and Skill Requirements: Unlike CT or MRI, where image quality depends primarily on equipment calibration and patient cooperation, ultrasound image quality depends heavily on operator skill. The sonographer or physician performing the study must understand anatomy, recognize normal and abnormal appearances, optimize machine settings for different body habitus, and adapt scanning techniques for challenging patients.

This operator dependency explains why ultrasound codes often specify "complete" versus "limited" examinations and why proper training and certification are essential for accurate diagnostic ultrasound. The skill required to obtain diagnostic-quality images justifies the professional reimbursement associated with ultrasound services.

Ultrasound's Unique Advantages: Real-time imaging allows assessment of organ function and blood flow patterns that can't be evaluated with static imaging modalities. No ionizing radiation makes ultrasound safe for pregnant patients and children, and suitable for repeated follow-up examinations. Portability allows bedside imaging in intensive care units, emergency departments, and other clinical settings where patient transport might be dangerous or impractical.

Cost-effectiveness makes ultrasound accessible for screening and diagnostic applications where more expensive imaging might not be justified. These advantages explain ultrasound's broad clinical applications and the importance of accurate ultrasound coding.

Obstetrical and Gynecological Ultrasound

Obstetrical ultrasound represents one of medicine's most emotionally significant imaging applications, providing expectant parents their first glimpse of their developing baby while ensuring healthy fetal development and identifying potential complications early.

First Trimester Obstetrical Ultrasound (76801): First trimester ultrasound serves multiple critical functions in early pregnancy management. The primary goals include confirming fetal viability by documenting fetal cardiac activity, accurate pregnancy dating through crown-rump length measurements, determining the number of fetuses and their chorionicity in multiple pregnancies, and evaluating the uterus and adnexa for abnormalities that might affect pregnancy.

Early pregnancy ultrasound can identify miscarriage, ectopic pregnancy, molar pregnancy, and other complications that require immediate medical attention. The ability to document fetal cardiac activity provides reassurance to expectant parents while identifying pregnancies at risk for miscarriage.

Coding Considerations: 76801 represents a complete first trimester study that includes all standard measurements and documentation. Limited studies for specific indications use different codes and require clear documentation of the limited nature of the examination.

Second and Third Trimester Obstetrical Ultrasound (76805): Later pregnancy ultrasound provides comprehensive assessment of fetal growth and development, anatomical evaluation for birth defects and genetic conditions, placental location and function assessment, and amniotic fluid volume evaluation.

These studies require systematic evaluation of fetal anatomy including the brain, spine, heart, kidneys, limbs, and other organ systems. Biometric measurements track fetal growth and estimate gestational age and fetal weight. Placental evaluation determines location relative to the cervix and assesses for abnormalities that might affect delivery.

The complexity of these examinations requires specialized training and equipment capable of detailed anatomical evaluation. Many facilities employ maternal-fetal medicine specialists or specially trained sonographers for these critical studies.

Detailed Fetal Anatomical Ultrasound (76811): When routine obstetrical ultrasound identifies potential abnormalities or when patients have risk factors for fetal anomalies, detailed anatomical ultrasound provides comprehensive evaluation of fetal organ systems. These studies require specialized expertise and equipment capable of detailed anatomical assessment.

Detailed anatomical ultrasound might identify cardiac defects, neural tube defects, kidney abnormalities, skeletal disorders, and other conditions that affect pregnancy management and delivery planning. Early identification of these conditions allows for appropriate specialist consultation and delivery planning at facilities equipped to handle complex neonatal care.

Gynecological Ultrasound Applications: Pelvic ultrasound evaluates the uterus, ovaries, and surrounding structures for a wide range of gynecological conditions. Common indications include evaluation of abnormal uterine bleeding, pelvic pain, suspected ovarian cysts or masses, and infertility evaluation.

Transvaginal ultrasound provides detailed evaluation of pelvic organs using a specialized probe placed in the vagina, allowing closer proximity to structures of interest and improved image resolution. This technique is particularly valuable for early pregnancy evaluation and detailed assessment of ovarian and uterine abnormalities.

Non-Obstetrical Ultrasound Applications

Complete Abdominal Ultrasound (76700): Complete abdominal ultrasound provides comprehensive evaluation of multiple organ systems including the liver, gallbladder, common bile duct, pancreas, spleen, kidneys, and aorta. This study requires systematic evaluation of each organ with documentation of normal and abnormal findings.

Abdominal ultrasound is commonly used to evaluate right upper quadrant pain (possible gallbladder disease), abnormal liver function tests, suspected kidney stones, abdominal aortic aneurysm screening, and follow-up of known abnormalities. The non-invasive nature and lack of radiation exposure make abdominal ultrasound an excellent first-line imaging study for many abdominal complaints.

Technical Requirements: Complete abdominal ultrasound requires evaluation of all specified organs with adequate visualization and documentation. If certain organs cannot be visualized due to patient factors (obesity, bowel gas), this should be documented and may justify use of limited study codes.

Limited Abdominal Ultrasound (76705): Limited abdominal ultrasound focuses on specific organs or regions rather than providing comprehensive abdominal evaluation. This might include focused gallbladder evaluation for suspected cholecystitis, kidney evaluation for suspected stones, or follow-up of previously identified abnormalities.

Limited studies must be clearly documented as such, with specific indication for the focused examination. Simply performing a complete study but documenting only certain organs doesn't justify limited study coding—the billing must reflect the actual scope of the examination performed.

Retroperitoneal Ultrasound (76770): Retroperitoneal ultrasound specifically evaluates structures behind the peritoneum, including the kidneys, abdominal aorta, inferior vena cava, and any abnormal fluid collections or masses. This study is often used for kidney evaluation, aortic aneurysm assessment, and evaluation of retroperitoneal masses.

The retroperitoneal space presents unique imaging challenges due to overlying bowel gas and the deep location of structures of interest. Successful retroperitoneal ultrasound requires specialized techniques and expertise to obtain diagnostic-quality images.

Vascular Ultrasound Studies: Doppler ultrasound adds functional information to structural imaging by evaluating blood flow patterns, vessel patency, and hemodynamic function. This technology is essential for evaluating peripheral arterial disease, deep vein thrombosis, carotid artery stenosis, and other vascular conditions.

Extremity Arterial Studies (76820): Evaluate arterial blood flow in arms or legs, commonly used to assess peripheral arterial disease, monitor bypass graft function, or evaluate circulation in patients with diabetes or other conditions affecting blood flow.

Extremity Venous Studies (76821): Focus on venous circulation, most commonly used to evaluate suspected deep vein thrombosis, chronic venous insufficiency, or complications of venous access devices.

Vascular ultrasound requires specialized training and equipment capable of detecting blood flow and measuring flow velocities. The combination of anatomical and functional information provided by vascular ultrasound makes it invaluable for diagnosing and monitoring vascular conditions.

Radiologic Guidance: Precision Through Imaging

Modern medicine increasingly relies on imaging guidance to perform procedures with precision and safety that would be impossible with blind techniques. Understanding radiologic guidance coding requires appreciating how different imaging modalities provide guidance for various procedures and when guidance codes can be reported separately.

The Evolution of Image-Guided Procedures

From Blind to Guided Procedures: Historically, many medical procedures were performed using anatomical landmarks and palpation to guide needle or catheter placement. While experienced physicians could achieve reasonable success rates with these techniques, complications from inaccurate placement were significant and success rates were limited.

Image guidance revolutionized these procedures by allowing real-time visualization of needle advancement, confirmation of accurate placement, and immediate detection of complications. This technological advancement improved success rates, reduced complications, and allowed procedures to be performed on patients who wouldn't have been candidates for blind techniques.

Types of Imaging Guidance: Different imaging modalities offer unique advantages for procedure guidance. Fluoroscopy provides real-time X-ray imaging that's excellent for visualizing needles, catheters, and contrast-filled structures. CT provides cross-sectional imaging that's ideal for targeting small lesions and avoiding critical structures. Ultrasound offers real-time imaging without radiation exposure, making it perfect for many soft tissue procedures.

The choice of guidance modality depends on the procedure being performed, the structures involved, patient factors, and available equipment. Understanding these factors helps you appreciate why certain guidance codes are used in specific situations.

Fluoroscopic Guidance Applications

Central Venous Access Guidance (77001): Central venous catheter placement represents one of the most common applications of fluoroscopic guidance in modern medicine. These procedures involve placing large-bore catheters into major veins near the heart for medication administration, blood sampling, hemodialysis, or other therapeutic purposes.

Fluoroscopic guidance dramatically improves the safety and success of central venous access by allowing real-time visualization of needle advancement, confirmation of intravascular placement, detection of complications like pneumothorax or arterial puncture, and verification of proper catheter tip position.

The guidance includes real-time imaging during needle insertion, contrast injection to confirm venous access, imaging during catheter advancement, and final imaging to confirm appropriate catheter tip position. This comprehensive guidance justifies the additional reimbursement provided by guidance codes.

Needle Placement Guidance (77002): Fluoroscopic needle guidance is used for a wide variety of procedures including joint injections, nerve blocks, biopsies, drainage procedures, and other interventions requiring precise needle placement. The real-time imaging allows physicians to guide needles accurately while avoiding critical structures.

Joint injections, for example, benefit significantly from fluoroscopic guidance that ensures intra-articular placement and confirms that therapeutic medications are delivered to the intended location. Without guidance, some injections might miss the joint space entirely, providing no therapeutic benefit while exposing patients to medication risks.

Documentation and Billing Requirements: Fluoroscopic guidance codes require documentation of the imaging performed, including the number of images obtained, the reason for guidance, and how the guidance affected the procedure. Simply having fluoroscopic equipment available doesn't justify guidance billing—the imaging must actually be used to guide the procedure.

CT Guidance for Precision Procedures

CT-Guided Needle Placement (77012): CT guidance offers unparalleled precision for targeting small lesions, avoiding critical structures, and accessing difficult anatomical locations. The cross-sectional imaging allows visualization of needles in relation to organs, blood vessels, and other structures that might not be visible with fluoroscopy.

CT-guided biopsies can sample lesions as small as a few millimeters in diameter, often providing diagnostic information that prevents the need for surgical biopsy. The precision of CT guidance allows procedures to be performed safely even when lesions are located near critical structures like major blood vessels or the spinal cord.

The CT Guidance Process: CT-guided procedures typically begin with pre-procedure planning using recent CT images to determine the optimal approach, identify potential complications, and select appropriate needle types and sizes. During the procedure, limited CT scans guide needle advancement with periodic imaging to confirm progress and adjust direction as needed.

The procedure concludes with final imaging to confirm needle placement and evaluate for immediate complications. This systematic approach ensures optimal results while minimizing radiation exposure and procedure time.

Tissue Ablation Monitoring (77013): CT guidance for tissue ablation procedures requires continuous monitoring to ensure adequate treatment while protecting surrounding normal tissues. Ablation procedures use heat, cold, or other energy sources to destroy abnormal tissue, typically for cancer treatment or pain management.

During ablation, CT monitoring shows the extent of tissue destruction, confirms adequate treatment margins, and detects complications like bleeding or damage to adjacent organs. This intensive monitoring requires multiple imaging sessions throughout the procedure and justifies the specialized guidance code.

Ultrasound Guidance Benefits

Real-Time Ultrasound Guidance (76942): Ultrasound guidance provides real-time visualization without radiation exposure, making it ideal for many procedures, especially those requiring multiple needle passes or prolonged procedure times. The real-time nature allows continuous needle visualization and immediate adjustment of needle direction.

Ultrasound guidance is particularly valuable for procedures involving fluid collections, soft tissue masses, and vascular access. The ability to visualize blood flow using Doppler techniques helps avoid vascular complications during needle procedures.

Procedures Commonly Using Ultrasound Guidance: Paracentesis (abdominal fluid drainage) benefits from ultrasound guidance that identifies fluid collections, avoids bowel and other organs, and confirms adequate drainage. Thyroid biopsies use ultrasound guidance to target specific nodules while avoiding critical neck structures.

Vascular access procedures increasingly use ultrasound guidance, particularly for difficult access situations or when patient anatomy makes landmark-based techniques unreliable. The ability to visualize vessels and confirm placement reduces complications and improves success rates.

Bundled vs. Separate Guidance Billing: Many procedure codes include imaging guidance as part of the global service. When guidance is included in the procedure description, separate guidance billing is inappropriate and represents unbundling that violates coding guidelines.

However, when procedure codes don't specifically include guidance, separate guidance billing is appropriate and ensures proper recognition of the additional work involved in image-guided procedures. Understanding which procedures include guidance requires careful review of code descriptions and coding guidelines.

Breast Mammography: Early Detection Through Expert Imaging

Breast imaging represents one of radiology's most socially important applications, providing early detection of breast cancer that can be life-saving when identified in its earliest stages. Understanding breast imaging coding requires appreciating both the technical complexity of mammographic imaging and the interpretive expertise required for accurate diagnosis.

The Clinical and Social Impact of Mammography

Mammography as a Public Health Tool: Mammographic screening has dramatically reduced breast cancer mortality by detecting cancers before they can be felt by clinical examination. Studies consistently show that regular mammographic screening reduces breast cancer deaths by 20-40% in women over age 50, with emerging evidence suggesting benefits in younger women as well.

This public health impact depends on high-quality mammographic imaging combined with expert interpretation by radiologists trained in breast imaging. The combination of sophisticated technology and specialized expertise justifies the specific coding structure for mammographic services.

Technical Advances in Mammography: Modern mammography uses low-dose X-ray systems specifically designed for breast imaging, with specialized compression devices that spread breast tissue for optimal visualization while minimizing patient discomfort. Digital mammography provides improved image quality and manipulation capabilities compared to older film-based systems.

Tomosynthesis (3D mammography) represents the latest advance, creating multiple thin-section images through the breast that can be viewed individually or as a reconstructed 3D volume. This technology reduces false-positive rates by separating overlapping tissue layers and improves cancer detection, particularly in women with dense breast tissue.

Computer-Aided Detection (CAD): CAD systems use sophisticated algorithms to analyze mammographic images and highlight areas that might represent cancer, serving as a "second reader" to help radiologists identify subtle abnormalities. While CAD doesn't replace radiologist interpretation, it provides additional quality assurance that can improve cancer detection rates.

CAD technology is included in mammography codes when performed, recognizing that this technology represents an additional service that improves diagnostic accuracy. The integration of CAD into routine mammographic interpretation reflects the evolution of breast imaging toward increasingly sophisticated diagnostic tools.

Screening vs. Diagnostic Mammography

Understanding the distinction between screening and diagnostic mammography is crucial for accurate coding and appropriate patient care. These represent fundamentally different clinical scenarios with different coding requirements.

Screening Mammography (77067): Screening mammography is performed in asymptomatic women as part of routine health maintenance, similar to other screening tests like Pap smears or colonoscopy. The goal is early detection of breast cancer before symptoms develop, when treatment is most likely to be successful.

Screening mammography typically includes standard views of both breasts: craniocaudal (top-to-bottom) and mediolateral oblique (angled side-to-side) views that provide comprehensive visualization of breast tissue. The examination is performed according to standardized protocols that ensure consistent image quality and complete breast coverage.

Patient Preparation and Technique: Patients are instructed to avoid deodorants, powders, and lotions that might create artifacts on mammographic images. The mammographic technologist positions the patient carefully to ensure optimal breast compression and tissue separation while minimizing discomfort.

The bilateral nature of screening mammography is reflected in the code description (77067), recognizing that screening inherently involves comparison between breasts and evaluation of both breasts for abnormalities.

Diagnostic Mammography (77065-77066): Diagnostic mammography is performed to evaluate specific breast symptoms, follow up on previous abnormalities, or investigate clinical findings discovered during physical examination. This represents problem-focused imaging rather than routine screening.

Diagnostic mammography often requires additional views beyond the standard screening views, including spot compression views, magnification views, or special projections designed to evaluate specific areas of concern. The radiologist may be involved in real-time image acquisition, directing additional views based on initial findings.

Unilateral vs. Bilateral Diagnostic Studies: Diagnostic mammography can be unilateral (77065) when evaluating a specific breast symptom or bilateral (77066) when symptoms are bilateral or when comparison views are needed for complete evaluation.

The distinction between unilateral and bilateral coding depends on whether imaging of both breasts is medically necessary for the diagnostic evaluation, not simply whether both breasts are imaged for comparison purposes.

Clinical Scenarios Requiring Diagnostic Mammography: Palpable breast lumps require diagnostic evaluation to determine whether the palpable abnormality corresponds to a mammographic finding and to evaluate the remainder of the breast for additional abnormalities. Breast pain, nipple discharge, skin changes, or other breast symptoms might warrant diagnostic mammography depending on patient age and clinical circumstances.

Follow-up of previous abnormalities uses diagnostic mammography to monitor known benign findings, evaluate response to treatment, or detect changes that might indicate malignancy.

Advanced Breast Imaging Techniques

Breast Ultrasound (76641-76642): Breast ultrasound serves as an important adjunct to mammography, particularly for evaluating palpable abnormalities, characterizing mammographic findings, and screening high-risk women. Ultrasound can distinguish between solid masses and fluid-filled cysts, guide biopsy procedures, and evaluate areas that are difficult to assess mammographically.

Complete Breast Ultrasound (76641): Involves systematic evaluation of both breasts and regional lymph nodes, typically performed as a screening study in high-risk women or as comprehensive diagnostic evaluation of breast symptoms.

Limited Breast Ultrasound (76642): Focuses on specific areas of concern, such as evaluation of a palpable lump or characterization of a mammographic finding. Limited studies require clear documentation of the focused nature of the examination.

Breast MRI (77046-77047): Breast MRI provides the most sensitive imaging for breast cancer detection and is particularly valuable for high-risk screening, extent of disease evaluation in newly diagnosed breast cancer patients, and monitoring response to chemotherapy.

MRI Without Contrast (77046): Limited to specific indications where contrast enhancement isn't necessary or contraindicated. Less commonly performed than contrast-enhanced studies.

MRI Without and With Contrast (77047): The most comprehensive breast MRI examination, using dynamic contrast enhancement to evaluate tissue perfusion patterns that help distinguish benign from malignant lesions.

Breast MRI requires specialized protocols, dedicated breast coils, and radiologists with expertise in breast MRI interpretation. The high sensitivity of breast MRI can also lead to false-positive results, requiring careful patient selection and expert interpretation.

Bone and Joint Studies: Imaging the Musculoskeletal System

Musculoskeletal imaging encompasses a wide range of studies from simple plain radiographs to sophisticated cross-sectional imaging that reveals both bones and soft tissues in exquisite detail. Understanding bone and joint coding requires appreciating how different imaging modalities complement each other and provide different types of diagnostic information.

Plain Film Radiography: The Foundation of Musculoskeletal Imaging

The Enduring Value of Plain Radiographs: Despite advances in CT and MRI technology, plain radiographs remain the cornerstone of musculoskeletal imaging due to their excellent bone detail, wide availability, low cost, and rapid acquisition times. Plain films provide fundamental information about bone structure, joint alignment, and pathological changes that guide further diagnostic workup.

Plain radiography excels at demonstrating fractures, joint space narrowing, bone destruction, and calcifications that might not be apparent on other imaging modalities. The high contrast between bone and soft tissue makes plain films ideal for initial evaluation of musculoskeletal complaints.

Understanding Radiographic Views and Projections: Radiographic coding depends partly on the number and type of views obtained during each examination. Standard views are designed to provide comprehensive evaluation while minimizing radiation exposure and examination time.

Two-View Studies: Typically include anteroposterior (front-to-back) and lateral (side-to-side) projections that provide perpendicular views of the anatomical area. These views are sufficient for most initial evaluations and follow-up studies.

Complete Studies: Include additional views beyond the standard two projections, such as oblique projections or specialized views designed to visualize specific anatomical areas or pathological conditions. Complete studies provide more comprehensive evaluation but take longer and expose patients to additional radiation.

Complete Radiographic Examinations Examples:

Wrist, Complete (73110): Includes anteroposterior, lateral, and oblique views that provide comprehensive evaluation of all carpal bones, their articulations, and the surrounding soft tissues. The oblique view is particularly valuable for detecting subtle fractures that might be missed on standard AP and lateral views.

Consider a patient who falls on an outstretched hand—a mechanism commonly associated with scaphoid fractures. The scaphoid bone has a complex three-dimensional shape that may not be adequately visualized on just two views. The oblique view in a complete wrist examination provides additional perspective that can reveal occult fractures, potentially preventing missed diagnoses that could lead to complications like avascular necrosis.

Knee, Complete (73060): A complete knee examination typically includes anteroposterior, lateral, and sunrise (patellofemoral) views. The sunrise view provides unique visualization of the patellofemoral joint space and can reveal patellar tracking abnormalities, chondromalacia, or other conditions affecting the kneecap's relationship with the femur.

Athletes presenting with anterior knee pain might have normal-appearing AP and lateral views, but the sunrise view could reveal patellar maltracking or cartilage abnormalities that explain their symptoms. This additional diagnostic information justifies the complete examination coding and demonstrates why comprehensive imaging is valuable in appropriate clinical situations.

Specialized Views and Their Clinical Significance: Some anatomical areas require specialized projections that capture specific anatomical relationships or pathological processes. These views demonstrate the sophistication of radiographic imaging and the importance of proper technique in diagnostic accuracy.

Cervical Spine Flexion/Extension Views: Evaluate spinal stability by having patients bend their neck forward and backward during imaging. These dynamic views can reveal ligamentous injuries, spinal instability, or abnormal movement patterns that aren't apparent on static radiographs.

Weight-Bearing Views: Some joint examinations require patients to bear weight during imaging to evaluate joint alignment under physiological stress. Weight-bearing knee X-rays can reveal joint space narrowing that's hidden when patients lie down, providing more accurate assessment of arthritic changes.

Cross-Sectional Imaging: CT and MRI of Bones and Joints

CT Imaging of Musculoskeletal System: CT excels at demonstrating bone detail and is particularly valuable for evaluating complex fractures, joint alignment, and bone destruction from tumors or infections. The cross-sectional nature of CT imaging allows visualization of anatomical relationships that can't be appreciated on plain radiographs.

CT Without Contrast (73200-73206): Provides excellent bone detail and is sufficient for most musculoskeletal applications. Bone fractures, joint alignment, and bone destruction are typically well-demonstrated without the need for intravenous contrast material.

Trauma Applications: CT is invaluable for evaluating complex trauma, particularly in areas like the pelvis, spine, and skull where overlapping bones can obscure fractures on plain radiographs. CT can reveal the exact extent of fractures, displacement of bone fragments, and involvement of nearby soft tissues.

For example, a patient involved in a motor vehicle accident might have a complex acetabular fracture that's difficult to fully characterize on plain pelvic X-rays. CT examination can show the exact fracture pattern, degree of joint involvement, and presence of loose bone fragments within the joint space. This detailed information is crucial for surgical planning and determining whether operative fixation is necessary.

CT With Contrast (73201-73207): Enhanced studies are used when soft tissue evaluation is important or when vascular assessment is needed. Contrast enhancement can help differentiate between various soft tissue masses, evaluate the blood supply to bones and joints, and assess for complications like infection or tumor.

MRI of Musculoskeletal System: MRI provides unparalleled soft tissue detail and is particularly valuable for evaluating muscles, tendons, ligaments, cartilage, and bone marrow. The ability to obtain images in multiple planes and use different pulse sequences makes MRI extremely versatile for musculoskeletal diagnosis.

MRI Without Contrast (73218-73223): Many musculoskeletal conditions can be adequately evaluated without contrast enhancement. Ligament tears, meniscal injuries, muscle strains, and many bone and joint abnormalities are well-demonstrated on non-contrast MRI studies.

Sports Medicine Applications: MRI has revolutionized sports medicine by allowing precise diagnosis of internal joint derangements, ligament injuries, and other conditions that affect athletes. A football player with knee pain might have normal X-rays, but MRI could reveal an anterior cruciate ligament tear, meniscal damage, or bone contusions that explain the symptoms and guide treatment decisions.

The ability to visualize cartilage, ligaments, and other soft tissues that don't show up on X-rays makes MRI invaluable for athletes whose careers depend on precise diagnosis and optimal treatment of injuries.

MRI With Contrast (73219-73225): Contrast-enhanced studies are used when evaluating tumors, infections, or other conditions where contrast enhancement provides additional diagnostic information. Gadolinium contrast can help differentiate between various soft tissue masses and evaluate the extent of inflammatory or infectious processes.

Joint-Specific MRI Considerations: Different joints present unique imaging challenges and clinical questions that affect MRI technique and interpretation. Understanding these differences helps explain why joint-specific codes exist and why imaging protocols vary.

Shoulder MRI: The shoulder's complex anatomy and wide range of motion create unique imaging challenges. Rotator cuff tears, labral injuries, and impingement syndrome are common conditions that require specialized MRI techniques for accurate diagnosis. Some shoulder studies use arthrography (contrast injection into the joint) to better visualize internal joint structures.

Knee MRI: The knee's complex internal anatomy—including menisci, cruciate ligaments, and cartilage—makes MRI particularly valuable for this joint. Different pulse sequences highlight different anatomical structures, allowing comprehensive evaluation of all internal joint components.

Spine MRI: Spinal imaging requires specialized techniques to evaluate the spinal cord, nerve roots, and intervertebral discs. Different pulse sequences can highlight disc degeneration, nerve compression, or inflammatory conditions affecting the spine.

Radiation Oncology: Precision in Cancer Treatment

Radiation oncology represents one of medicine's most sophisticated applications of imaging technology, using precisely targeted radiation beams to destroy cancer cells while sparing surrounding normal tissues. Understanding radiation oncology coding requires appreciating both the complexity of treatment planning and the precision required for safe, effective cancer treatment.

The Science and Art of Radiation Therapy

How Radiation Therapy Works: Radiation therapy uses high-energy beams to damage cancer cell DNA, preventing these cells from reproducing and ultimately causing them to die. Normal cells can typically repair radiation damage better than cancer cells, allowing therapeutic doses that preferentially affect malignant tissue.

Modern radiation therapy uses sophisticated computer planning systems to calculate optimal beam angles, intensities, and dose distributions that maximize cancer cell kill while minimizing damage to nearby normal organs. This treatment planning process is as critical as the actual radiation delivery and represents a significant component of radiation oncology services.

Treatment Planning and Simulation: Before any radiation treatment can begin, patients undergo comprehensive treatment planning that may take several days or weeks to complete. This process involves detailed imaging studies, computerized dose calculations, and quality assurance procedures that ensure safe, accurate treatment delivery.

Simulation (77280-77295): Treatment simulation uses specialized CT scanners or other imaging equipment to determine optimal patient positioning and beam arrangements. Patients are positioned exactly as they will be for daily treatments, and imaging is performed to map internal anatomy and identify critical structures that must be protected.

During simulation, patients may have immobilization devices created—such as custom masks for head and neck treatments or body molds for other anatomical areas. These devices ensure reproducible positioning for every treatment session, which is critical for treatment accuracy.

Treatment Planning (77300-77370): After simulation, medical physicists and dosimetrists use sophisticated computer systems to calculate radiation dose distributions. This planning process considers tumor location, size, and shape, as well as the location of critical normal organs that must be protected.

Simple planning might involve basic beam arrangements for straightforward treatments, while complex planning could involve dozens of beams with varying intensities and shapes. Intensity-modulated radiation therapy (IMRT) represents the most sophisticated planning approach, using computer-controlled beam modulation to create highly conformal dose distributions.

Treatment Delivery Systems: Modern radiation therapy uses sophisticated linear accelerators that can deliver precisely shaped radiation beams from multiple angles around the patient. These machines are capable of modulating beam intensity in real-time and can adjust for patient movement during treatment.

Image-Guided Radiation Therapy (IGRT): Many modern treatments use daily imaging to verify patient positioning and internal anatomy before each treatment session. This may involve cone-beam CT scans, portal imaging, or other techniques that ensure accurate treatment delivery despite potential changes in patient anatomy or positioning.

Stereotactic Radiosurgery and Radiotherapy: These techniques use extremely precise targeting to deliver very high radiation doses to small targets, often in single or few treatment sessions. The precision required for these treatments necessitates specialized equipment, extensive quality assurance, and highly trained personnel.

Treatment Delivery Coding

Simple Radiation Treatment Delivery (77402-77407): Simple treatments typically involve basic beam arrangements treating straightforward anatomical areas. These might include palliative treatments for bone metastases, simple skin cancer treatments, or other situations where complex planning isn't required.

Simple treatments still require careful attention to patient positioning, dose calculation, and safety procedures, but they don't involve the sophisticated computer planning used for more complex cases. The reduced complexity is reflected in lower reimbursement rates compared to more complex delivery techniques.

Intermediate Radiation Treatment Delivery (77407-77412): Intermediate treatments involve more complex beam arrangements or treatment techniques that require additional planning and quality assurance. These might include treatments using multiple beam angles, custom blocking to protect normal tissues, or other techniques that increase treatment complexity.

Complex Radiation Treatment Delivery (77412-77417): Complex treatments represent the most sophisticated radiation delivery techniques, often involving computer-controlled beam modulation, multiple beam angles, and extensive quality assurance procedures. These treatments require the highest level of technical expertise and equipment sophistication.

Intensity-Modulated Radiation Therapy (IMRT): Uses computer-controlled beam modulation to create highly conformal dose distributions that closely match tumor shapes while sparing nearby normal tissues. IMRT requires extensive quality assurance and represents the most complex form of conventional radiation therapy.

Stereotactic Body Radiation Therapy (SBRT): Delivers very high doses to small targets with extreme precision, often completing treatment in 1-5 sessions rather than the conventional 25-40 sessions. The precision required for SBRT necessitates specialized equipment and extensive quality assurance procedures.

Quality Assurance and Safety

Physics and Dosimetry Services: Radiation therapy requires extensive physics support to ensure safe, accurate treatment delivery. Medical physicists are responsible for equipment calibration, dose calculations, treatment plan verification, and quality assurance procedures that maintain treatment accuracy and safety.

Daily Quality Assurance: Linear accelerators undergo daily checks to verify proper function before any patients are treated. These checks include beam output verification, alignment checks, and safety system testing.

Patient-Specific Quality Assurance: Complex treatments like IMRT require individual verification that planned dose distributions can be accurately delivered. This may involve measuring dose distributions in phantoms or using other verification techniques.

Brachytherapy Services: Brachytherapy involves placing radioactive sources directly into or adjacent to tumors, allowing very high doses to be delivered to small volumes while sparing distant normal tissues. This technique requires specialized expertise in radioactive source handling, dose calculation, and radiation safety.

High-Dose Rate (HDR) Brachytherapy: Uses highly radioactive sources that can deliver therapeutic doses in minutes rather than hours or days. HDR systems require sophisticated afterloading equipment and extensive safety procedures.

Low-Dose Rate (LDR) Brachytherapy: Uses less radioactive sources that remain in place for longer periods. LDR treatments may involve temporary implants removed after several days or permanent implants that remain in place as radioactivity decays.

Nuclear Medicine: Functional Imaging and Targeted Therapy

Nuclear medicine represents a unique branch of radiology that evaluates organ function rather than just anatomy. By administering small amounts of radioactive materials and detecting their distribution throughout the body, nuclear medicine provides information about physiological processes that can't be obtained with other imaging modalities.

The Principles of Nuclear Medicine

How Nuclear Medicine Works: Nuclear medicine uses radioactive tracers—typically very small amounts of radioactive materials attached to substances that naturally accumulate in specific organs or tissues. After administration, usually by injection, these tracers distribute throughout the body according to physiological processes like blood flow, metabolism, or receptor binding.

Specialized cameras detect the radiation emitted by these tracers and create images that show functional activity rather than anatomical structure. Areas of increased tracer uptake appear brighter on nuclear medicine images, indicating increased functional activity, while areas of decreased uptake suggest reduced function.

Radiopharmaceuticals and Targeting: Different radiopharmaceuticals target different physiological processes or anatomical structures. Bone scans use tracers that accumulate in areas of increased bone metabolism, making them valuable for detecting bone metastases, fractures, or infections. Heart scans use tracers that evaluate cardiac blood flow or heart muscle viability.

The sophistication of modern radiopharmaceuticals allows targeted evaluation of specific physiological processes. For example, tracers used in brain imaging can evaluate blood flow, glucose metabolism, or neurotransmitter function, providing information about various neurological and psychiatric conditions.

SPECT and PET Imaging: Single Photon Emission Computed Tomography (SPECT) and Positron Emission Tomography (PET) represent advanced nuclear medicine techniques that provide cross-sectional images with improved anatomical localization compared to traditional planar nuclear medicine images.

SPECT Imaging: Uses rotating cameras to create cross-sectional images that show radiotracer distribution in three dimensions. SPECT is commonly used for cardiac imaging, brain imaging, and bone scanning applications where improved anatomical localization is valuable.

PET Imaging: Uses special tracers that emit positrons, creating very high-quality images that can be combined with CT or MRI scans for precise anatomical localization. PET is particularly valuable for cancer imaging, where it can detect metabolic activity that indicates malignancy.

Diagnostic Nuclear Medicine Procedures

Bone and Joint Studies (78300-78399): Nuclear medicine bone scanning remains one of the most commonly performed nuclear medicine procedures, particularly valuable for detecting bone metastases in cancer patients and evaluating unexplained bone pain.

Whole Body Bone Scan (78315): Provides comprehensive evaluation of the entire skeleton and is particularly valuable for detecting bone metastases that might be too small to see on conventional X-rays. The bone scan can identify abnormal bone metabolism weeks or months before changes become visible on plain radiographs.

Cancer patients often undergo bone scans to evaluate for metastatic disease, as many cancers commonly spread to bone. The ability to evaluate the entire skeleton in a single examination makes bone scanning invaluable for cancer staging and follow-up.

SPECT Bone Imaging (78320): Provides cross-sectional images that improve anatomical localization and can help distinguish between benign and malignant bone abnormalities. SPECT is particularly valuable for evaluating the spine, where improved anatomical detail can help identify the specific anatomical structures involved in abnormal uptake.

Cardiac Nuclear Medicine (78414-78499): Nuclear cardiology provides unique information about heart function, blood flow, and viability that can't be obtained with other imaging modalities. These studies are particularly valuable for evaluating coronary artery disease and heart muscle function.

Myocardial Perfusion Imaging (78451-78454): Evaluates blood flow to heart muscle under both rest and stress conditions. These studies can identify areas of heart muscle that don't receive adequate blood flow, indicating coronary artery disease that might require intervention.

Stress testing may involve exercise on a treadmill or bicycle, or pharmacological stress using medications that simulate the effects of exercise. The comparison between rest and stress images allows identification of coronary artery disease even when resting heart function appears normal.

Cardiac Function Studies (78472-78473): Evaluate heart muscle function by measuring how effectively the heart pumps blood. These studies can identify areas of heart muscle damage from heart attacks and monitor changes in heart function over time.

Pulmonary Studies (78580-78599): Nuclear medicine lung scanning can evaluate both lung ventilation (airflow) and perfusion (blood flow), providing information about various lung conditions including pulmonary embolism, chronic lung disease, and other conditions affecting lung function.

Ventilation/Perfusion Scans (78580-78588): These studies evaluate both airflow and blood flow to different parts of the lungs and are particularly valuable for diagnosing pulmonary embolism. Areas of lung that receive adequate airflow but poor blood flow suggest blood clots blocking lung circulation.

The ventilation portion involves inhaling radioactive gas or aerosol, while the perfusion study uses injected tracers that follow lung blood flow. The combination of these studies provides comprehensive evaluation of lung function.

Therapeutic Nuclear Medicine

Radioiodine Therapy: Thyroid tissue naturally concentrates iodine, making radioactive iodine an effective treatment for thyroid cancer and hyperthyroidism. The radioactive iodine selectively accumulates in thyroid tissue, delivering targeted radiation therapy while sparing other organs.

Thyroid Cancer Treatment: Uses high doses of radioactive iodine to destroy remaining thyroid tissue after surgical removal of thyroid cancer. This treatment can eliminate microscopic thyroid cancer cells that might not be removed by surgery alone.

Hyperthyroidism Treatment: Uses lower doses of radioactive iodine to reduce thyroid hormone production in patients with overactive thyroid glands. This treatment offers an alternative to long-term medication or surgical thyroid removal.

Radiopharmaceutical Therapy for Bone Metastases: Certain radiopharmaceuticals concentrate in areas of increased bone metabolism, making them valuable for treating pain from bone metastases. These treatments can provide significant pain relief while potentially slowing the progression of bone metastases.

Targeted Radiotherapy: Emerging radiopharmaceutical therapies target specific receptors or antigens found on cancer cells, allowing delivery of radiation directly to tumor sites while sparing normal tissues. These treatments represent a rapidly evolving area of nuclear medicine with exciting potential for cancer treatment.

Comprehensive Radiology Coding Practice Questions

Test your mastery of radiology coding principles across all modalities:

Question 1: A radiologist interprets a chest CT performed at a hospital where the radiologist is not employed. How should the radiologist bill this service?

A) 71250 (chest CT without contrast) B) 71250-26 (chest CT, professional component) C) 71250-TC (chest CT, technical component) D) Cannot bill separately from hospital

Answer: B Explanation: When a radiologist provides only professional interpretation of a study performed at another facility, use modifier -26 for professional component billing. The hospital bills the technical component (-TC) separately.

Question 2: Complete abdominal ultrasound examining liver, gallbladder, pancreas, spleen, and kidneys should be coded as:

A) 76700 (complete abdominal ultrasound) B) 76705 (limited abdominal ultrasound) C) Multiple organ-specific ultrasound codes D) 76770 (retroperitoneal ultrasound)

Answer: A Explanation: 76700 represents complete abdominal ultrasound that includes systematic evaluation of liver, gallbladder, common bile duct, pancreas, spleen, kidneys, and aorta. Don't code multiple organ-specific studies when complete examination is performed.

Question 3: Bilateral screening mammography in an asymptomatic 52-year-old woman should be coded as:

A) 77065 (diagnostic mammography, unilateral) B) 77066 (diagnostic mammography, bilateral) C) 77067 (screening mammography, bilateral) D) 77065 with modifier -50 (bilateral)

Answer: C Explanation: 77067 specifically represents bilateral screening mammography performed in asymptomatic patients for early cancer detection. Diagnostic codes (77065-77066) are used when specific symptoms or findings are being evaluated.

Question 4: CT guidance for percutaneous needle biopsy should be coded:

A) 77012 (CT guidance) only if biopsy code doesn't include guidance B) 77012 (CT guidance) plus biopsy code in all cases C) Never separately - always included in biopsy D) Only when multiple needle passes are required

Answer: A Explanation: Check the biopsy procedure code description. If it includes imaging guidance, don't code guidance separately. If guidance is not included in the procedure description, code both the biopsy and 77012 for CT guidance.

Question 5: Obstetrical ultrasound at 32 weeks gestation for routine prenatal care should be coded as:

A) 76801 (obstetrical ultrasound, first trimester) B) 76805 (obstetrical ultrasound, after first trimester) C) 76811 (obstetrical ultrasound, detailed anatomic examination) D) 76700 (abdominal ultrasound, complete)

Answer: B Explanation: 76805 covers routine obstetrical ultrasound after the first trimester (after 14 weeks). 32 weeks gestation falls into this category for routine prenatal evaluation.

Question 6: Wrist X-ray with anteroposterior, lateral, and oblique views should be coded as:

A) 73100 (wrist, 2 views) B) 73110 (wrist, complete, minimum 3 views) C) Three separate single-view wrist codes D) 73100 with modifier indicating additional views

Answer: B Explanation: 73110 represents complete wrist examination with minimum of 3 views, which includes the AP, lateral, and oblique views described. Use this code when more than the standard 2 views are obtained.

Question 7: Knee MRI without contrast material should be coded as:

A) 73721 (MRI any joint of lower extremity, without contrast) B) 73722 (MRI any joint of lower extremity, with contrast) C) 73723 (MRI any joint of lower extremity, without and with contrast) D) 73700 (CT lower extremity, without contrast)

Answer: A Explanation: 73721 represents MRI of any joint of the lower extremity without contrast material. The knee is a lower extremity joint, and no contrast was administered.

Question 8: Nuclear medicine bone scan of the entire skeleton should be coded as:

A) 78300 (bone imaging, limited area) B) 78305 (bone imaging, multiple areas) C) 78315 (bone imaging, 3-phase study) D) 78306 (bone imaging, whole body)

Answer: D Explanation: 78306 represents whole body bone imaging that evaluates the entire skeleton. This is the appropriate code for comprehensive bone scanning, commonly performed for cancer staging.

Question 9: Radiation treatment delivery using IMRT (intensity-modulated radiation therapy) should be coded as:

A) 77402 (radiation treatment delivery, simple) B) 77407 (radiation treatment delivery, intermediate) C) 77418 (intensity-modulated radiation treatment delivery) D) 77412 (radiation treatment delivery, complex)

Answer: C Explanation: 77418 specifically represents intensity-modulated radiation treatment delivery (IMRT), which uses computer-controlled beam modulation. This technique requires separate coding from conventional radiation delivery methods.

Question 10: Ultrasound guidance for needle biopsy that includes real-time imaging should be coded as:

A) 76942 (ultrasonic guidance for needle placement) B) 77002 (fluoroscopic guidance for needle placement) C) 77012 (CT guidance for needle placement) D) Guidance codes not separately reportable

Answer: A Explanation: 76942 represents ultrasonic guidance for needle placement with real-time imaging. This code is used when ultrasound guidance is provided for biopsy or other needle procedures, assuming the primary procedure code doesn't include guidance.

Chapter 13 Summary: Mastering Radiology Coding Excellence

You have now achieved comprehensive mastery of radiology coding across all major imaging modalities and clinical applications. Your expertise encompasses:

Technical and Professional Component Mastery: You understand the fundamental split between technical and professional components and can apply modifiers correctly in various practice settings, from hospital-based radiologists to private practice imaging centers.

Modality-Specific Expertise: You've mastered the unique coding requirements for ultrasound, CT, MRI, mammography, nuclear medicine, and radiation oncology, understanding how each modality answers different clinical questions and requires different coding approaches.

Clinical Integration: You understand why different imaging studies are performed, how they complement each other in diagnostic workups, and how clinical indications affect code selection and modifier usage.

Guidance and Supervision Coding: You can distinguish between procedures that include imaging guidance and those requiring separate guidance coding, preventing both undercoding and inappropriate unbundling.

Complex Scenario Management: You can handle challenging situations like component billing in different practice settings, multiple imaging studies performed during single encounters, and billing for both diagnostic and interventional procedures.

The Foundation You've Built

Your radiology coding expertise represents more than just knowing which codes to assign—you've developed a deep understanding of medical imaging technology, clinical applications, and the business relationships that drive healthcare delivery. This knowledge positions you as a valuable specialist who can:

Support Quality Patient Care: By ensuring accurate coding and appropriate billing, you help maintain the financial viability of imaging services that are essential for modern medical diagnosis and treatment.

Navigate Complex Healthcare Relationships: Understanding how radiologists, hospitals, imaging centers, and referring physicians work together helps you apply coding rules correctly in various practice settings.

Adapt to Technological Advances: Your foundation in imaging principles prepares you to understand and code new technologies as they emerge and become incorporated into medical practice.

Provide Expert Consultation: Your comprehensive knowledge allows you to train others, resolve coding disputes, and serve as a resource for complex radiology coding questions.

Professional Development Opportunities

This radiology coding mastery opens several career advancement opportunities:

Radiology Practice Specialization: Many radiology practices seek coders with deep imaging expertise who can handle complex billing scenarios and ensure optimal reimbursement.

Hospital Imaging Department Roles: Hospitals value coders who understand both technical and professional component billing and can manage the complex relationships between hospital services and contracted radiologists.

Imaging Center Management: Freestanding imaging centers need coders who understand both the business and clinical aspects of imaging services.

Consulting and Education: Your expertise qualifies you to provide consulting services to imaging practices and to train other coders in radiology principles.

Integration with Complete Medical Coding

Your radiology expertise integrates seamlessly with your other coding skills:

Surgical Integration: Understanding imaging studies helps you appreciate why certain procedures require imaging guidance and how surgical planning depends on diagnostic imaging.

Diagnostic Integration: Radiology findings often drive diagnosis coding decisions and help explain the medical necessity for various procedures and treatments.

Clinical Context: Your understanding of imaging applications enhances your appreciation of clinical decision-making across all medical specialties.

Remember: Radiology coding excellence comes from understanding both the technology and the medicine behind the images. You've mastered both aspects, making you a complete radiology coding professional who can handle any challenge with confidence and accuracy.

Your next step involves applying these analytical skills to pathology and laboratory coding, where understanding test methodologies and clinical laboratory medicine becomes key to accurate code selection. The systematic approach you've developed here—understanding technology, clinical applications, and billing relationships—will serve you well as you complete your comprehensive CPT® education.

The foundation you've built in radiology coding will serve you throughout your career, as imaging technology continues to evolve and play an increasingly important role in modern healthcare delivery.

Chapter 14: Pathology and Laboratory Coding (80047-89398)

"In medicine, there are only two types of data: that which helps the patient, and that which you haven't collected yet." - Anonymous Pathologist

Welcome to the world where medicine meets mathematics, where tiny specimens reveal life-changing diagnoses, and where objective data drives critical treatment decisions. Pathology and laboratory coding represents the foundation of evidence-based medicine—every blood test, tissue biopsy, and molecular analysis that guides physicians in making accurate diagnoses and monitoring treatment effectiveness.

You're about to master one of healthcare's most essential yet complex coding areas. Laboratory medicine touches every patient, every day, providing the objective evidence that confirms clinical suspicions, monitors disease progression, and ensures medication safety. From routine cholesterol checks to sophisticated genetic testing, your coding accuracy directly impacts both patient care and healthcare economics.

This chapter transforms the seemingly overwhelming world of laboratory testing into logical, manageable coding concepts. You'll discover how different test methodologies affect code selection, learn to navigate complex panel structures and bundling rules, and develop the confidence to handle even the most challenging pathology scenarios that appear on the CPC exam.

Your clinical knowledge becomes crucial here—understanding why tests are ordered, how results are interpreted, and what follow-up testing might be indicated helps you select the most appropriate codes and avoid common coding pitfalls.

By the end of this chapter, you'll think like a laboratory medicine specialist who understands not just what codes to assign, but the sophisticated science and clinical reasoning behind every test order. You'll appreciate how laboratory medicine has evolved from simple chemistry tests to complex molecular diagnostics that can predict disease risk and guide personalized treatment decisions.

Understanding Laboratory Medicine as the Foundation of Modern Healthcare

Before diving into specific coding rules, it's essential to understand the pivotal role laboratory medicine plays in modern healthcare and why accurate coding of these services is so critical to both patient care and healthcare economics.

Laboratory Medicine: Where Science Meets Patient Care

The Evolution of Laboratory Testing: Laboratory medicine has transformed from simple visual inspection of urine and blood to sophisticated automated systems that can perform hundreds of tests simultaneously with remarkable precision. Modern clinical laboratories use robotics, artificial intelligence, and molecular techniques that would have seemed like science fiction just decades ago.

This evolution reflects medicine's increasing reliance on objective data to guide clinical decisions. Where physicians once depended primarily on physical examination and clinical intuition, today's medical practice integrates laboratory results, imaging studies, and clinical assessment to achieve diagnostic accuracy that was impossible in earlier eras.

Understanding this evolution helps explain why laboratory coding has become increasingly complex. Simple blood chemistry tests have given way to comprehensive metabolic panels, genetic testing, and molecular diagnostics that require sophisticated coding rules to capture the work involved accurately.

The Laboratory's Role in Patient Care: Every patient encounter potentially generates laboratory testing needs. Emergency department visits often require immediate blood work to guide urgent treatment decisions. Routine office visits might include screening tests for early disease detection. Hospital patients typically have daily laboratory monitoring to assess response to treatment and detect complications.

Consider a patient presenting to the emergency department with chest pain. Within minutes, laboratory tests for cardiac enzymes, blood gases, and metabolic function provide critical information that helps physicians distinguish between heart attack, lung problems, anxiety, and other conditions. The speed and accuracy of these tests can literally save lives, while their cost-effectiveness helps control healthcare expenses.

This clinical significance explains why laboratory coding requires such precision. Undercoding fails to capture the complexity and value of sophisticated testing, while overcoding inflates healthcare costs and may trigger compliance concerns. Accurate coding ensures laboratories receive appropriate compensation while maintaining the financial sustainability of essential diagnostic services.

The Business of Laboratory Medicine: Clinical laboratories represent a significant component of healthcare infrastructure, employing thousands of medical technologists, pathologists, and support staff who operate sophisticated equipment worth millions of dollars. Understanding the business aspects of laboratory medicine helps explain why coding rules exist and how they affect different practice settings.

Hospital laboratories often operate as cost centers that support the overall patient care mission, while independent commercial laboratories must maintain profitability to continue serving patients. Reference laboratories provide specialized testing that smaller facilities can't perform economically, creating complex billing relationships that require careful attention to coding accuracy.

These different business models affect how laboratory services are coded and billed. Hospital-employed pathologists might bill only professional interpretation services, while independent laboratories bill global fees that include both technical and professional components. Understanding these relationships prevents coding errors and ensures appropriate billing.

Quality Assurance and Regulatory Environment

Laboratory Regulation and Accreditation: Clinical laboratories operate under extensive federal and state regulations designed to ensure accurate, reliable test results. The Clinical Laboratory Improvement Amendments (CLIA) establish quality standards for laboratory testing, while organizations like the College of American Pathologists (CAP) provide accreditation programs that ensure laboratories meet high standards for accuracy and reliability.

These regulatory requirements significantly impact laboratory operations and costs. Laboratories must maintain extensive quality control programs, participate in proficiency testing, and employ qualified personnel who meet specific education and training requirements. Understanding these requirements helps explain why certain laboratory codes include quality assurance activities and why professional interpretation is often separately billable.

Test Complexity and Personnel Requirements: CLIA regulations classify laboratory tests into three complexity levels—waived, moderate complexity, and high complexity—based on factors like ease of performance, interpretation requirements, and potential for harm from inaccurate results. Higher complexity tests require more qualified personnel and extensive quality control, justifying higher reimbursement levels.

For example, simple glucose testing using modern point-of-care devices might be performed by nursing staff with minimal training, while complex genetic testing requires specially trained technologists and pathologist oversight. This complexity gradient is reflected in laboratory coding structures that recognize different levels of technical and professional work.

Organ or Disease-Oriented Panels: Efficient Testing Through Standardization

Laboratory panels represent one of medicine's most successful applications of standardization to improve efficiency while controlling costs. Understanding panel coding requires appreciating both the clinical logic behind panel design and the economic benefits of grouping related tests.

The Science Behind Panel Development

Clinical Correlation and Test Grouping: Laboratory panels group tests that are commonly ordered together for specific clinical situations, reflecting decades of clinical experience about which tests provide complementary diagnostic information. These groupings aren't arbitrary—they represent evidence-based approaches to efficient diagnostic testing.

Consider the comprehensive metabolic panel (CMP), which includes tests for kidney function, liver function, electrolyte balance, and glucose metabolism. A physician evaluating a patient with weakness and fatigue might order this panel because abnormalities in any of these areas could explain the symptoms. Rather than ordering individual tests and potentially missing important relationships, the panel provides comprehensive screening with a single order.

Panel development involves input from practicing physicians, laboratory medicine specialists, and health economists who evaluate both clinical utility and cost-effectiveness. The goal is creating test combinations that provide maximum diagnostic information while minimizing both cost and patient inconvenience.

Standardization Benefits: Standardized panels improve healthcare efficiency by reducing ordering errors, streamlining laboratory workflows, and enabling more accurate cost comparisons between providers. When physicians know that a "basic metabolic panel" includes the same eight tests regardless of which laboratory performs the analysis, they can make more informed decisions about testing strategies.

Standardization also enables more efficient laboratory operations. Automated analyzers can be programmed to perform panel tests simultaneously, reducing per-test costs and improving turnaround times. These operational efficiencies benefit both providers and patients through reduced costs and faster results.

Understanding Panel Structure and Coding Rules

Complete Panel Requirements: The fundamental rule of panel coding is that all tests included in the panel description must be performed to justify panel billing. This seems straightforward, but it creates important implications for clinical practice and coding accuracy.

If a physician orders a comprehensive metabolic panel but the laboratory cannot perform one of the included tests due to equipment malfunction or specimen problems, the panel code cannot be used. Instead, each successfully performed test must be coded individually. This requirement ensures that panel billing accurately reflects the work performed and prevents inappropriate cost savings from incomplete testing.

Real-World Panel Scenarios:

Scenario 1: Complete Basic Metabolic Panel (80048) A 65-year-old patient with diabetes and hypertension comes for routine follow-up. The physician orders a basic metabolic panel to monitor kidney function, electrolyte balance, and glucose control.

Tests Performed:

- Glucose: 145 mg/dL
- Blood urea nitrogen (BUN): 22 mg/dL
- Creatinine: 1.1 mg/dL
- Sodium: 140 mEq/L
- Potassium: 4.2 mEq/L
- Chloride: 102 mEq/L
- Carbon dioxide: 24 mEq/L

- Calcium, total: 9.8 mg/dL

Correct Coding: 80048 (Basic metabolic panel, calcium total)

Clinical Significance: All eight required tests were performed, providing comprehensive assessment of the patient's metabolic status. The slightly elevated glucose and BUN suggest the need for closer diabetes management and continued monitoring of kidney function.

Scenario 2: Incomplete Panel Due to Specimen Issues A patient's blood specimen clots before analysis, making potassium measurement unreliable. The laboratory performs seven of the eight basic metabolic panel tests.

Tests Performed:

- Glucose, BUN, creatinine, sodium, chloride, carbon dioxide, calcium (7 tests)
- Potassium: Unable to perform due to specimen clotting

Correct Coding: Individual codes for each test performed **Incorrect Coding:** 80048 (basic metabolic panel) - cannot use panel code when any test is missing

Clinical Significance: The missing potassium result requires either specimen recollection or alternative testing method, as electrolyte balance assessment is incomplete without this critical measurement.

Comprehensive Metabolic Panel: The Workhorse of Clinical Chemistry

80053 - Comprehensive Metabolic Panel: The Most Frequently Ordered Laboratory Panel

The comprehensive metabolic panel represents one of modern medicine's most valuable diagnostic tools, providing broad screening for common medical conditions while serving as a baseline for monitoring chronic diseases. Understanding this panel's components and clinical applications helps you appreciate why it appears so frequently in medical coding.

Panel Components and Clinical Significance:

Glucose: Screening for diabetes and monitoring blood sugar control. Elevated levels suggest diabetes or prediabetes, while low levels might indicate hypoglycemia from medication effects or other causes.

Blood Urea Nitrogen (BUN) and Creatinine: Kidney function assessment. These tests evaluate the kidneys' ability to filter waste products from blood. Elevated levels suggest kidney dysfunction that might require medication adjustments or specialist referral.

Sodium, Potassium, Chloride, and Carbon Dioxide: Electrolyte balance assessment. These minerals are crucial for nerve function, muscle contraction, and fluid balance. Abnormalities can cause symptoms ranging from weakness to life-threatening heart rhythm disturbances.

Albumin and Total Protein: Nutritional status and liver function assessment. Low protein levels might indicate malnutrition, liver disease, or kidney problems. These tests help evaluate overall health status and guide nutritional interventions.

Bilirubin, Total: Liver function and red blood cell breakdown assessment. Elevated bilirubin causes jaundice and might indicate liver disease, bile duct obstruction, or excessive red blood cell destruction.

Alkaline Phosphatase, ALT (Alanine Aminotransferase), and AST (Aspartate Aminotransferase): Liver enzyme assessment. These enzymes leak into blood when liver cells are damaged, providing early detection of liver problems from medications, alcohol, infections, or other causes.

Clinical Applications: The comprehensive metabolic panel serves multiple clinical purposes that explain its widespread use in medical practice:

Routine Health Screening: Annual physical examinations often include CMP testing to detect common conditions like diabetes, kidney disease, and liver problems before symptoms develop. Early detection enables preventive interventions that can prevent progression to more serious conditions.

Chronic Disease Monitoring: Patients with diabetes, hypertension, heart disease, and other chronic conditions require regular CMP monitoring to assess disease progression and medication effects. For example, ACE inhibitors used for blood pressure control can affect kidney function and electrolyte balance, requiring periodic monitoring.

Medication Safety: Many medications can affect liver function, kidney function, or electrolyte balance. Regular CMP monitoring helps detect these effects early, allowing medication adjustments before serious complications develop.

Hospital Patient Management: Hospitalized patients often receive daily CMP testing to monitor their response to treatment and detect complications. Surgical patients might have CMP testing before surgery to ensure they're stable for anesthesia, and again after surgery to monitor for complications.

Lipid Panel: Cardiovascular Risk Assessment

80061 - Lipid Panel: Essential for Heart Disease Prevention

The lipid panel represents one of medicine's most successful preventive screening tools, enabling early detection and management of cardiovascular risk factors that can prevent heart attacks and strokes. Understanding lipid testing helps you appreciate its crucial role in preventive medicine.

Panel Components and Cardiovascular Significance:

Total Cholesterol: Overall cholesterol measurement that provides general cardiovascular risk assessment. While total cholesterol has limitations, it remains a useful screening tool and is often the first lipid measurement patients learn about.

High-Density Lipoprotein (HDL) Cholesterol: "Good" cholesterol that helps remove cholesterol from artery walls, transporting it to the liver for disposal. Higher HDL levels are associated with lower cardiovascular risk, while low HDL levels increase risk even when total cholesterol is normal.

Triglycerides: Blood fats that increase cardiovascular risk when elevated. High triglyceride levels are often associated with diabetes, obesity, and metabolic syndrome. Very high levels can also cause pancreatitis, a serious inflammatory condition.

Low-Density Lipoprotein (LDL) Cholesterol: "Bad" cholesterol that contributes to artery plaque formation. LDL is typically calculated from other lipid measurements rather than measured directly, though direct measurement is available when triglycerides are very high.

Clinical Guidelines and Risk Assessment: Lipid panel interpretation involves more than just comparing results to reference ranges. Current guidelines consider multiple risk factors including age, gender, blood pressure, diabetes status, smoking history, and family history to calculate overall cardiovascular risk.

For example, a 45-year-old male with diabetes might need more aggressive cholesterol management than a healthy 30-year-old female with the same cholesterol levels. This individualized approach to risk assessment explains why lipid panels are often ordered along with other tests that evaluate cardiovascular risk factors.

Treatment Monitoring: Lipid panels are essential for monitoring cholesterol-lowering medications like statins, which can reduce cardiovascular events by 25-50% when used appropriately. Patients starting cholesterol medications typically need follow-up lipid testing after 6-12 weeks to assess treatment effectiveness and guide dose adjustments.

The combination of cardiovascular risk reduction and medication monitoring makes lipid panels one of the most frequently ordered laboratory tests, particularly in primary care settings where cardiovascular prevention is a major focus.

Hepatic Function Panel: Liver Health Assessment

80076 - Hepatic Function Panel: Comprehensive Liver Evaluation

The hepatic function panel provides systematic evaluation of liver health, combining tests that assess different aspects of liver function including protein synthesis, enzyme activity, and waste processing. Understanding liver function testing helps you appreciate the complexity of this vital organ and the multiple ways disease can affect its function.

Panel Components and Liver Function Assessment:

Albumin: The most abundant protein produced by the liver, albumin helps maintain blood volume and transports substances throughout the body. Low albumin levels suggest chronic liver disease, malnutrition, or kidney problems that cause protein loss.

Total Protein: Includes albumin plus other proteins like globulins that are produced by the liver and immune system. The ratio between albumin and globulins can provide additional information about liver function and immune system activity.

Bilirubin, Total and Direct: Bilirubin is produced when red blood cells break down and must be processed by the liver for elimination. Elevated bilirubin causes jaundice and can indicate liver disease, bile duct obstruction, or excessive red blood cell destruction.

Alkaline Phosphatase: An enzyme found in liver cells and bile ducts. Elevated levels can indicate liver disease, bile duct obstruction, or bone disease. Additional testing might be needed to determine which organ system is causing elevation.

ALT (Alanine Aminotransferase) and AST (Aspartate Aminotransferase): Liver enzymes that leak into blood when liver cells are damaged. ALT is more specific for liver damage, while AST can also be elevated with heart or muscle damage. The pattern and degree of elevation help determine the cause and severity of liver injury.

Clinical Applications: Hepatic function panels are used in multiple clinical scenarios that demonstrate the liver's central role in health and disease:

Medication Monitoring: Many medications can cause liver damage, particularly when used long-term or in high doses. Medications like acetaminophen, statins, and some antibiotics require periodic liver function monitoring to detect problems early.

Chronic Disease Management: Conditions like hepatitis, fatty liver disease, and cirrhosis require regular monitoring to assess disease progression and treatment effectiveness. The pattern of abnormalities can help distinguish between different types of liver disease.

Surgical Risk Assessment: Liver function affects surgical risk because the liver metabolizes anesthetic medications and produces proteins necessary for blood clotting. Patients with liver disease might need special precautions during surgery.

Alcohol Assessment: Liver function testing can help evaluate the effects of alcohol use and monitor patients in recovery programs. Certain patterns of liver enzyme elevation are characteristic of alcohol-related liver damage.

Drug Assay and Therapeutic Drug Monitoring: Precision Medicine Through Measurement

Therapeutic drug monitoring represents one of laboratory medicine's most direct applications to patient care, ensuring medications achieve therapeutic benefit while avoiding toxic effects. Understanding drug monitoring helps you appreciate how laboratory testing enables safe, effective medication use.

The Science of Pharmacokinetics and Drug Monitoring

Why Drug Levels Matter: Most medications have a "therapeutic window"—a range of blood concentrations that provides beneficial effects without causing toxicity. Below this range, medications don't work effectively. Above this range, side effects and toxicity become problematic. Therapeutic drug monitoring helps ensure patients stay within this optimal range.

Individual patients can have dramatically different responses to the same medication dose due to genetic differences in drug metabolism, kidney and liver function variations, drug interactions, and other factors. A dose that's perfect for one patient might be ineffective for another or cause serious side effects in a third patient.

Consider digoxin, a heart medication with a very narrow therapeutic window. Too little digoxin fails to improve heart function, while too much can cause dangerous heart rhythm abnormalities. Regular blood level monitoring allows physicians to adjust doses for optimal benefit with minimal risk.

Factors Affecting Drug Levels: Understanding factors that influence drug concentrations helps explain why monitoring is necessary and how results should be interpreted:

Kidney Function: Many medications are eliminated through the kidneys. When kidney function declines, drug levels can accumulate to toxic levels unless doses are reduced. Elderly patients and those with diabetes or hypertension often have reduced kidney function requiring dose adjustments.

Liver Function: The liver metabolizes many medications, converting them to inactive forms that can be eliminated safely. Liver disease can dramatically affect medication levels, requiring dose adjustments or alternative medications.

Drug Interactions: Multiple medications can interact in ways that affect drug levels. Some medications inhibit enzymes that metabolize other drugs, causing levels to rise. Others can speed up metabolism, causing levels to fall below therapeutic ranges.

Genetic Variations: Individuals have genetic differences in drug-metabolizing enzymes that can cause dramatic variations in drug levels. Some people are "rapid metabolizers" who need higher doses, while others are "poor metabolizers" who need lower doses to avoid toxicity.

Common Therapeutic Drug Monitoring Applications

80162 - Digoxin: Classic Example of Narrow Therapeutic Window

Digoxin monitoring demonstrates the principles of therapeutic drug monitoring better than perhaps any other medication. This heart medication has been used for over 200 years, but its narrow therapeutic window makes blood level monitoring essential for safe use.

Clinical Applications: Digoxin is used primarily for heart failure and certain heart rhythm disorders. It works by increasing the force of heart muscle contractions and slowing rapid heart rates. However, the difference between therapeutic and toxic doses is small, making monitoring crucial.

Monitoring Protocol: Digoxin levels are typically checked 5-7 days after starting treatment or changing doses, allowing time for steady-state levels to develop. Levels are drawn immediately before the next dose (trough levels) to assess the lowest concentration during the dosing interval.

Interpreting Results: Therapeutic digoxin levels typically range from 1.0-2.0 ng/mL, though some patients benefit from lower levels. Levels above 2.0 ng/mL increase toxicity risk, while levels below 1.0 ng/mL might not provide adequate therapeutic benefit.

Toxicity Signs: Digoxin toxicity can cause nausea, confusion, visual disturbances, and dangerous heart rhythm abnormalities. Blood level monitoring helps detect toxicity before symptoms develop, allowing dose adjustments that prevent serious complications.

80176 - Lithium: Mood Stabilization with Careful Monitoring

Lithium monitoring demonstrates the challenges of managing psychiatric medications that require ongoing laboratory surveillance for safe use.

Clinical Applications: Lithium is primarily used for bipolar disorder treatment and prevention of manic episodes. It's one of the most effective medications for this condition, but requires careful monitoring due to potential side effects affecting kidneys, thyroid, and other organs.

Monitoring Requirements: Lithium requires initial monitoring every few days until stable levels are achieved, then periodic monitoring throughout treatment. The frequency depends on patient factors, dose changes, and concurrent medical conditions.

Complex Interactions: Lithium levels can be affected by dehydration, kidney function changes, salt intake variations, and interactions with other medications. Patients need education about maintaining consistent fluid and salt intake to prevent level fluctuations.

Long-term Considerations: Long-term lithium use requires monitoring of kidney function, thyroid function, and other parameters beyond just lithium levels. This comprehensive monitoring ensures early detection of side effects that might require treatment adjustments.

80200 - Phenytoin: Anticonvulsant with Complex Pharmacokinetics

Phenytoin monitoring illustrates the complexity of medications with nonlinear pharmacokinetics, where small dose changes can cause large changes in blood levels.

Nonlinear Pharmacokinetics: Unlike most medications that have proportional relationships between dose and blood level, phenytoin has saturable metabolism. At lower doses, the body can metabolize phenytoin efficiently, but at higher doses, the metabolic system becomes saturated and small dose increases cause disproportionate level increases.

This nonlinear relationship makes phenytoin dosing challenging and explains why careful monitoring is essential. A dose increase that seems modest might push levels from therapeutic to toxic ranges.

Protein Binding Considerations: Phenytoin is highly bound to blood proteins, and only the unbound (free) fraction is pharmacologically active. Conditions that affect protein binding—such as kidney disease, liver disease, or pregnancy—can change the relationship between total and free phenytoin levels.

In some cases, free phenytoin levels provide more accurate assessment of drug effect than total levels, particularly in patients with conditions that affect protein binding.

Presumptive vs. Definitive Drug Testing

Understanding Different Testing Methodologies: Drug testing uses different analytical methods depending on the clinical situation, required accuracy, and available resources. Understanding these differences helps explain why different codes exist for seemingly similar tests.

Presumptive Testing (80305-80377): Presumptive testing provides rapid screening results but has limitations in specificity and accuracy. These tests are valuable for initial screening but may require confirmatory testing for legal or critical clinical decisions.

Immunoassays: Use antibody-based detection that can cross-react with similar substances, potentially causing false-positive results. However, immunoassays are rapid, relatively inexpensive, and suitable for most clinical screening applications.

Point-of-Care Testing: Allows immediate results in clinical settings but may have lower accuracy than laboratory-based methods. These tests are valuable for urgent clinical decisions but shouldn't be used as the sole basis for critical treatment decisions.

Definitive Testing (80320-80377): Definitive testing uses sophisticated analytical methods that provide high specificity and accuracy. These methods are more expensive and time-consuming but are necessary when precise identification and quantification are required.

Chromatography-Mass Spectrometry: Combines separation techniques with mass spectrometry to provide definitive identification and quantification of specific substances. This method is considered the gold standard for drug testing accuracy.

Legal and Forensic Applications: Definitive testing is often required for legal proceedings, employment testing, or other situations where high accuracy is essential. The additional cost and time are justified by the need for defensible results.

Evocative/Suppression Testing: Dynamic Assessment of Endocrine Function

Evocative and suppression testing represents some of the most sophisticated approaches to diagnosing endocrine disorders, using carefully controlled stimuli to assess gland function under dynamic conditions rather than relying on single-point-in-time measurements.

Understanding Dynamic Endocrine Testing

Why Static Testing Has Limitations: Many endocrine disorders involve subtle abnormalities in hormone regulation that aren't apparent from single hormone measurements. Hormone levels fluctuate throughout the day, respond to stress and other factors, and may appear normal even when significant dysfunction exists.

For example, a patient with early adrenal insufficiency might have normal morning cortisol levels but fail to increase cortisol appropriately in response to stress. Static testing might miss this important dysfunction, while dynamic testing can reveal the problem clearly.

Stimulation vs. Suppression Testing: The choice between stimulation and suppression testing depends on the suspected disorder. If hormone deficiency is suspected, stimulation testing challenges the gland to produce hormones and demonstrates whether it can respond appropriately. If hormone excess is suspected, suppression testing challenges the body's feedback mechanisms to determine whether hormone production can be turned off normally.

Clinical Integration: Dynamic testing requires careful integration with clinical assessment, imaging studies, and other diagnostic information. The tests are often technically complex and require specialized interpretation, justifying separate coding recognition for the comprehensive evaluation they provide.

ACTH Stimulation Testing: Adrenal Function Assessment

80400 - ACTH Stimulation Panel: The Gold Standard for Adrenal Assessment

ACTH stimulation testing provides definitive assessment of adrenal gland function by challenging the adrenals to produce cortisol in response to synthetic ACTH (cosyntropin) injection.

The Physiology Behind the Test: The hypothalamic-pituitary-adrenal axis normally works like a sophisticated feedback system. The hypothalamus produces corticotropin-releasing hormone (CRH), which stimulates the pituitary to produce ACTH, which stimulates the adrenals to produce cortisol. When this system is working properly, ACTH injection should cause a robust cortisol response.

Testing Protocol: Baseline cortisol is measured, then synthetic ACTH is injected, and cortisol levels are measured at specific intervals (typically 30 and 60 minutes post-injection). Normal adrenal glands should double or triple cortisol production in response to ACTH stimulation.

Clinical Applications: ACTH stimulation testing is used to diagnose primary adrenal insufficiency (Addison's disease), assess adrenal function in patients taking steroid medications, and evaluate patients with symptoms suggesting adrenal dysfunction like fatigue, weakness, or abnormal blood pressure responses.

Interpreting Results: A normal response demonstrates adequate adrenal reserve and rules out significant adrenal insufficiency. A blunted response suggests adrenal dysfunction that might require hormone replacement therapy. The degree of impairment helps guide treatment decisions and monitoring requirements.

Clinical Significance: Undiagnosed adrenal insufficiency can be life-threatening, particularly during stress situations like illness or surgery. ACTH stimulation testing provides definitive diagnosis that enables appropriate treatment and prevents adrenal crises.

Dexamethasone Suppression Testing: Evaluating Cortisol Excess

80422 - Dexamethasone Suppression Panel: Diagnosing Cushing's Syndrome

Dexamethasone suppression testing evaluates the body's ability to suppress cortisol production in response to synthetic steroid administration, helping diagnose conditions involving excess cortisol production.

The Suppression Principle: Normal feedback mechanisms should suppress cortisol production when synthetic steroids like dexamethasone are administered. Autonomous cortisol-producing tumors or other causes of Cushing's syndrome fail to suppress appropriately, maintaining high cortisol levels despite dexamethasone administration.

Testing Variations: Low-dose dexamethasone suppression (1 mg overnight) is used for initial screening, while high-dose suppression (8 mg) can help distinguish between different causes of Cushing's syndrome. The choice of protocol depends on clinical suspicion and initial test results.

Clinical Context: Cushing's syndrome causes multiple serious health problems including diabetes, osteoporosis, hypertension, and increased infection risk. Early diagnosis enables treatment that can reverse many of these complications and prevent progression to more serious conditions.

Diagnostic Challenges: Cortisol levels can be affected by stress, medications, depression, and other factors that can complicate interpretation. Careful clinical correlation and sometimes repeat testing are necessary to reach accurate diagnoses.

Growth Hormone and Other Specialized Testing

Growth Hormone Stimulation Testing: Growth hormone deficiency in children can cause significant growth retardation that responds dramatically to hormone replacement therapy. However, growth hormone levels fluctuate widely, making single measurements unreliable for diagnosis.

Growth hormone stimulation testing uses various stimuli (exercise, insulin-induced hypoglycemia, or pharmacological agents) to challenge the pituitary to produce growth hormone. Normal responses rule out growth hormone deficiency, while blunted responses support the diagnosis and justify treatment.

Glucose Tolerance Testing: While often considered a diabetes test, glucose tolerance testing can also evaluate hormone responses to glucose loads. The test measures not just glucose levels but also insulin responses, helping diagnose conditions like insulin resistance, reactive hypoglycemia, or other disorders of glucose metabolism.

The complexity of interpreting multiple hormone responses over time justifies the comprehensive panel coding approach used for these sophisticated diagnostic procedures.

Consultations (Clinical Pathology): Expert Interpretation and Guidance

Clinical pathology consultations represent one of medicine's most valuable but underutilized resources, providing expert interpretation of complex laboratory results and guidance for additional testing strategies.

The Role of Clinical Pathology Consultations

Beyond Simple Result Interpretation: While most laboratory results can be interpreted using reference ranges and clinical guidelines, complex cases often benefit from expert consultation that considers multiple factors including test interactions, clinical context, analytical limitations, and alternative testing strategies.

Clinical pathologists bring specialized expertise in laboratory medicine, understanding not just what tests measure but how analytical methods work, what factors can affect results, and how to design testing strategies that provide maximum diagnostic information efficiently.

80500 - Clinical Pathology Consultation: Comprehensive Case Review

Comprehensive clinical pathology consultations involve detailed review of patient history, clinical findings, and laboratory results to provide diagnostic recommendations and testing strategies.

Consultation Components:

- Review of patient clinical history and symptoms
- Analysis of existing laboratory results and their relationships
- Identification of additional testing that might provide diagnostic information
- Interpretation of unusual or conflicting results
- Recommendations for follow-up monitoring
- Communication with attending physicians about findings and recommendations

Clinical Scenarios Requiring Consultation: Complex cases involving multiple abnormal results that don't fit typical disease patterns often benefit from pathology consultation. For example, a patient with unusual blood cell abnormalities might need expert interpretation to distinguish between various blood disorders and determine appropriate follow-up testing.

Medication effects can cause complex laboratory abnormalities that require expert interpretation. A patient taking multiple medications might have laboratory changes that could represent drug interactions, underlying disease, or normal medication effects.

80502 - Clinical Pathology Consultation, Limited: Focused Expert Input

Limited consultations focus on specific questions or particular aspects of laboratory results rather than comprehensive case review.

Focused Applications:

- Interpretation of specific unusual results
- Recommendations for additional testing for particular conditions
- Assessment of laboratory findings in context of specific medications
- Evaluation of specimen adequacy or analytical issues

Efficiency and Cost-Effectiveness: Limited consultations provide expert input for specific questions without the time and expense of comprehensive review. This approach allows efficient use of pathology expertise while controlling costs.

Integration with Clinical Care

Multidisciplinary Collaboration: Clinical pathology consultations work best when integrated with broader clinical teams including attending physicians, specialists, and other healthcare providers. The consultation process involves ongoing communication rather than just written reports.

Educational Component: Consultations often include educational components that help referring physicians understand laboratory principles and interpret similar cases independently in the future. This educational aspect extends the value of consultation beyond individual cases.

Quality Improvement: Pattern recognition from multiple consultations can identify systematic issues in testing strategies, result interpretation, or analytical methods that benefit broader patient populations through quality improvement initiatives.

Urinalysis: The Original Laboratory Test with Modern Applications

Urinalysis represents one of medicine's oldest laboratory tests, yet it remains relevant in modern practice due to its simplicity, low cost, and valuable diagnostic information for a wide range of conditions.

The Evolution and Continued Relevance of Urinalysis

Historical Significance: Urinalysis predates most modern laboratory tests by centuries, with ancient physicians recognizing that urine appearance, odor, and other characteristics could provide information about health and disease. The development of chemical and microscopic testing transformed urinalysis into a sophisticated diagnostic tool.

Modern Applications: Contemporary urinalysis combines visual inspection, chemical testing, and microscopic examination to provide information about kidney function, urinary tract infections, diabetes, liver disease, and other conditions. The combination of simplicity and diagnostic value makes urinalysis one of the most cost-effective laboratory tests available.

Urinalysis Components and Coding

81001 - Urinalysis, Automated with Microscopy: Modern urinalysis typically uses automated analyzers that perform multiple chemical tests simultaneously, followed by microscopic examination when abnormalities are detected or clinical circumstances warrant detailed evaluation.

Chemical Testing Components:

- **Protein:** Detects kidney damage or disease
- **Glucose:** Screens for diabetes
- **Ketones:** Identifies metabolic disorders
- **Blood:** Detects urinary tract bleeding
- **Leukocyte esterase:** Screens for white blood cells (infection)
- **Nitrites:** Detects certain bacteria
- **pH and specific gravity:** Assess kidney concentration ability

Microscopic Examination: When chemical testing reveals abnormalities or clinical circumstances suggest urinary tract disease, microscopic examination provides additional diagnostic information:

- **Red blood cells:** Confirm hematuria and assess source
- **White blood cells:** Evaluate for infection or inflammation

- **Bacteria:** Assess for urinary tract infection
- **Casts:** Detect kidney disease
- **Crystals:** Identify stone-forming tendency

81002 - Urinalysis,Non-automated Dipstick or Tablet Reagent: Non-automated urinalysis uses manual methods that might be more appropriate for small-volume testing or when automated equipment isn't available. While less efficient than automated methods, manual testing can provide equivalent diagnostic information when performed properly.

81003 - Urinalysis, by Microscopy Only: In some clinical situations, microscopic examination is the primary diagnostic need. This might occur when chemical testing has already been performed or when specific microscopic findings are the focus of clinical concern.

Microscopic urinalysis requires significant technical expertise to identify and enumerate various formed elements accurately. Proper specimen handling, preparation techniques, and systematic examination protocols are essential for reliable results.

Clinical Applications and Diagnostic Value

Urinary Tract Infection Diagnosis: Urinalysis remains the cornerstone of urinary tract infection diagnosis, providing rapid screening that can guide immediate treatment decisions. The combination of chemical testing (leukocyte esterase and nitrites) with microscopic examination (white blood cells and bacteria) provides excellent diagnostic accuracy for most UTIs.

However, urinalysis interpretation requires understanding its limitations. Some bacteria don't produce nitrites, and white blood cell counts can be elevated for reasons other than infection. Clinical correlation with symptoms and risk factors is essential for accurate diagnosis.

Kidney Disease Screening: Proteinuria (protein in urine) is often the first sign of kidney disease, appearing before patients develop symptoms or abnormal blood tests. Regular urinalysis screening can detect kidney problems years before they become clinically apparent, enabling early intervention that can slow disease progression.

The presence of cellular casts in urine provides specific information about kidney damage location and severity. Red blood cell casts indicate glomerular bleeding, while white blood cell casts suggest interstitial inflammation. These findings help guide further diagnostic workup and treatment decisions.

Diabetes Monitoring: While blood glucose testing has largely replaced urine glucose testing for diabetes diagnosis and management, urinalysis still provides valuable information about diabetes complications. Proteinuria can indicate diabetic kidney disease, while ketones in urine might suggest inadequate diabetes control.

The combination of routine blood glucose monitoring with periodic urinalysis provides comprehensive diabetes assessment that can detect complications early and guide treatment adjustments.

Molecular Pathology: The Future of Precision Medicine

Molecular pathology represents one of medicine's most rapidly evolving fields, using sophisticated genetic and molecular techniques to diagnose disease, predict treatment responses, and guide personalized therapy decisions.

Understanding Molecular Diagnostics

The Molecular Revolution in Medicine: Molecular pathology has transformed our understanding of disease from organ-based classifications to molecular-based categories that often cross traditional boundaries. Cancer that looks identical under the microscope might have completely different molecular characteristics that require different treatments.

This molecular understanding has enabled precision medicine approaches where treatment decisions are based on specific molecular characteristics of each patient's disease rather than one-size-fits-all approaches. The result is more effective treatments with fewer side effects and better outcomes.

Technology Behind Molecular Testing: Modern molecular pathology uses sophisticated techniques like polymerase chain reaction (PCR), next-generation sequencing (NGS), and mass spectrometry to analyze DNA, RNA, and proteins at the molecular level. These techniques can detect single nucleotide changes, gene rearrangements, and protein modifications that affect disease behavior and treatment response.

The complexity and cost of these techniques require specialized equipment, highly trained personnel, and extensive quality control procedures. Understanding this complexity helps explain why molecular pathology codes often have higher reimbursement rates than traditional laboratory tests.

Genetic Testing Applications

Inherited Disease Testing: Genetic testing can identify mutations that cause inherited diseases, enabling early diagnosis, family screening, and reproductive counseling. Tests for conditions like cystic fibrosis, sickle cell disease, and hereditary cancer syndromes can provide life-changing information for patients and families.

Pharmacogenomics: Understanding how genetic variations affect drug metabolism allows personalized medication selection and dosing. For example, genetic testing can identify patients who metabolize certain medications rapidly (requiring higher doses) or slowly (requiring lower doses or alternative medications).

Cancer Genetics: Molecular testing of tumors can identify specific mutations that predict treatment response, enabling selection of targeted therapies that are more likely to be effective. This approach has revolutionized cancer treatment, with many patients achieving remarkable responses to therapies selected based on their tumor's molecular characteristics.

Infectious Disease Molecular Testing

Rapid Pathogen Identification: Molecular techniques can identify infectious organisms within hours rather than days required for traditional culture methods. This speed can be crucial for guiding appropriate antibiotic therapy and infection control measures.

Antimicrobial Resistance Testing: Molecular methods can detect resistance genes that predict antibiotic effectiveness, enabling selection of appropriate therapy before culture results are available. This capability is particularly important for serious infections where delayed appropriate therapy can be life-threatening.

Viral Load Monitoring: Quantitative molecular tests can measure viral levels in patients with chronic infections like HIV or hepatitis, guiding treatment decisions and monitoring response to antiviral therapy.

Microbiology: Identifying the Invisible Threats

Microbiology laboratory services focus on identifying microorganisms that cause infection and determining their susceptibility to antimicrobial agents. This information is crucial for selecting appropriate treatment and implementing infection control measures.

Understanding Microbiological Testing

The Challenge of Microorganism Identification: Microorganisms are diverse, numerous, and often difficult to distinguish from each other using traditional methods. Bacteria that cause different diseases might look similar under the microscope, while similar-appearing symptoms might be caused by completely different organisms.

Modern microbiology combines traditional culture methods with sophisticated identification techniques including automated systems, molecular methods, and mass spectrometry to provide rapid, accurate organism identification and antimicrobial susceptibility testing.

Clinical Significance of Rapid Results: Microbiological results directly impact patient care decisions, often determining which antibiotics are prescribed and how long treatment continues. Rapid identification of organisms and their antimicrobial susceptibilities can mean the difference between effective treatment and treatment failure.

Consider a patient with pneumonia: identifying whether the infection is caused by bacteria, viruses, or fungi determines whether antibiotics are appropriate and which specific agents are most likely to be effective. This information guides treatment decisions that can be life-saving.

Culture and Sensitivity Testing

87040-87158 - Culture Procedures: Microbiological cultures involve growing organisms from patient specimens under controlled laboratory conditions, allowing identification and antimicrobial susceptibility testing.

Specimen Collection and Processing: Proper specimen collection is crucial for accurate microbiological results. Different specimen types require different collection techniques, transport conditions, and processing methods. Blood cultures require strict sterile technique, while respiratory specimens need rapid processing to maintain organism viability.

Culture Media and Conditions: Different organisms require different growth conditions including specific nutrients, atmospheric conditions, and incubation temperatures. Skilled microbiologists select appropriate culture media and conditions based on suspected organisms and specimen types.

Identification Methods: Once organisms grow in culture, various methods are used for identification including biochemical tests, automated identification systems, and molecular techniques. The choice of identification method depends on the organism type, clinical urgency, and available technology.

87181-87190 - Antimicrobial Susceptibility Testing: Determining which antibiotics are effective against specific organisms is crucial for selecting appropriate therapy and avoiding treatment failures.

Testing Methods: Susceptibility testing uses standardized methods to determine minimum inhibitory concentrations (MICs) of various antibiotics against isolated organisms. These results are interpreted using established criteria to categorize organisms as susceptible, intermediate, or resistant to specific antibiotics.

Clinical Correlation: Susceptibility results must be interpreted in context of patient factors including infection site, antibiotic penetration characteristics, and patient immune status. An organism might be "susceptible" in the laboratory but still cause treatment failure if the antibiotic doesn't reach adequate concentrations at the infection site.

Molecular Microbiology

87470-87801 - Infectious Agent Detection by Nucleic Acid: Molecular methods can detect organisms directly from specimens without requiring culture, providing rapid results that can guide immediate treatment decisions.

Advantages of Molecular Methods:

- Rapid results (hours instead of days)
- Detection of organisms that don't grow in culture
- Quantitative results for monitoring treatment response
- Simultaneous detection of multiple organisms

Limitations and Considerations:

- Higher cost than traditional methods
- May detect non-viable organisms
- Requires sophisticated equipment and expertise
- May not provide antimicrobial susceptibility information

Clinical Applications: Molecular microbiology is particularly valuable for detecting organisms that are difficult to culture, identifying organisms in patients who have already received antibiotics, and providing rapid results for critically ill patients where immediate treatment decisions are necessary.

Anatomic Pathology: Where Tissue Tells the Story

Anatomic pathology involves microscopic examination of tissues and cells to diagnose disease, determine prognosis, and guide treatment decisions. This field represents one of medicine's most direct applications of visual pattern recognition and morphologic expertise.

Understanding Tissue Diagnosis

The Art and Science of Microscopic Diagnosis: Anatomic pathology combines sophisticated technical methods with expert pattern recognition to translate tissue appearances into clinically meaningful diagnoses. Pathologists must understand normal tissue architecture, recognize disease patterns, and correlate morphologic findings with clinical information.

This expertise requires extensive training including medical school, residency, and often fellowship training in subspecialty areas. The combination of medical knowledge and technical expertise justifies the professional fees associated with anatomic pathology services.

Tissue Processing and Preparation: Before microscopic examination can occur, tissues must undergo complex processing including fixation, dehydration, embedding, sectioning, and staining. This process typically takes 12-24 hours and requires skilled technologists and quality control procedures to ensure optimal results.

Understanding tissue processing helps explain why pathology results often take several days and why expedited processing (for urgent cases) might require additional fees. The technical complexity of tissue preparation represents a significant component of anatomic pathology services.

Surgical Pathology Services

88300-88309 - Level of Service Coding: Surgical pathology uses a level-of-service coding system that reflects the complexity of specimens and the expertise required for accurate diagnosis.

88300 - Level I: Simple Specimens Level I includes specimens that rarely require extensive gross examination or microscopic evaluation. Examples include skin tags, hemorrhoids, or other benign lesions where the diagnosis is usually straightforward.

88302 - Level II: Straightforward Specimens Level II specimens require systematic examination but generally have straightforward diagnostic possibilities. Examples include simple skin biopsies, benign cysts, or routine appendectomy specimens.

88304 - Level III: Moderate Complexity Level III represents the most commonly submitted specimens that require careful examination and consideration of multiple diagnostic possibilities. Examples include skin lesions with concern for malignancy, prostate biopsies, or endometrial biopsies.

88305 - Level IV: Complex Specimens Level IV includes specimens that require extensive examination, multiple sections, and consideration of complex diagnostic possibilities. Examples include cancer resection specimens, complex biopsies, or specimens requiring special studies.

88307 - Level V: Highly Complex Specimens Level V represents the most complex specimens requiring extensive examination, multiple sampling, and sophisticated diagnostic expertise. Examples include major cancer resections, transplant biopsies, or specimens requiring complex staging.

88309 - Level VI: Extremely Complex Specimens Level VI is reserved for the most complex specimens requiring extraordinary examination and expertise. Examples might include complex tumor resections requiring extensive sampling and staging.

Cytopathology Services

88104-88199 - Cytopathology Procedures: Cytopathology involves examination of individual cells rather than intact tissues, providing diagnostic information through cellular morphology and architecture.

88150 - Cervical or Vaginal Cytology (Pap Smears): Cervical cytology represents one of medicine's most successful cancer screening programs, dramatically reducing cervical cancer incidence and mortality through early detection of precancerous changes.

Specimen Preparation: Modern cervical cytology uses liquid-based preparation methods that improve specimen quality and enable additional testing like HPV detection from the same specimen.

Screening and Interpretation: Cytology specimens undergo initial screening by cytotechnologists who identify abnormal cells requiring pathologist review. This two-level review system ensures quality while controlling costs.

88160-88162 - Other Cytology Specimens: Non-cervical cytology includes specimens from various body sites including respiratory tract, urinary tract, body fluids, and fine needle aspirations.

Clinical Applications: Cytology provides diagnostic information that can guide treatment decisions without requiring surgical biopsy. For example, fine needle aspiration of a thyroid nodule can often determine whether surgical removal is necessary.

Special Studies and Advanced Techniques

88311-88365 - Immunohistochemistry and Special Stains: Special staining techniques can highlight specific cellular components, organisms, or molecular markers that aren't visible with routine staining methods.

Immunohistochemistry: Uses antibodies to detect specific proteins in tissues, enabling precise diagnosis of tumors, identification of infectious organisms, and assessment of prognostic markers.

Molecular Pathology in Tissue Diagnosis: Increasingly, tissue diagnosis incorporates molecular techniques that detect genetic alterations, gene expression patterns, or other molecular characteristics that guide treatment decisions.

88371-88399 - In Situ Hybridization: Detects specific DNA or RNA sequences within tissue sections, enabling identification of genetic alterations or infectious agents with precise localization.

Comprehensive Pathology and Laboratory Coding Practice Questions

Test your mastery of pathology and laboratory coding across all areas:

Question 1: A patient has blood drawn for glucose, BUN, creatinine, sodium, potassium, chloride, CO2, and total calcium. How should this be coded?

A) 80048 (Basic metabolic panel, calcium total) B) 80053 (Comprehensive metabolic panel) C) Individual codes for each test D) 80047 (Basic metabolic panel, ionized calcium)

Answer: A Explanation: All eight tests in the basic metabolic panel (calcium, total) were performed: glucose, BUN, creatinine, sodium, potassium, chloride, CO2, and total calcium. When all tests in a panel are performed, use the panel code rather than individual test codes.

Question 2: Digoxin level monitoring in a patient taking digoxin for heart failure should be coded as:

A) 80162 (Digoxin, total) B) 80299 (Quantitation of therapeutic drug, not elsewhere specified) C) 80305 (Drug test, presumptive) D) 80320 (Drug test, definitive)

Answer: A Explanation: 80162 specifically represents digoxin quantitation for therapeutic drug monitoring. Use specific drug codes when available rather than general drug testing codes.

Question 3: ACTH stimulation test with cortisol measurements before and after stimulation should be coded as:

A) 80400 (ACTH stimulation panel) B) 82533 (Cortisol, free) × 2 C) 80418 (Chorionic gonadotropin stimulation panel) D) Individual cortisol codes plus ACTH injection

Answer: A Explanation: 80400 represents the complete ACTH stimulation panel including baseline and post-stimulation cortisol measurements. Panel codes should be used when the complete protocol is performed.

Question 4: Automated urinalysis with microscopic examination when indicated should be coded as:

A) 81001 (Urinalysis, automated with microscopy) B) 81002 (Urinalysis, non-automated) C) 81003 (Urinalysis, microscopy only) D) 81025 (Urine pregnancy test)

Answer: A Explanation: 81001 represents automated urinalysis that includes microscopic examination when clinically indicated or when abnormalities are detected on chemical testing.

Question 5: Clinical pathology consultation for interpretation of complex laboratory results should be coded as:

A) 80500 (Clinical pathology consultation) B) 80502 (Clinical pathology consultation, limited) C) Depends on extent of consultation required D) Cannot be coded separately

Answer: C Explanation: Use 80500 for comprehensive consultation involving detailed case review, or 80502 for limited consultation focusing on specific questions. The choice depends on the scope and complexity of the consultation provided.

Question 6: Prostate needle biopsy examination should be coded as:

A) 88302 (Level II surgical pathology) B) 88304 (Level III surgical pathology) C) 88305 (Level IV surgical pathology) D) 88307 (Level V surgical pathology)

Answer: C Explanation: Prostate needle biopsies are specifically listed as Level IV (88305) specimens due to their complexity and the expertise required for accurate interpretation, particularly regarding cancer diagnosis and grading.

Question 7: Cervical cytology (Pap smear) using liquid-based preparation should be coded as:

A) 88150 (Cervical or vaginal cytology) B) 88152 (Cervical or vaginal cytology, collected in preservative fluid) C) 88153 (Cervical or vaginal cytology, with manual screening) D) 88160 (Cytopathology, other source)

Answer: B Explanation: 88152 specifically represents cervical/vaginal cytology using liquid-based preparation methods (collected in preservative fluid), which is the current standard of care for Pap smears.

Question 8: Blood culture with organism identification and antimicrobial susceptibility testing should be coded as:

A) 87040 (Blood culture) only B) 87040 + 87181 (Susceptibility testing) C) 87040 + 87076 (Bacterial identification) + 87181 D) Depends on organisms isolated

Answer: C Explanation: When organisms are isolated from blood culture, code the culture (87040), identification (87076 or other appropriate identification code), and susceptibility testing (87181) separately as these represent distinct services.

Question 9: Comprehensive metabolic panel plus lipid panel should be coded as:

A) 80053 (CMP) + 80061 (Lipid panel) B) 80053 (CMP) only C) Individual codes for all tests D) 80076 (Hepatic function panel) + 80061 (Lipid panel)

Answer: A Explanation: When multiple panels are performed, code each panel separately. The comprehensive metabolic panel and lipid panel contain different tests and can be coded together when both are performed.

Question 10: Immunohistochemistry staining for tumor markers on tissue biopsy should be coded as:

A) Included in surgical pathology code B) 88342 (Immunohistochemistry, each antibody) C) 88360 (Morphometric analysis) D) 88365 (In situ hybridization)

Answer: B Explanation: Immunohistochemistry is coded separately from the surgical pathology examination using 88342 for each antibody used. These are additional studies that provide diagnostic information beyond routine microscopic examination.

Chapter 14 Summary: Mastering Laboratory Medicine Coding Excellence

You have now achieved comprehensive mastery of pathology and laboratory coding across the full spectrum of clinical laboratory medicine. Your expertise encompasses:

Panel Mastery: You understand the clinical logic behind laboratory panels and can apply panel coding rules correctly, distinguishing between complete and incomplete panels while recognizing when individual test coding is appropriate.

Therapeutic Drug Monitoring: You've mastered the principles of pharmacokinetics and can code drug monitoring services accurately, understanding the clinical significance of drug level testing and the factors that affect interpretation.

Dynamic Testing Expertise: You understand the sophisticated protocols used for endocrine function testing and can code complex stimulation and suppression tests that require specialized interpretation.

Molecular Medicine Knowledge: You appreciate how molecular diagnostics is transforming medicine and can navigate the complex coding requirements for genetic testing, molecular pathology, and other advanced diagnostic techniques.

Microbiology Proficiency: You understand how microbiological testing identifies infectious agents and guides antimicrobial therapy, enabling accurate coding of culture, identification, and susceptibility testing services.

Anatomic Pathology Mastery: You've learned the sophisticated level-of-service system used for surgical pathology and understand how tissue complexity affects coding decisions.

The Clinical Foundation You've Built

Your laboratory medicine expertise represents more than technical coding knowledge—you've developed a deep understanding of how laboratory testing drives medical decision-making and supports quality patient care. This knowledge positions you as a valuable specialist who can:

Support Evidence-Based Medicine: By ensuring accurate coding of sophisticated diagnostic tests, you help maintain the financial viability of laboratory services that are essential for modern medical practice.

Navigate Complex Testing Relationships: Understanding how different laboratory specialties interact helps you code complex cases involving multiple testing modalities and interpret billing relationships between different providers.

Adapt to Technological Innovation: Your foundation in laboratory principles prepares you to understand and code new testing technologies as they emerge and become incorporated into clinical practice.

Provide Expert Consultation: Your comprehensive knowledge allows you to resolve complex coding disputes, train other coders, and serve as a resource for challenging laboratory coding questions.

Integration with Complete Medical Coding Practice

Your laboratory medicine expertise integrates seamlessly with your other coding specialties:

Surgical Integration: Understanding which laboratory tests support surgical decision-making helps you appreciate the complete patient care process and code related services appropriately.

Radiology Correlation: Laboratory results often complement imaging studies, and understanding both areas enhances your appreciation of comprehensive diagnostic workups.

Clinical Decision Support: Your knowledge of why tests are ordered and how results are interpreted enhances your understanding of medical necessity and appropriate utilization.

Professional Development and Career Advancement

This laboratory medicine coding mastery opens several career advancement opportunities:

Laboratory Management: Clinical laboratories value coders who understand both the technical and business aspects of laboratory medicine.

Pathology Practice Specialization: Pathology groups need coders who can handle complex anatomic pathology, molecular diagnostics, and clinical consultation services.

Healthcare Consulting: Your expertise qualifies you to provide consulting services to laboratories, pathology practices, and healthcare systems.

Education and Training: You can develop and deliver educational programs for other coders, technologists, and healthcare professionals.

The Future of Laboratory Medicine

Your expertise positions you to adapt to the rapidly evolving field of laboratory medicine:

Precision Medicine: Understanding molecular diagnostics prepares you for the increasing use of genetic testing and personalized medicine approaches.

Point-of-Care Testing: Knowledge of testing complexity helps you understand and code the growing trend toward decentralized testing.

Artificial Intelligence: Understanding test interpretation principles helps you appreciate how AI will augment but not replace human expertise in laboratory medicine.

Global Health Applications: Laboratory medicine principles apply worldwide, opening opportunities in international healthcare consulting and development.

Remember: Laboratory medicine coding excellence comes from understanding both the science and the business of diagnostic testing. You've mastered both aspects, making you a complete laboratory medicine coding professional who can handle any challenge with confidence and accuracy.

Your final step in mastering CPT® coding involves Chapter 15: Medicine Coding, where you'll apply your comprehensive coding knowledge to the diverse world of non-surgical procedures and services. The analytical skills and systematic approach you've developed throughout this study guide will serve you well as you complete your comprehensive CPT® education.

The foundation you've built in laboratory medicine coding will serve you throughout your career, as diagnostic testing continues to evolve and play an increasingly sophisticated role in modern healthcare delivery. You're now equipped to grow with the field and contribute to its continued advancement through accurate, professional coding practices.

Chapter 15: Medicine Coding (90281-99607)

"Medicine is not only a science; it is also an art. It does not consist of compounding pills and plasters; it deals with the very processes of life, which must be understood before they may be guided." - Paracelsus

Welcome to the final frontier of CPT® coding mastery—the Medicine section. Here, you'll discover the vast landscape of non-surgical medical services that keep patients healthy, manage chronic conditions, and provide specialized care across dozens of medical subspecialties. This isn't just about memorizing codes; you're learning to navigate the complex ecosystem of modern medical practice.

The Medicine section represents the evolution of healthcare from purely surgical interventions to sophisticated medical management, preventive care, and targeted therapies. Every injection that prevents disease, every therapy session that restores function, and every specialized procedure that improves quality of life finds its coding home in this comprehensive section.

This chapter empowers you with the knowledge to handle everything from routine immunizations to complex chemotherapy protocols, from cardiac rehabilitation to neurological monitoring. You'll master the coding principles that ensure healthcare providers are appropriately compensated for the full spectrum of medical services they provide.

Your journey through the previous CPT® sections has prepared you for this moment. Your surgical knowledge helps you understand when medical management might be preferred over operative intervention. Your radiology expertise helps you appreciate the diagnostic studies that guide medical treatment decisions. Your laboratory understanding supports the monitoring that ensures medical therapies are working safely and effectively.

By the end of this chapter, you'll possess complete CPT® coding mastery—the confidence to handle any medical coding challenge with professional expertise and systematic precision. You're about to become the coding professional that healthcare organizations seek and medical practices depend upon.

Understanding the Medicine Section's Unique Role

The Medicine section serves as healthcare's Swiss Army knife, containing the tools needed for preventive care, medical management, rehabilitation, and specialized procedures that don't fit neatly into other CPT® sections. Understanding this section requires appreciating its breadth, flexibility, and the diverse medical specialties it serves.

The Evolution of Medical Practice

From Treatment to Prevention: Modern medicine has evolved from primarily treating illness to preventing disease and managing chronic conditions. This evolution is reflected in the Medicine section's emphasis on immunizations, screenings, health assessments, and ongoing care management. Where historical medicine focused on crisis intervention, today's practice emphasizes wellness maintenance and early intervention.

Consider the transformation in diabetes care over the past decades. Previously, diabetic patients were treated episodically when complications arose—emergency department visits for diabetic ketoacidosis, surgical interventions for complications, and reactive care for end-stage complications. Modern diabetes management emphasizes continuous glucose monitoring, regular ophthalmologic surveillance, nutritional counseling, and proactive complication prevention.

This shift from reactive to proactive care creates new coding challenges and opportunities. The Medicine section captures the value of prevention, early intervention, and ongoing management that keeps patients out of hospitals and maintains their quality of life.

Integration of Technology and Personalized Medicine: The Medicine section reflects medicine's technological revolution, incorporating codes for telemedicine, remote monitoring, computer-assisted analysis, and precision medicine approaches. These advances require new coding paradigms that capture both traditional hands-on medical care and innovative technological interventions.

Cardiac monitoring exemplifies this integration. Traditional cardiac care relied on intermittent electrocardiograms and periodic office visits. Modern cardiac monitoring uses implantable devices that continuously monitor heart rhythm, smartphone apps that track symptoms, and artificial intelligence algorithms that detect dangerous patterns before they become life-threatening emergencies.

Subspecialty Medicine and Team-Based Care: The Medicine section accommodates the increasing subspecialization of medical practice and the recognition that optimal patient care often requires coordinated efforts from multiple healthcare professionals. Rather than expecting primary care physicians to manage all aspects of complex conditions, modern medicine uses specialist expertise and multidisciplinary teams.

A patient with heart failure might receive care from cardiologists, cardiac rehabilitation specialists, clinical pharmacists, nutritionists, and behavioral health professionals. Each contributes specialized expertise, and the Medicine section provides codes that recognize these diverse contributions to patient care.

The Structure and Logic of Medicine Coding

Preventive vs. Therapeutic Services: The Medicine section distinguishes between services designed to prevent illness and those intended to treat existing conditions. This distinction affects not only code selection but also medical necessity documentation, insurance coverage, and patient education requirements.

Preventive services include immunizations, screenings, and health assessments performed in healthy individuals to prevent disease or detect conditions in their earliest stages. These services often have different coverage rules, don't require copayments under many insurance plans, and focus on population health rather than individual illness.

Therapeutic services treat existing medical conditions, manage symptoms, or restore function. These services require medical necessity documentation, may require preauthorization, and focus on individual patient needs rather than population-wide prevention.

Diagnostic vs. Therapeutic Procedures: Many Medicine section procedures serve dual purposes—providing diagnostic information while simultaneously offering therapeutic benefits. Understanding this duality helps explain why some procedures seem to overlap with diagnostic testing while providing clear patient benefits.

Cardiac stress testing exemplifies this duality. The procedure provides diagnostic information about coronary artery function and exercise tolerance while simultaneously serving as a therapeutic intervention that can improve cardiac conditioning and patient confidence in their physical capabilities.

Individual vs. Group Services: The Medicine section recognizes that some medical services are more effectively delivered in group settings, while others require individual attention. This recognition reflects both the economics of healthcare delivery and the therapeutic benefits of peer support in certain clinical situations.

Diabetes education often benefits from group settings where patients learn from each other's experiences, share problem-solving strategies, and develop peer support networks. In contrast, individual psychotherapy requires privacy and personalized attention that group settings cannot provide.

Immune Globulins and Immunizations: The Foundation of Public Health

Immunization represents one of medicine's greatest success stories, preventing millions of deaths and reducing disease burden across the globe. Understanding immunization coding requires appreciating both the public health impact of vaccination programs and the complex logistics of vaccine administration, storage, and documentation.

The Science and Impact of Immunization

How Vaccines Work: Vaccines stimulate the immune system to develop protection against specific diseases without causing the diseases themselves. This protection occurs through various mechanisms—some vaccines contain weakened or killed versions of disease-causing organisms, others contain only specific parts of organisms that trigger immunity, and newer vaccines use messenger RNA to instruct cells to produce proteins that trigger immune responses.

The immune system's response to vaccination creates both immediate protection through antibody production and long-term protection through immune memory. When exposed to actual disease-causing organisms, vaccinated individuals can mount rapid, effective immune responses that prevent illness or reduce disease severity.

Understanding these mechanisms helps explain why vaccination schedules exist, why booster doses are sometimes necessary, and why population-wide vaccination creates community immunity that protects even unvaccinated individuals.

Population Health Impact: Vaccination programs have eliminated smallpox globally, nearly eliminated polio, and dramatically reduced the incidence of measles, mumps, rubella, and other vaccine-preventable diseases. The economic impact extends beyond healthcare savings to include reduced lost productivity, decreased healthcare utilization, and improved quality of life.

The COVID-19 pandemic demonstrated both the power of vaccine development and the challenges of vaccine distribution and acceptance. The rapid development of effective vaccines showcased modern biotechnology capabilities, while implementation challenges highlighted the complexity of vaccination programs.

Vaccination Administration Complexities: Successful vaccination programs require sophisticated logistics including cold chain management to maintain vaccine potency, trained personnel to administer vaccines safely, surveillance systems to monitor adverse effects, and documentation systems to track vaccination status and provide reminders for follow-up doses.

Each of these components represents potential points of failure that can compromise vaccination effectiveness. Understanding these complexities helps explain why vaccination administration involves more than simply giving injections and why appropriate coding recognition is important for maintaining effective programs.

Immunization Product and Administration Coding

The Two-Code System: Immunization billing requires two types of codes—one for the vaccine product itself and another for the administration service. This separation recognizes that vaccines represent significant product costs while administration requires professional expertise, time, and oversight.

Vaccine Product Codes (90476-90749): These codes represent the actual vaccines, immune globulins, or other immunization products administered to patients. The codes distinguish between different vaccine types, combinations, and formulations that may have different costs, storage requirements, or administration considerations.

Single vs. Combination Vaccines: Single-component vaccines contain protection against one disease, while combination vaccines provide protection against multiple diseases in a single injection. Combination vaccines often improve patient compliance and reduce the number of injections required, but they may cost more than individual components.

For example, MMR vaccine (90707) provides protection against measles, mumps, and rubella in a single injection. While this costs more than individual vaccines might, the improved compliance and reduced number of injections often justify the additional expense.

Age-Specific Formulations: Some vaccines have different formulations for different age groups, reflecting differences in immune system development, disease risk, and safety considerations. Influenza vaccines, for instance, have specific formulations for children under 3 years, children 3-17 years, and adults.

These age-specific formulations aren't just marketing distinctions—they reflect real differences in vaccine composition, dosing, and safety profiles that affect clinical decision-making and regulatory approval.

Administration Codes (90460-90474): Administration codes capture the professional work involved in vaccine administration including patient assessment, vaccine preparation, injection technique, patient education, adverse reaction monitoring, and documentation requirements.

Age-Based Administration: Administration codes distinguish between services provided to patients under 19 years old and those 19 years and older. This distinction reflects different counseling requirements, different adverse reaction risks, and different documentation standards for pediatric vs. adult vaccination.

Counseling Component: Pediatric administration codes include vaccine counseling and education as part of the service, recognizing that parents need information about vaccine benefits, risks, and expected reactions. Adult administration codes may or may not include counseling depending on the specific circumstances.

Multiple Vaccine Administration: When multiple vaccines are administered during the same encounter, each vaccine and each administration is coded separately. However, the second and subsequent administrations often use different codes that reflect the reduced work involved in additional administrations.

Special Immunization Scenarios

Post-Exposure Prophylaxis: Some immunizations are administered after potential exposure to prevent disease development. These situations require different decision-making processes, different urgency levels, and often different products than routine preventive vaccination.

Rabies Post-Exposure Prophylaxis: When individuals are bitten by potentially rabid animals, they require both rabies immune globulin (passive immunity) and rabies vaccine (active immunity) administered according to specific protocols. The urgency of this situation and the high cost of products involved make accurate coding critical for both patient care and practice sustainability.

Hepatitis B Post-Exposure: Healthcare workers exposed to hepatitis B through needlestick injuries may require both hepatitis B immune globulin and accelerated hepatitis B vaccination schedules. The timing and coordination of these interventions can be critical for preventing chronic hepatitis B infection.

Travel Medicine: International travel may require vaccinations against diseases not commonly found in the United States, such as yellow fever, Japanese encephalitis, or typhoid. These vaccines often have special storage requirements, limited availability, and specific administration timing related to travel dates.

Travel medicine also involves complex decision-making about which vaccines are necessary based on travel destinations, planned activities, traveler health status, and current disease outbreak information. This specialized knowledge justifies separate recognition of travel medicine services.

Immunocompromised Patients: Patients with weakened immune systems due to disease or medical treatment may require modified vaccination schedules, special vaccine formulations, or additional monitoring for adverse reactions. These patients may not respond normally to standard vaccines and may require alternative approaches to achieve protection.

For example, organ transplant recipients taking immunosuppressive medications may not develop adequate immunity from standard vaccines and may require higher doses, additional doses, or different vaccine types. The complexity of managing immunization in these patients requires specialized expertise and additional time.

Therapeutic, Prophylactic, and Diagnostic Injections

Injectable medications represent a cornerstone of modern medical treatment, offering rapid drug delivery, precise dosing, and therapeutic options not available through oral medications. Understanding injection coding requires appreciating the diversity of injectable treatments and the professional expertise required for safe, effective administration.

The Art and Science of Injection Therapy

Why Injectable Medications Matter: Injectable medications bypass the digestive system, providing faster onset of action, more predictable blood levels, and treatment options for patients who cannot take oral medications. Some medications—like insulin, many antibiotics, and most vaccines—can only be given by injection due to their chemical properties or therapeutic requirements.

The route of injection affects drug absorption, onset of action, and potential side effects. Intravenous injections provide immediate drug delivery for emergency situations, while intramuscular injections offer sustained release for medications like long-acting antibiotics. Subcutaneous injections provide convenient self-administration for medications like insulin or biologics.

Professional Expertise Requirements: Safe injection administration requires understanding of anatomy, sterile technique, drug properties, patient assessment, and adverse reaction management. Healthcare providers must select appropriate injection sites, use proper techniques to minimize discomfort and complications, and monitor patients for immediate and delayed reactions.

The complexity varies significantly among different types of injections. Simple vitamin B12 injections require basic technical skills, while chemotherapy administration requires specialized training, extensive safety protocols, and sophisticated monitoring equipment.

Patient Safety and Monitoring: All injection procedures carry risks including allergic reactions, injection site complications, medication errors, and systemic adverse effects. Healthcare providers must be prepared to recognize and manage these complications, which requires training, equipment, and protocols that extend beyond the simple act of giving an injection.

Serious allergic reactions can occur with any injection and may progress rapidly to life-threatening anaphylaxis. Healthcare facilities that administer injections must maintain emergency equipment and trained personnel capable of managing these emergencies effectively.

Injection Administration Coding Structure

Route-Based Coding: Injection codes are organized by the route of administration, recognizing that different routes require different techniques, carry different risks, and achieve different therapeutic goals.

Subcutaneous Injections (96372): Subcutaneous injections deliver medications into the tissue layer between skin and muscle, providing relatively slow absorption and sustained drug levels. This route is commonly used for insulin, growth hormones, and some biologics that patients can learn to self-administer.

The subcutaneous route requires proper site selection, rotation of injection sites to prevent tissue damage, and patient education about self-administration techniques. While technically simpler than other injection routes, subcutaneous administration still requires professional oversight to ensure safety and effectiveness.

Intramuscular Injections (96372): Intramuscular injections deliver medications directly into muscle tissue, providing faster absorption than subcutaneous administration while avoiding the immediate systemic effects of intravenous delivery. This route is commonly used for vaccines, antibiotics, and medications that require depot effects.

Proper intramuscular injection requires knowledge of muscle anatomy, appropriate needle selection, and techniques to minimize discomfort and complications. Site selection must consider muscle size, patient age, medication volume, and potential for nerve or vascular injury.

Intravenous Injections (96365-96368): Intravenous administration delivers medications directly into the bloodstream, providing immediate drug availability and precise control over drug levels. This route is essential for emergency medications, many hospital treatments, and drugs that cannot be absorbed through other routes.

Intravenous injection requires vascular access, sterile technique, and continuous monitoring for complications including infiltration, phlebitis, and systemic reactions. The immediacy of intravenous drug effects means that adverse reactions can develop rapidly and may be more severe than with other administration routes.

Infusion vs. Push Administration: The duration and complexity of intravenous drug administration affects coding. Simple "push" injections involve rapid administration of small medication volumes, while infusions involve slower administration of larger volumes over extended time periods.

Infusion therapy often requires specialized equipment including infusion pumps, multiple medications, and extended monitoring. The additional complexity and time requirements justify separate coding recognition for infusion services.

Complex Injection Scenarios

Biologics and Specialty Medications: Biologic medications represent some of the most expensive and complex injectable treatments in modern medicine. These medications often require special handling, storage, and administration protocols that extend far beyond routine injection services.

Monoclonal Antibodies: These targeted therapies for cancer, autoimmune diseases, and other conditions often require premedication to prevent allergic reactions, extended infusion times, and intensive monitoring for adverse effects. The complexity and cost of these treatments require careful documentation and coding to ensure appropriate reimbursement.

Growth Factors and Hormones: Injectable hormones like growth hormone or fertility medications require precise dosing, patient education, and ongoing monitoring for effectiveness and side effects. Many of these medications are self-administered by patients who require initial training and ongoing support.

Joint and Soft Tissue Injections: Therapeutic injections into joints, trigger points, or other anatomical structures require specialized training, precise needle placement, and often imaging guidance to ensure accurate delivery and optimal therapeutic effects.

Corticosteroid Injections: Joint injections with corticosteroids can provide dramatic pain relief and functional improvement for patients with arthritis, bursitis, or other inflammatory conditions. However, these injections require proper patient selection, sterile technique, and monitoring for complications including infection and systemic steroid effects.

Hyaluronic Acid Injections: Viscosupplementation for knee arthritis involves injecting gel-like substances into joints to improve lubrication and reduce pain. These procedures require precise needle placement and may involve multiple injections over several weeks.

Nerve Blocks and Pain Management: Therapeutic injections for pain management often require specialized training, fluoroscopic or ultrasound guidance, and multidisciplinary care coordination. These procedures bridge the gap between Medicine section services and more invasive pain management interventions.

Epidural Injections: Spinal injections for back pain require specialized training, imaging guidance, and careful patient selection. While these procedures are often performed by anesthesiologists or pain management specialists, they represent important therapeutic options for patients with chronic pain conditions.

Trigger Point Injections: Injections into muscle trigger points can provide relief for patients with myofascial pain syndromes. While technically simpler than spinal injections, these procedures require understanding of muscle anatomy and trigger point identification.

Psychiatry: Healing the Mind

Mental health services represent one of healthcare's most important and challenging areas, requiring specialized training, complex therapeutic relationships, and innovative treatment approaches. Understanding psychiatry coding requires appreciating both the science of mental health treatment and the unique characteristics of psychiatric practice.

The Evolution of Mental Health Treatment

From Institutional to Community-Based Care: Mental health treatment has undergone dramatic transformation from primarily institutional care to community-based treatment that emphasizes patient autonomy, evidence-based interventions, and integration with primary care. This evolution affects both treatment approaches and coding requirements.

Historical psychiatric treatment often involved long-term hospitalization with limited therapeutic interventions. Modern mental health care emphasizes outpatient treatment, medication management, psychotherapy, and social support services that help patients maintain independent functioning while managing their conditions.

Integration of Biological and Psychological Approaches: Contemporary psychiatry recognizes that mental health conditions result from complex interactions between biological, psychological, and social factors. Treatment approaches often combine medication management with psychotherapy, lifestyle interventions, and social support services.

This integrated approach requires healthcare providers who understand both the biological aspects of mental illness and the psychological and social factors that influence treatment outcomes. The complexity of this integration is reflected in psychiatric coding that recognizes different types of services and varying levels of complexity.

Evidence-Based Treatment Approaches: Modern psychiatry increasingly relies on evidence-based treatments that have been proven effective through rigorous research. These approaches include specific psychotherapy techniques, medication protocols, and combined treatments that have demonstrated superior outcomes compared to traditional approaches.

The sophistication of evidence-based psychiatric treatment requires specialized training, ongoing education, and careful monitoring of treatment outcomes. This expertise justifies the professional recognition provided by psychiatric coding systems.

Psychotherapy Services

Individual Psychotherapy (90834-90837): Individual psychotherapy represents the foundation of many mental health treatments, providing a therapeutic relationship where patients can explore thoughts, feelings, and behaviors in a safe, confidential environment.

Time-Based Coding: Psychotherapy codes are organized by session duration, recognizing that different therapeutic approaches and patient needs require different amounts of time. Shorter sessions may be appropriate for medication management or brief interventions, while longer sessions allow for more intensive therapeutic work.

90834 (45 minutes): This duration allows for substantial therapeutic work while fitting efficiently into clinical schedules. Many psychotherapy approaches can be effectively delivered in 45-minute sessions, making this a common session length for routine psychotherapy.

90837 (60 minutes): Longer sessions provide more time for complex therapeutic work, processing of difficult emotions, or addressing multiple issues within single sessions. Some therapeutic approaches, such as certain trauma treatments, may benefit from extended session times.

Therapeutic Techniques and Approaches: Modern psychotherapy encompasses numerous evidence-based approaches, each with specific techniques, training requirements, and therapeutic applications. Understanding these approaches helps explain why psychotherapy requires specialized expertise and justifies professional recognition.

Cognitive Behavioral Therapy (CBT): CBT focuses on identifying and changing thought patterns and behaviors that contribute to mental health problems. This approach has strong evidence for treating depression, anxiety disorders, and many other conditions.

Psychodynamic Therapy: This approach explores how unconscious thoughts and past experiences influence current behavior and relationships. While requiring longer treatment duration, psychodynamic therapy can provide lasting changes in personality and relationship patterns.

Trauma-Focused Therapies: Specialized approaches for treating post-traumatic stress disorder and other trauma-related conditions often require specific training and may involve techniques like eye movement desensitization and reprocessing (EMDR) or exposure therapy.

Group Psychotherapy (90853): Group therapy provides therapeutic benefits that can't be achieved in individual sessions, including peer support, social learning, and opportunities to practice interpersonal skills in a therapeutic environment.

Group therapy requires specialized skills in group dynamics, managing multiple therapeutic relationships simultaneously, and creating safe environments where all participants can benefit. The complexity of managing group processes justifies separate coding recognition.

Different Group Approaches: Support groups focus on mutual aid and shared experiences, while therapy groups emphasize psychological change and skill development. The therapeutic goals and leader qualifications differ significantly between these approaches.

Psychiatric Diagnostic Services

Diagnostic Evaluations (90791-90792): Comprehensive psychiatric evaluation requires specialized interview techniques, mental status examination, risk assessment, and integration of information from multiple sources to develop accurate diagnoses and treatment plans.

90791 (Without Medical Services): Focuses primarily on psychiatric assessment without significant medical evaluation. This evaluation includes detailed psychiatric history, mental status examination, and initial treatment planning.

90792 (With Medical Services): Includes medical evaluation as part of the psychiatric assessment, recognizing that many psychiatric symptoms have medical causes or medical conditions that influence psychiatric treatment.

The distinction between these codes reflects the reality that some psychiatric evaluations require extensive medical assessment, while others focus primarily on psychological and social factors.

Psychological Testing and Assessment: Psychological testing provides objective measurement of cognitive functioning, personality characteristics, and symptom severity that supplement clinical interviews and observations.

Neuropsychological Testing: Evaluates cognitive functions like memory, attention, and executive functioning to identify brain-related causes of behavioral or emotional problems. These evaluations often require several hours and specialized training in test administration and interpretation.

Personality Testing: Assesses personality characteristics, coping styles, and psychological dynamics that influence treatment planning and prognosis. These evaluations help clarify diagnoses and guide therapeutic approaches.

Medication Management

Pharmacotherapy Services (90862-90863): Psychiatric medication management requires specialized knowledge of psychopharmacology, drug interactions, side effect monitoring, and the complex relationships between medications and psychotherapy.

Modern psychiatric medications include numerous classes of drugs with different mechanisms of action, side effect profiles, and therapeutic applications. Selecting appropriate medications requires understanding of individual patient factors, previous treatment responses, and potential drug interactions.

Medication Monitoring: Many psychiatric medications require ongoing monitoring for therapeutic effectiveness, side effects, and potential medical complications. Some medications require regular laboratory testing, while others need careful assessment of cardiovascular or metabolic effects.

Complex Medication Regimens: Some patients require multiple psychiatric medications, creating complex interactions and monitoring requirements. Managing these regimens requires specialized expertise and careful coordination with other healthcare providers.

Dialysis: Life-Sustaining Technology

Dialysis represents one of medicine's most dramatic life-sustaining technologies, providing artificial kidney function for patients whose own kidneys have failed. Understanding dialysis coding requires appreciating both the complex technology involved and the comprehensive medical management required for dialysis patients.

The Science and Impact of Dialysis

How Dialysis Works: Dialysis removes waste products and excess fluid from the blood when kidneys can no longer perform these functions. Two main approaches exist: hemodialysis, which filters blood through an artificial kidney machine, and peritoneal dialysis, which uses the patient's abdominal lining as a natural filter.

Hemodialysis Process: Patient blood is pumped through tubes to an artificial kidney (dialyzer) where waste products and excess fluid are removed. The cleaned blood is then returned to the patient. This process typically takes 3-4 hours and is performed 3 times per week.

Peritoneal Dialysis Process: Dialysis solution is infused into the patient's abdominal cavity, where it absorbs waste products and excess fluid. The solution is then drained and replaced with fresh solution. This process can be performed continuously or intermittently, often at home.

Patient Population and Outcomes: Dialysis serves patients with end-stage kidney disease who would die within days or weeks without treatment. The dialysis population includes patients awaiting kidney transplantation, those who are not transplant candidates, and some patients who choose dialysis over transplantation.

Dialysis patients typically have multiple medical conditions including diabetes, hypertension, heart disease, and bone disorders. Managing these complex patients requires multidisciplinary teams and comprehensive care coordination that extends far beyond the dialysis procedure itself.

Quality of Life Considerations: While dialysis is life-sustaining, it significantly impacts patient quality of life through time requirements, dietary restrictions, fluid limitations, and treatment-related symptoms. Understanding these impacts helps explain why dialysis coding recognizes both the technical procedure and the comprehensive medical management required.

Dialysis Service Components

Monthly Dialysis Services (90960-90962): Dialysis coding recognizes that optimal patient care requires comprehensive monthly management that includes the dialysis procedures themselves plus extensive medical oversight, care planning, and coordination.

90960 (End-Stage Renal Disease Services, Age 12-19): Recognizes that adolescent dialysis patients have unique medical and psychosocial needs requiring specialized expertise. This population faces challenges related to growth, development, education, and transition to adult care.

90961 (End-Stage Renal Disease Services, Age 20 and older): Covers comprehensive monthly management for adult dialysis patients including treatment planning, complication management, and care coordination.

Comprehensive Care Components: Monthly dialysis services include much more than the dialysis procedures themselves. Comprehensive care encompasses medication management, nutritional counseling, vascular access monitoring, laboratory test interpretation, complication prevention, and coordination with other healthcare providers.

Medication Management: Dialysis patients typically require complex medication regimens including phosphate binders, vitamin supplements, blood pressure medications, and treatments for bone disease. Many medications require dose adjustments based on dialysis schedules and residual kidney function.

Nutritional Management: Dialysis patients have complex nutritional requirements including protein needs, phosphorus restrictions, fluid limitations, and vitamin supplementation. Nutritional management requires specialized expertise and ongoing monitoring.

Vascular Access Management: Hemodialysis requires vascular access through arteriovenous fistulas, grafts, or catheters. Maintaining functional vascular access requires ongoing monitoring, preventive care, and prompt intervention when problems arise.

Dialysis Setting and Service Variations

In-Center Hemodialysis: Most hemodialysis patients receive treatment in specialized dialysis centers staffed by trained nurses and technicians under physician supervision. These facilities provide the complex equipment, water treatment systems, and safety protocols required for safe hemodialysis.

In-center treatment allows for professional supervision, immediate response to complications, and social interaction with other patients. However, it requires patients to travel to facilities 3 times per week and limits scheduling flexibility.

Home Hemodialysis: Some patients can be trained to perform hemodialysis at home, providing greater scheduling flexibility and potentially better outcomes. However, home hemodialysis requires extensive patient training, home modification for equipment, and ongoing support from healthcare teams.

Home dialysis requires highly motivated patients who can master complex technical procedures and respond appropriately to complications. The training and ongoing support required for home dialysis represent significant resource investments.

Peritoneal Dialysis: Peritoneal dialysis offers greater patient independence and can often be performed at home or work. This approach may provide better preservation of residual kidney function and avoid some complications associated with hemodialysis.

Patient Training Requirements: Peritoneal dialysis requires extensive patient education about sterile technique, solution exchanges, complication recognition, and equipment management. The training process may take weeks and requires ongoing reinforcement.

Complication Management: Peritoneal dialysis patients face risks including peritonitis (abdominal infection), catheter problems, and inadequate dialysis. Managing these complications requires specialized expertise and prompt intervention.

Gastroenterology: Digestive Health and Disease

Gastroenterology encompasses the diagnosis and treatment of conditions affecting the entire digestive system, from the esophagus to the rectum, plus related organs including the liver, pancreas, and gallbladder. Understanding gastroenterology coding requires appreciating both the diagnostic procedures that visualize internal anatomy and the therapeutic interventions that treat digestive diseases.

The Scope and Complexity of Digestive Medicine

Digestive System Impact on Health: The digestive system affects overall health through nutrient absorption, immune function, and the production of hormones that regulate metabolism and appetite. Digestive diseases can have systemic effects that influence cardiovascular health, mental health, and quality of life.

Understanding these relationships helps explain why gastroenterology often involves complex diagnostic workups, multidisciplinary treatment approaches, and long-term management strategies that extend beyond simple symptom relief.

Technology and Innovation in Gastroenterology: Modern gastroenterology relies heavily on sophisticated imaging and therapeutic technologies including flexible endoscopes, ultrasound systems, and minimally invasive surgical techniques. These technologies enable both detailed visualization of internal anatomy and therapeutic interventions that were impossible just decades ago.

Endoscopic Capabilities: Modern endoscopes include high-definition imaging, narrow-band imaging for enhanced tissue visualization, and working channels that allow therapeutic interventions during diagnostic procedures. These capabilities transform endoscopy from purely diagnostic procedures to therapeutic interventions.

Therapeutic Endoscopy: Advanced endoscopic techniques can remove polyps, stop bleeding, dilate strictures, place stents, and even perform complex procedures like endoscopic submucosal dissection for early cancer treatment. These therapeutic capabilities often eliminate the need for surgical intervention.

Endoscopic Procedures

Upper Endoscopy (43235-43259): Upper endoscopy allows direct visualization of the esophagus, stomach, and duodenum, providing diagnostic information that can't be obtained through other imaging modalities while offering therapeutic options during the same procedure.

Diagnostic Upper Endoscopy (43235): Provides comprehensive evaluation of upper digestive tract symptoms including difficulty swallowing, abdominal pain, nausea, and bleeding. The procedure can identify inflammation, ulcers, tumors, and other abnormalities that explain patient symptoms.

Upper Endoscopy with Biopsy (43239): Tissue sampling during endoscopy provides definitive diagnosis of many conditions including infections, inflammatory diseases, and malignancies. Biopsy capabilities transform endoscopy from a purely observational procedure to a diagnostic tool that can provide definitive answers.

Therapeutic Upper Endoscopy: Various therapeutic interventions can be performed during upper endoscopy including treatment of bleeding ulcers, removal of foreign objects, dilation of strictures, and placement of feeding tubes. These therapeutic capabilities often prevent the need for surgical intervention.

Lower Endoscopy (45330-45398): Lower endoscopy includes sigmoidoscopy and colonoscopy procedures that evaluate the colon and rectum for various conditions including cancer screening, inflammatory diseases, and evaluation of symptoms like bleeding or changes in bowel habits.

Colonoscopy for Screening (45378): Colonoscopy represents the gold standard for colorectal cancer screening, providing both visualization of the entire colon and the ability to remove precancerous polyps during the same procedure. This combination of screening and treatment makes colonoscopy uniquely effective for cancer prevention.

Colonoscopy with Polypectomy (45385): The ability to remove polyps during screening colonoscopy transforms a diagnostic procedure into a therapeutic intervention that can prevent cancer development. Different polypectomy techniques are used depending on polyp size, location, and characteristics.

Diagnostic vs. Screening Colonoscopy: The distinction between diagnostic and screening colonoscopy affects both coding and insurance coverage. Screening procedures are performed in asymptomatic individuals for cancer prevention, while diagnostic procedures evaluate specific symptoms or follow up on previous abnormalities.

Specialized GI Procedures

Capsule Endoscopy (91110): Capsule endoscopy involves swallowing a pill-sized camera that takes thousands of pictures as it travels through the digestive tract. This technology allows visualization of the small intestine, which is difficult to reach with conventional endoscopes.

Small Bowel Evaluation: The small intestine represents the longest portion of the digestive tract but has been difficult to evaluate with conventional techniques. Capsule endoscopy provides comprehensive small bowel visualization that can identify bleeding sources, inflammatory conditions, and tumors.

Patient Preparation and Monitoring: Capsule endoscopy requires bowel preparation similar to colonoscopy plus dietary restrictions during the procedure. Patients wear monitoring equipment that records capsule location and ensures proper function during the 8-12 hour procedure.

Motility Studies (91020-91040): Gastrointestinal motility studies evaluate how well the digestive tract moves food and liquids, providing information about functional disorders that don't show structural abnormalities on imaging studies.

Esophageal Motility (91010): Evaluates swallowing function and esophageal muscle coordination using pressure sensors placed in the esophagus. These studies can diagnose conditions like achalasia, esophageal spasm, and other motility disorders.

Gastric Emptying Studies: Measure how quickly food leaves the stomach, helping diagnose gastroparesis and other conditions that affect stomach function. These studies often use radioactive markers to track food movement through the digestive system.

Cardiovascular Procedures: Heart Health and Function

Cardiovascular medicine encompasses the prevention, diagnosis, and treatment of heart and blood vessel diseases—the leading cause of death in the United States. Understanding cardiovascular coding requires appreciating both the sophisticated diagnostic technologies that evaluate heart function and the diverse therapeutic interventions that treat cardiovascular conditions.

The Scope of Cardiovascular Medicine

Cardiovascular Disease Burden: Heart disease and stroke affect millions of Americans and consume enormous healthcare resources. The complexity of cardiovascular conditions ranges from simple hypertension management to complex interventional procedures and heart transplantation.

Understanding this disease burden helps explain why cardiovascular medicine requires sophisticated diagnostic and therapeutic approaches. Early detection and intervention can prevent heart attacks, strokes, and other cardiovascular emergencies that consume enormous resources and cause significant disability and death.

Prevention and Risk Modification: Modern cardiovascular medicine emphasizes prevention through risk factor modification, lifestyle interventions, and early detection of asymptomatic disease. This approach requires comprehensive assessment, patient education, and long-term management strategies that extend far beyond treating acute cardiovascular events.

Understanding prevention strategies helps explain why cardiovascular coding includes services like cardiac rehabilitation, lifestyle counseling, and comprehensive risk assessments that might seem less dramatic than emergency interventions but provide enormous long-term benefits.

Technological Innovation: Cardiovascular medicine has been at the forefront of medical technology development, incorporating sophisticated imaging, minimally invasive interventions, and implantable devices that can monitor and treat cardiovascular conditions continuously.

These technological advances require specialized training, expensive equipment, and complex support systems that justify the coding recognition provided for cardiovascular services.

Diagnostic Cardiovascular Procedures

Electrocardiography (93000-93010): The electrocardiogram (ECG) remains fundamental to cardiovascular diagnosis despite being over a century old. Modern ECG technology provides detailed analysis of cardiac electrical activity that can detect heart attacks, rhythm abnormalities, and other conditions affecting heart function.

12-Lead ECG (93000): The standard 12-lead ECG provides comprehensive assessment of cardiac electrical activity from multiple perspectives, allowing detection of conditions affecting different areas of the heart. This non-invasive test can provide critical diagnostic information within minutes and is essential for emergency cardiac care.

Rhythm Strips (93040-93042): Continuous cardiac monitoring provides information about heart rhythm patterns over extended periods, detecting intermittent abnormalities that might be missed on routine ECGs. This monitoring is essential for patients with suspected rhythm disorders or those at risk for dangerous arrhythmias.

Echocardiography (93303-93350): Echocardiography uses ultrasound technology to create detailed images of heart structure and function, providing information about heart muscle strength, valve function, and blood flow patterns that can't be obtained through other non-invasive methods.

Transthoracic Echocardiography (93306): Standard echocardiography performed through the chest wall provides comprehensive assessment of heart structure and function. This study can evaluate heart muscle strength, valve function, chamber sizes, and blood flow patterns, making it invaluable for diagnosing and monitoring various heart conditions.

Stress Echocardiography (93350): Combines echocardiography with exercise or pharmacological stress to evaluate how the heart responds to increased demands. This testing can detect coronary artery disease that might not be apparent when the heart is at rest, providing crucial information for treatment planning.

Transesophageal Echocardiography (93312): Uses an ultrasound probe placed in the esophagus to obtain high-quality images of heart structures, particularly useful for evaluating the atria, heart valves, and suspected blood clots. This technique provides superior image quality compared to standard echocardiography but requires conscious sedation and specialized expertise.

Cardiac Stress Testing (93015-93018): Stress testing evaluates heart function during exercise or pharmacological stress, detecting coronary artery disease and assessing exercise capacity in patients with known or suspected heart disease.

Exercise Stress Testing: Patients exercise on a treadmill or bicycle while heart rhythm and blood pressure are monitored. This testing can detect coronary artery disease, evaluate treatment effectiveness, and assess safe activity levels for patients with heart conditions.

Pharmacological Stress Testing: For patients who cannot exercise adequately, medications can simulate the effects of exercise on the heart. This approach allows stress testing in patients with mobility limitations, arthritis, or other conditions that prevent adequate exercise.

Nuclear Stress Testing: Combines stress testing with nuclear imaging to provide detailed information about blood flow to different areas of the heart muscle. This comprehensive assessment can identify specific coronary arteries that are blocked and guide decisions about interventional procedures.

Therapeutic Cardiovascular Interventions

Cardiac Rehabilitation (93797-93798): Cardiac rehabilitation provides supervised exercise training, education, and counseling for patients recovering from heart attacks, cardiac surgery, or other cardiovascular events. This comprehensive approach can improve outcomes, reduce hospital readmissions, and enhance quality of life.

Supervised Exercise Training: Cardiac rehabilitation includes medically supervised exercise sessions that help patients safely increase their activity levels while monitoring for complications. This supervised approach allows patients to regain confidence in their physical abilities while ensuring safety.

Education and Counseling: Cardiac rehabilitation programs provide education about heart disease, risk factor modification, medication management, and lifestyle changes that can prevent future cardiovascular events. This education component is as important as the exercise training for long-term outcomes.

Psychosocial Support: Many cardiac patients experience depression, anxiety, and fear about their prognosis. Cardiac rehabilitation programs address these psychological aspects of recovery, providing counseling and support groups that help patients cope with their conditions.

Cardiovascular Device Services (93279-93299): Modern cardiovascular medicine increasingly relies on implantable devices that can monitor heart rhythm, provide life-saving therapies, and collect data about heart function continuously.

Pacemaker Services: Pacemakers treat slow heart rhythms by providing electrical stimulation when the heart's natural pacemaker fails. These devices require initial programming, ongoing monitoring, and periodic adjustments to ensure optimal function.

Implantable Cardioverter Defibrillator (ICD) Services: ICDs monitor heart rhythm continuously and can deliver life-saving shocks when dangerous rhythms are detected. These sophisticated devices require complex programming and regular monitoring to ensure they function properly when needed.

Cardiac Resynchronization Therapy (CRT): CRT devices coordinate the pumping action of different heart chambers in patients with heart failure, improving symptoms and potentially extending life. These devices require specialized expertise for implantation and ongoing management.

Remote Monitoring: Many modern cardiac devices can transmit data wirelessly to healthcare providers, allowing continuous monitoring without requiring office visits. This technology enables early detection of problems and reduces the need for routine device checks.

Pulmonary Medicine: Breathing and Lung Health

Pulmonary medicine focuses on the respiratory system, which provides oxygen to the body and removes carbon dioxide waste. Understanding pulmonary coding requires appreciating both the complex physiology of breathing and the diverse conditions that can affect respiratory function.

The Critical Nature of Respiratory Function

Respiratory System Physiology: The respiratory system performs the essential function of gas exchange—bringing oxygen from the environment into the bloodstream and removing carbon dioxide waste from the body. This process involves complex interactions between the lungs, chest wall muscles, nervous system, and cardiovascular system.

Understanding these interactions helps explain why respiratory conditions can have systemic effects and why pulmonary medicine often involves comprehensive assessment and multidisciplinary treatment approaches.

Common Respiratory Conditions: Respiratory diseases affect millions of people and range from acute conditions like pneumonia to chronic diseases like asthma and chronic obstructive pulmonary disease (COPD). These conditions can significantly impact quality of life, work productivity, and healthcare utilization.

Asthma: Affects over 25 million Americans and involves inflammation and narrowing of airways that can cause breathing difficulties, wheezing, and coughing. Asthma management requires understanding of triggers, medication management, and patient education about self-management techniques.

COPD: Includes emphysema and chronic bronchitis and primarily results from smoking exposure. COPD is progressive and can severely limit physical activity and quality of life. Management involves medication, pulmonary rehabilitation, and lifestyle modifications.

Sleep Disorders: Sleep-related breathing disorders like sleep apnea affect millions of people and can have serious cardiovascular and neurological consequences. These conditions require specialized diagnostic testing and treatment approaches.

Pulmonary Function Testing

Spirometry (94010-94070): Spirometry measures lung volumes and flow rates, providing objective assessment of respiratory function that can detect various lung diseases and monitor treatment effectiveness.

Basic Spirometry (94010): Measures fundamental lung functions including total lung capacity, forced vital capacity, and airflow rates. These measurements can detect restrictive lung diseases (where lung volumes are reduced) and obstructive diseases (where airflow is limited).

Spirometry Before and After Bronchodilator (94060): Compares lung function before and after administering medications that open airways. This testing can distinguish between reversible airway obstruction (like asthma) and fixed obstruction (like emphysema), guiding treatment decisions.

Complete Pulmonary Function Testing (94070): Comprehensive assessment that includes lung volumes, diffusion capacity, and other specialized measurements. This testing provides detailed information about lung function that can help diagnose specific lung diseases and monitor disease progression.

Interpretation Requirements: Pulmonary function testing requires specialized training to interpret results correctly and relate findings to clinical symptoms and other diagnostic information. The complexity of interpretation justifies professional component billing for these services.

Sleep Studies (95805-95811): Sleep studies evaluate breathing patterns during sleep, detecting conditions like sleep apnea that can have serious health consequences if left untreated.

Polysomnography (95810): Comprehensive sleep study that monitors brain waves, eye movements, muscle activity, heart rhythm, and breathing patterns throughout the night. This study can diagnose various sleep disorders and determine appropriate treatment approaches.

Home Sleep Studies (95800): Simplified sleep monitoring that can be performed at home for patients with suspected sleep apnea. While less comprehensive than laboratory studies, home testing provides a convenient alternative for appropriate patients.

CPAP Titration (95811): Once sleep apnea is diagnosed, patients often require continuous positive airway pressure (CPAP) therapy. Titration studies determine the optimal pressure settings for individual patients to ensure effective treatment.

Therapeutic Pulmonary Interventions

Pulmonary Rehabilitation (94625): Pulmonary rehabilitation provides comprehensive treatment for patients with chronic lung diseases, combining exercise training, education, and behavioral interventions to improve symptoms and quality of life.

Exercise Training Component: Supervised exercise programs help patients with lung disease improve their exercise tolerance and reduce shortness of breath. These programs must be carefully designed to accommodate individual limitations while providing therapeutic benefits.

Education Component: Pulmonary rehabilitation includes education about lung disease, medication management, breathing techniques, and energy conservation strategies. This education helps patients manage their conditions more effectively and prevent exacerbations.

Psychosocial Support: Chronic lung diseases can significantly impact mental health and social functioning. Pulmonary rehabilitation programs address these aspects of disease management through counseling and support groups.

Bronchoscopy Services (31622-31654): Bronchoscopy allows direct visualization of the airways and lungs, providing both diagnostic information and therapeutic capabilities for various respiratory conditions.

Diagnostic Bronchoscopy: Can identify infections, tumors, inflammation, and other conditions affecting the airways and lungs. The ability to directly visualize internal structures provides information that can't be obtained through other methods.

Therapeutic Bronchoscopy: Various therapeutic interventions can be performed during bronchoscopy including removal of foreign objects, treatment of bleeding, placement of stents, and laser therapy for tumors.

Bronchoscopic Biopsy: Tissue sampling during bronchoscopy can provide definitive diagnosis of lung cancer, infections, and inflammatory conditions. Different biopsy techniques are used depending on the location and nature of abnormalities.

Allergy and Clinical Immunology: Understanding Immune Responses

Allergy and immunology medicine addresses disorders of the immune system, including allergic reactions, immunodeficiencies, and autoimmune diseases. Understanding this specialty requires appreciating both the complexity of immune system function and the diverse ways immune dysfunction can affect health.

The Immune System in Health and Disease

Immune System Functions: The immune system protects the body from infectious diseases, cancer, and other threats while maintaining tolerance to the body's own tissues. This complex system involves multiple cell types, chemical mediators, and regulatory mechanisms that must be precisely balanced to maintain health.

Allergic Diseases: Result from immune system overreactions to normally harmless substances like foods, pollens, or medications. These reactions can range from mild symptoms like sneezing to life-threatening anaphylaxis that requires emergency treatment.

Immunodeficiency Diseases: Occur when the immune system fails to function properly, leaving patients vulnerable to infections, cancers, and other complications. These conditions may be inherited or acquired and often require specialized treatments to support immune function.

Autoimmune Diseases: Develop when the immune system mistakenly attacks the body's own tissues, causing conditions like rheumatoid arthritis, lupus, and type 1 diabetes. These diseases often require immunosuppressive treatments that must be carefully balanced to control disease while preserving protective immunity.

Allergy Testing and Evaluation

Skin Testing (95004-95071): Allergy skin testing provides rapid, cost-effective evaluation of allergic sensitivities by exposing small areas of skin to potential allergens and observing for reactions.

Scratch Testing (95004): Places small amounts of allergen extracts on scratched skin surfaces to test for immediate allergic reactions. This testing can evaluate multiple allergens simultaneously and provides results within 15-20 minutes.

Intradermal Testing (95024): Involves injecting small amounts of allergen extracts into the skin for patients who don't react to scratch testing but have clinical histories suggesting allergies. This more sensitive testing can detect allergies missed by scratch testing.

Patch Testing (95044): Evaluates delayed allergic reactions by applying allergens to patches placed on the skin for 48-72 hours. This testing is particularly useful for identifying contact allergies to substances like metals, fragrances, or chemicals.

In Vitro Allergy Testing (86003): Blood tests for specific allergen antibodies provide an alternative to skin testing for patients who cannot undergo skin testing due to medications, skin conditions, or other factors.

Advantages of Blood Testing: Can be performed on patients taking antihistamines, those with extensive skin disease, or patients at risk for severe allergic reactions. Blood testing also allows quantitative measurement of allergic sensitivity.

Limitations: Blood testing is more expensive than skin testing, takes longer to obtain results, and may be less sensitive for certain types of allergies. The choice between skin and blood testing depends on individual patient factors and clinical circumstances.

Immunotherapy and Treatment

Allergen Immunotherapy (95115-95199): Immunotherapy involves gradually exposing patients to increasing amounts of allergens to build tolerance and reduce allergic reactions. This treatment can provide long-lasting relief for patients with environmental allergies.

Subcutaneous Immunotherapy: Traditional allergy shots involve regular injections of allergen extracts over several years. This treatment requires careful dose escalation, monitoring for adverse reactions, and ongoing maintenance therapy.

Sublingual Immunotherapy: Places allergen extracts under the tongue, providing a convenient alternative to injections for certain allergies. This approach has lower risk of severe reactions but may be less effective than injection therapy.

Treatment Protocols: Immunotherapy requires specialized protocols for dose escalation, maintenance therapy, and adverse reaction management. The complexity of these protocols requires specialized training and ongoing patient monitoring.

Anaphylaxis Management: Severe allergic reactions require immediate recognition and treatment to prevent death. Healthcare providers involved in allergy care must be prepared to manage these emergencies effectively.

Emergency Medications: Epinephrine is the first-line treatment for anaphylaxis and must be available wherever allergen testing or immunotherapy is performed. Other medications like antihistamines and corticosteroids provide supportive care.

Patient Education: Patients at risk for anaphylaxis must be educated about trigger avoidance, emergency medication use, and when to seek emergency care. This education is literally life-saving and represents a critical component of allergy care.

Physical Medicine and Rehabilitation: Restoring Function

Physical medicine and rehabilitation (PM&R) focuses on restoring function and improving quality of life for patients with disabilities, injuries, or chronic conditions. Understanding PM&R coding requires appreciating both the comprehensive assessment required for rehabilitation planning and the diverse therapeutic interventions used to restore function.

The Philosophy and Approach of Rehabilitation

Functional Focus: Unlike medical specialties that focus primarily on diagnosing and treating diseases, PM&R emphasizes functional outcomes—helping patients achieve their maximum potential for independence and quality of life despite impairments or disabilities.

This functional focus requires comprehensive assessment of not just medical conditions but also social support, environmental factors, psychological adaptation, and individual goals that affect rehabilitation outcomes.

Interdisciplinary Team Approach: Effective rehabilitation usually requires coordinated efforts from multiple healthcare professionals including physicians, nurses, physical therapists, occupational therapists, speech therapists, social workers, and psychologists.

Understanding these team dynamics helps explain why rehabilitation coding often involves multiple providers and why coordination of care is such an important component of rehabilitation services.

Comprehensive Assessment and Planning: Rehabilitation planning requires detailed assessment of medical conditions, functional limitations, cognitive abilities, social support, and environmental factors that affect independence and quality of life.

This comprehensive approach distinguishes rehabilitation from other medical specialties and justifies the extensive evaluation and management codes often used in PM&R practice.

Rehabilitation Assessment and Planning

Comprehensive Rehabilitation Evaluation: Initial rehabilitation evaluations involve detailed assessment of multiple domains that affect functional outcomes, requiring specialized training and significant time investment.

Medical Assessment: Evaluates medical conditions, medications, and complications that might affect rehabilitation potential. This includes assessment of pain, muscle strength, range of motion, balance, coordination, and other physical factors.

Functional Assessment: Measures ability to perform activities of daily living, mobility, communication, and other functional tasks that determine independence levels. Standardized assessment tools provide objective measures of functional abilities.

Cognitive Assessment: Evaluates memory, attention, problem-solving, and other cognitive functions that affect learning and safety. Cognitive impairments can significantly impact rehabilitation outcomes and require specialized intervention approaches.

Psychosocial Assessment: Addresses motivation, coping skills, family support, and other psychological and social factors that influence rehabilitation success. These factors often determine whether patients can maintain gains achieved during formal rehabilitation programs.

Therapeutic Interventions

Therapeutic Exercise and Activities: Rehabilitation programs use specific exercises and activities designed to improve strength, range of motion, balance, coordination, and endurance while addressing individual functional goals.

Strengthening Programs: Target specific muscle groups or movement patterns that are important for functional activities. These programs must be carefully designed to avoid injury while providing therapeutic benefits.

Coordination Training: Helps patients relearn complex movement patterns required for activities like walking, reaching, or manipulating objects. This training often involves repetitive practice of functional movements.

Balance Training: Particularly important for fall prevention and safe mobility. Balance training uses various techniques including standing activities, weight shifting, and environmental challenges that improve stability.

Modalities and Therapeutic Technologies: Physical medicine uses various modalities and technologies to reduce pain, improve healing, and enhance therapeutic outcomes.

Electrical Stimulation: Can reduce pain, strengthen muscles, or facilitate healing depending on the specific parameters and application techniques used. Different types of electrical stimulation have different therapeutic applications.

Heat and Cold Therapy: Superficial heating can reduce muscle spasm and improve tissue flexibility, while cold therapy can reduce inflammation and pain. Deep heating techniques like ultrasound can affect deeper tissues.

Traction: Can relieve pressure on compressed nerves or joints, particularly in the spine. Different traction techniques are used for different conditions and anatomical areas.

Injection Procedures: PM&R physicians often perform injection procedures for pain management and functional improvement, using various injection techniques and medications.

Joint Injections: Can provide pain relief and improve function for patients with arthritis or other joint conditions. Different medications and injection approaches are used depending on the specific joint and condition.

Trigger Point Injections: Target specific muscle knots or tender points that contribute to pain and dysfunction. These injections can provide significant relief for patients with myofascial pain syndromes.

Nerve Blocks: Can provide diagnostic information about pain sources while simultaneously providing therapeutic relief. Different nerve block techniques target specific nerves or anatomical regions.

Comprehensive Medicine Coding Practice Questions

Test your mastery of Medicine section coding across all subspecialties:

Question 1: A patient receives DTaP vaccine (90700) with administration. How should this be coded for a 4-year-old patient?

A) 90700 + 90460 (vaccine product + administration through age 18) B) 90700 + 90471 (vaccine product + administration any age) C) 90460 only (administration includes vaccine) D) 90700 only (vaccine product includes administration)

Answer: A Explanation: Immunization requires two codes: vaccine product (90700) and administration (90460 for patients through age 18). These are separate services - the product and the professional administration service.

Question 2: A psychiatrist provides 60 minutes of individual psychotherapy with medical evaluation and management. The correct code is:

A) 90834 (45-minute psychotherapy) B) 90837 (60-minute psychotherapy) C) 90792 (psychiatric evaluation with medical services) D) 90837 + 99213 (psychotherapy + E/M)

Answer: B Explanation: 90837 represents 60 minutes of individual psychotherapy. When psychotherapy and E/M services are provided together, use the psychotherapy code that includes the time spent on both services, not separate codes.

Question 3: Monthly ESRD services for a 45-year-old dialysis patient should be coded as:

A) 90960 (ESRD services, age 12-19) B) 90961 (ESRD services, age 20 and older) C) 90962 (ESRD services, home dialysis) D) Individual dialysis session codes

Answer: B Explanation: 90961 covers monthly end-stage renal disease services for patients age 20 and older, including all dialysis sessions and comprehensive management for that month.

Question 4: Screening colonoscopy in a 55-year-old asymptomatic patient should be coded as:

A) 45378 (colonoscopy, diagnostic) B) 45380 (colonoscopy with biopsy) C) G0121 (colorectal cancer screening) D) 45378 with screening modifier

Answer: A Explanation: For screening colonoscopy, use 45378 (diagnostic colonoscopy). Some payers may have specific screening codes (like G0121), but the primary CPT® code for screening colonoscopy is 45378.

Question 5: Cardiac rehabilitation with ECG monitoring should be coded as:

A) 93797 (cardiac rehabilitation with ECG monitoring) B) 93798 (cardiac rehabilitation without ECG monitoring) C) 93000 (ECG) + 97110 (therapeutic exercise) D) 93015 (stress test)

Answer: A Explanation: 93797 specifically represents cardiac rehabilitation with continuous ECG monitoring. This is different from 93798, which is cardiac rehabilitation without ECG monitoring.

Question 6: Allergen immunotherapy injection of pre-mixed dose should be coded as:

A) 95115 (professional services for allergen immunotherapy) B) 95117 (allergen immunotherapy injection) C) 95144 (professional services for single stinging insect venom) D) 95165 (professional services for single or multiple antigens)

Answer: B Explanation: 95117 represents the injection of a pre-mixed allergen immunotherapy dose. The professional services codes (95115, 95144, 95165) are for the physician work in preparing and managing immunotherapy, not the injection itself.

Question 7: Pulmonary function test with spirometry before and after bronchodilator should be coded as:

A) 94010 (spirometry) B) 94060 (spirometry before and after bronchodilator) C) 94070 (complete pulmonary function study) D) 94010 × 2 (spirometry performed twice)

Answer: B Explanation: 94060 specifically represents spirometry performed before and after bronchodilator administration to assess airway reversibility. This is more comprehensive than simple spirometry (94010).

Question 8: Upper endoscopy with biopsy and control of bleeding should be coded as:

A) 43239 (EGD with biopsy) + 43255 (EGD with control of bleeding) B) 43255 (EGD with control of bleeding) only C) 43235 (EGD diagnostic) + 43239 + 43255 D) 43259 (EGD with endoscopic ultrasound)

Answer: B Explanation: When multiple endoscopic procedures are performed during the same session, code only the most extensive procedure. Control of bleeding (43255) is more extensive than biopsy and includes any biopsies performed.

Question 9: Comprehensive metabolic panel plus lipid panel should be coded as:

A) 80053 (comprehensive metabolic panel) + 80061 (lipid panel) B) 80053 only (includes lipid panel) C) Individual codes for each test D) 80048 (basic metabolic panel) + 80061 (lipid panel)

Answer: A Explanation: Comprehensive metabolic panel (80053) and lipid panel (80061) test different analytes and can be coded separately when both are performed. The CMP does not include lipid testing.

Question 10: Moderate sedation provided by the same physician performing a procedure should be coded as:

A) 99151-99153 (moderate sedation by same physician) B) 99155-99157 (moderate sedation by different physician) C) Usually bundled into the procedure code D) 00100-01999 (anesthesia codes)

Answer: C Explanation: Most procedures that typically require moderate sedation have the sedation bundled into the procedure code. Separate moderate sedation coding is only appropriate when specifically allowed by CPT® guidelines.

Chapter 15 Summary: Completing Your CPT® Mastery Journey

Congratulations! You have now achieved comprehensive mastery of the entire CPT® coding system. Your journey through the Medicine section completes a coding education that spans every aspect of modern medical practice, from routine office visits to complex surgical procedures, from diagnostic imaging to life-sustaining treatments.

The Foundation You've Built

Complete CPT® Expertise: You now possess working knowledge of all six CPT® sections—Evaluation and Management, Anesthesia, Surgery, Radiology, Pathology and Laboratory, and Medicine. This comprehensive foundation allows you to handle any coding challenge with confidence and accuracy.

Clinical Understanding: Beyond simply knowing codes, you understand the medical reasoning behind procedures, the technology that enables modern healthcare, and the clinical relationships that drive treatment decisions. This clinical context makes you a more valuable and insightful coding professional.

Systematic Approach: Throughout your journey, you've developed systematic approaches to complex coding scenarios. Whether analyzing surgical procedures, calculating anesthesia units, or applying modifier rules, you now have proven methods for handling challenging situations.

Professional Judgment: You've learned when to seek clarification, how to handle ambiguous documentation, and when to apply professional judgment to make appropriate coding decisions. These skills separate expert coders from those who simply follow rules.

The Medicine Section's Unique Contributions

The Medicine section has added several critical capabilities to your coding toolkit:

Preventive Care Understanding: You can now code the full spectrum of preventive services that keep patients healthy and detect diseases early, understanding both the public health impact and the coding complexities involved.

Chronic Disease Management: You understand how healthcare manages long-term conditions like diabetes, heart disease, and mental health disorders through ongoing medical interventions rather than episodic crisis care.

Subspecialty Medicine: You've gained insight into how medical subspecialists provide focused expertise for complex conditions, understanding both the sophisticated technology involved and the extensive training required.

Team-Based Care: You appreciate how modern healthcare uses multidisciplinary teams and understand the coding implications of care coordination, shared decision-making, and integrated treatment approaches.

Professional Development and Career Opportunities

Your comprehensive CPT® mastery opens numerous career advancement opportunities:

Multi-Specialty Expertise: You can work confidently in any medical specialty, understanding both the clinical context and coding requirements for diverse practice types.

Leadership Roles: Your broad knowledge base qualifies you for coding supervisor, compliance officer, or department manager positions where comprehensive understanding is essential.

Consulting and Training: You can provide expert consulting services to healthcare organizations and train other coding professionals across all specialties.

Revenue Cycle Management: Your understanding of how different services are coded and reimbursed makes you valuable for revenue cycle optimization and compliance initiatives.

Quality and Compliance: Your knowledge of coding accuracy requirements and clinical appropriateness makes you well-suited for quality assurance and compliance roles.

Integration with ICD-10-CM and HCPCS

Your CPT® expertise integrates seamlessly with your diagnostic coding and supply coding knowledge:

Complete Coding Scenarios: You can now handle complex patient encounters that require accurate diagnosis coding, procedure coding, and supply coding working together.

Medical Necessity: You understand the relationships between diagnoses and procedures that support medical necessity and appropriate care.

Compliance Excellence: Your comprehensive knowledge helps you identify and prevent coding errors that could create compliance issues or affect reimbursement.

The Continuous Learning Journey

Healthcare and coding continue to evolve, but you now have the foundation to adapt to changes:

New Technology Integration: As new medical technologies emerge, you can understand their clinical applications and coding implications.

Regulatory Changes: You can adapt to coding guideline updates, new regulations, and evolving healthcare practices.

Career Growth: Your comprehensive foundation supports continued learning and specialization in areas that interest you most.

Your Professional Identity

You are now a complete medical coding professional with expertise that spans the entire healthcare spectrum. This achievement represents:

Technical Excellence: You have mastered one of healthcare's most complex administrative systems.

Clinical Understanding: You appreciate the medicine behind the codes and can contribute meaningfully to healthcare teams.

Professional Integrity: You understand the ethical responsibilities of accurate coding and its impact on patient care and healthcare economics.

Continuous Improvement: You have the tools and mindset for lifelong learning in an evolving field.

Final Thoughts: Your Coding Future

The comprehensive CPT® knowledge you've gained is more than just a professional skill—it's your contribution to healthcare excellence. Every code you assign accurately helps ensure:

- Patients receive appropriate care
- Providers are fairly compensated
- Healthcare resources are used efficiently
- Quality measures reflect true clinical performance
- Healthcare data supports research and improvement

Remember that coding accuracy affects real people: patients who need their insurance to cover necessary care, providers who depend on fair reimbursement to maintain their practices, and healthcare organizations that must balance quality care with financial sustainability.

Your expertise makes you a guardian of healthcare's financial integrity and a contributor to quality patient care. This responsibility is both challenging and rewarding, offering opportunities for continuous learning, professional growth, and meaningful contribution to one of society's most important endeavors.

Welcome to the ranks of expert medical coding professionals. Your journey of learning continues, but you now have the foundation to handle whatever challenges and opportunities lie ahead.

Your next step: Apply this knowledge confidently in your chosen career path, whether that's working for a healthcare provider, insurance company, consulting firm, or other healthcare organization. Your comprehensive CPT® mastery will serve you well in any role you choose.

The healthcare industry needs professionals like you—those who combine technical expertise with clinical understanding and professional integrity. You're ready to make your mark!

Chapter 16: HCPCS Level II Fundamentals

"Success is where preparation and opportunity meet." - Bobby Unser

Welcome to your final coding system mastery—HCPCS Level II coding. You've conquered ICD-10-CM diagnosis coding and CPT® procedure coding. Now you're about to complete your comprehensive medical coding education by mastering the system that captures everything else healthcare providers need to bill for: supplies, equipment, drugs, transportation, and specialized services that keep patients healthy and healthcare systems functioning.

HCPCS Level II represents the practical side of healthcare—the wheelchairs that restore mobility, the oxygen that sustains life, the ambulance rides that provide emergency access to care, and the medications that manage chronic conditions. Every piece of medical equipment, every supply item, and every specialized service that doesn't have a CPT® code finds its home in the HCPCS Level II system.

This chapter completes your transformation into a comprehensive medical coding professional. You'll gain the knowledge to handle any coding scenario with confidence, whether it's a complex surgical procedure requiring multiple supply items, a diabetic patient needing continuous glucose monitoring equipment, or a cancer patient receiving expensive chemotherapy medications.

Your journey through ICD-10-CM taught you to think like a clinician who understands disease processes. Your CPT® mastery showed you how to think like healthcare providers who perform procedures and deliver services. Now HCPCS Level II will teach you to think like healthcare administrators who ensure patients have access to the equipment, supplies, and services they need to maintain their health and independence.

By the end of this chapter, you'll possess complete medical coding mastery—the confidence to walk into any healthcare organization and handle whatever coding challenges await. You're about to join the elite ranks of coding professionals who truly understand every aspect of healthcare billing and reimbursement.

Understanding HCPCS Level II's Critical Role in Healthcare

Before diving into specific coding rules, it's essential to understand why HCPCS Level II exists and how it complements the other coding systems you've mastered. This understanding provides the foundation for making good coding decisions and appreciating the broader healthcare ecosystem you're helping to support.

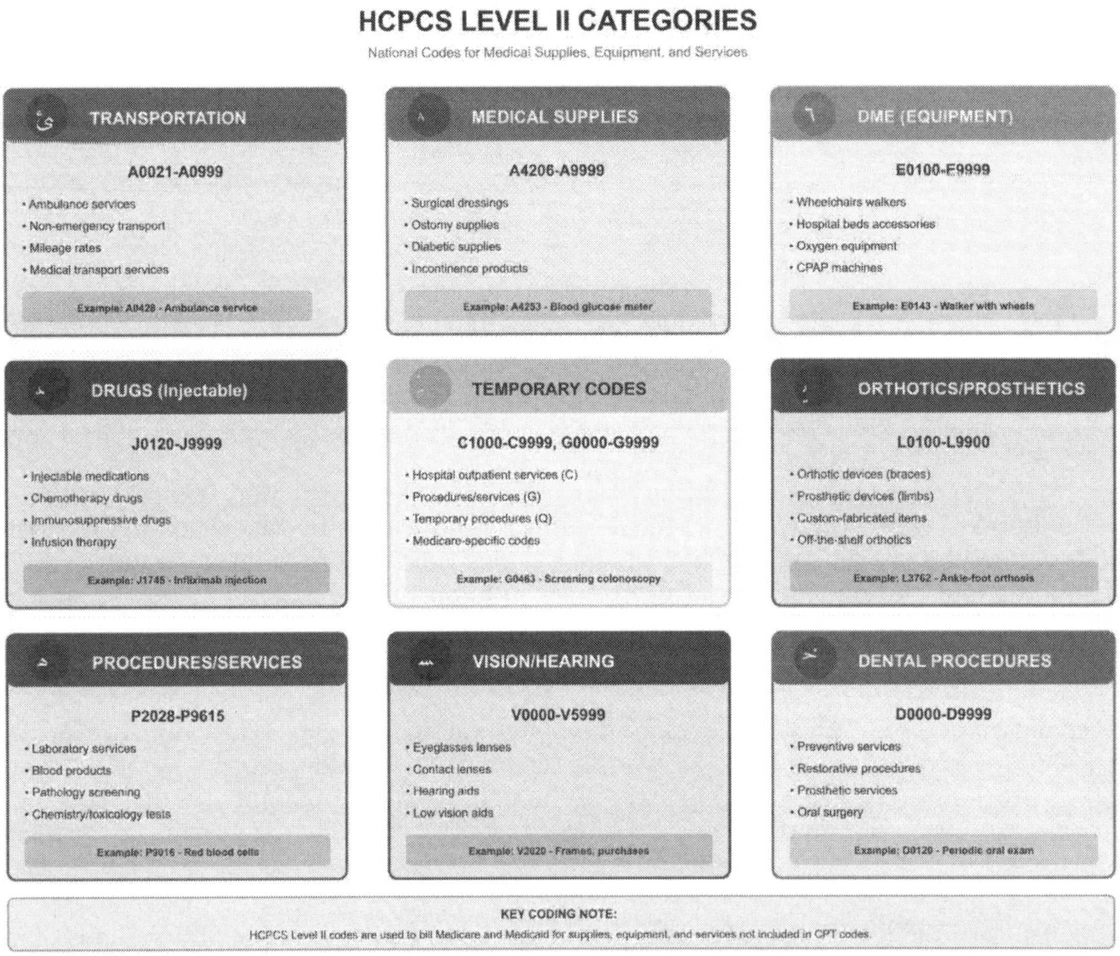

The Gap That HCPCS Level II Fills

Beyond Procedures to Products and Services: While CPT® codes capture the professional services and procedures that healthcare providers perform, they don't address the thousands of medical products, supplies, and specialized services that patients need. A patient receiving dialysis doesn't just need the professional service of dialysis management—they need the dialysis machine, the specialized tubing, the dialysis solution, and potentially transportation to and from the dialysis center.

Consider a diabetic patient managing their condition at home. CPT® codes capture the physician visits, the laboratory tests, and the diagnostic procedures. But the patient also needs a glucose meter, test strips, lancets, insulin, syringes, and potentially a continuous glucose monitor. Without HCPCS Level II codes, there would be no standardized way to bill for these essential items.

This example illustrates why HCPCS Level II is often called the "everything else" coding system—it captures all the non-physician services and products that make healthcare possible but don't fit into other coding systems.

Medicare's Innovation and National Adoption: HCPCS Level II was originally developed by the Centers for Medicare and Medicaid Services (CMS) to address Medicare's need for standardized codes for supplies, equipment, and services not covered by CPT®. However, the system proved so useful that most other insurance programs adopted it as well.

This Medicare origin explains several characteristics of HCPCS Level II coding: the emphasis on medical necessity, the detailed coverage guidelines, and the focus on cost-effective care delivery that serves the Medicare population's needs while controlling healthcare costs.

Understanding this origin helps explain why HCPCS Level II includes some codes that might seem unusual or overly specific—they address real-world situations that Medicare and other insurers encounter regularly in serving their beneficiaries.

The Intersection of Medicine and Economics: HCPCS Level II coding sits at the intersection of clinical care and healthcare economics. While ICD-10-CM codes describe what's wrong with patients and CPT® codes describe what providers do to help them, HCPCS Level II codes describe what resources are needed to deliver that care effectively.

This economic dimension means that HCPCS Level II coding directly affects healthcare accessibility and affordability. Accurate coding ensures that patients can obtain necessary equipment and supplies, while inaccurate coding can create barriers to care or inappropriate resource utilization.

The Scope and Diversity of HCPCS Level II

Temporary vs. Permanent Codes: One unique aspect of HCPCS Level II is its inclusion of both permanent codes and temporary codes that can be implemented quickly to address emerging healthcare needs. This flexibility allows the healthcare system to adapt rapidly to new technologies, changing regulations, or public health emergencies.

The COVID-19 pandemic demonstrated this flexibility when new HCPCS Level II codes were created rapidly to cover testing, treatments, and vaccines that didn't exist when the regular coding update cycle was established. This responsiveness ensures that healthcare providers can be reimbursed for new services without waiting for the next annual update cycle.

National vs. Local Codes: HCPCS Level II includes both national codes that are used throughout the United States and local codes that address regional variations in healthcare delivery or regulatory requirements. This dual structure recognizes that while most healthcare needs are universal, some variations exist based on geography, population characteristics, or state-specific regulations.

Understanding this distinction helps explain why some HCPCS Level II codes might not be familiar to coders in all regions and why it's important to verify coverage policies with specific insurance programs before assuming that a code will be accepted.

Integration with Quality and Outcome Measures: Modern healthcare increasingly emphasizes quality outcomes and value-based care, and HCPCS Level II codes play important roles in these initiatives. Some codes specifically capture quality reporting, outcome measurements, and performance metrics that help healthcare systems demonstrate their effectiveness.

This integration with quality initiatives means that accurate HCPCS Level II coding affects not just reimbursement but also quality scores, patient satisfaction measures, and healthcare system reputation. Understanding these broader implications helps explain why mastering HCPCS Level II coding is essential for healthcare organizations' success.

HCPCS Structure and Organization

Understanding how HCPCS Level II codes are structured and organized provides the foundation for efficient code lookup and ensures you understand the logic behind the coding system. This structure reflects decades of evolution to address changing healthcare needs while maintaining systematic organization.

The Alphabetic Code Structure

Letter-Based Category System: Unlike CPT® codes that use five-digit numbers, HCPCS Level II codes begin with a letter followed by four digits (e.g., A4100, E0143, J7050). This alphabetic structure allows for logical grouping of related items while providing enormous capacity for code expansion as new products and services are developed.

The letter categories aren't arbitrary—they reflect logical groupings that make sense for healthcare providers, suppliers, and billing personnel. Understanding these category meanings helps you locate codes more efficiently and ensures you're looking in the right section for specific items.

Systematic Code Assignment: Within each letter category, codes are generally assigned systematically to group related items together. For example, diabetic supplies are grouped together within their category, making it easier to find all related codes when coding for diabetic patients.

This systematic assignment means that understanding one code in a series often helps you understand related codes. If you know how to code basic wheelchairs, you can apply similar logic to power wheelchairs, wheelchair accessories, and wheelchair modifications.

Code Expansion and Updates: The HCPCS Level II system is updated more frequently than other coding systems, with quarterly updates that can add new codes, modify existing codes, or delete obsolete codes. This frequent updating ensures that the coding system keeps pace with rapidly changing healthcare technology and regulatory requirements.

These frequent updates mean that HCPCS Level II coding requires ongoing education and attention to changes. What was correct coding practice six months ago might not be correct today, making it essential to stay current with updates and changes.

Major Category Groupings and Their Logic

A Codes: Transportation Services, Medical and Surgical Supplies, and Administrative Services The A code section demonstrates HCPCS Level II's diversity by including everything from ambulance services to administrative fees. This category's breadth reflects healthcare's complexity and the need for codes that capture diverse services and supplies.

Transportation Services (A0021-A0999): These codes capture ambulance services, wheelchair van transportation, and other medical transportation that patients need to access healthcare services. Understanding these codes requires appreciating both medical necessity requirements and geographic considerations that affect transportation availability.

A typical ambulance call involves much more than simply driving a patient to the hospital. Advanced life support ambulances carry sophisticated medical equipment, employ trained paramedics who can provide emergency interventions, and coordinate with hospital emergency departments to ensure continuity of care. These complexities justify the detailed code structure for transportation services.

Medical and Surgical Supplies (A4000-A8999): This extensive subsection includes items like ostomy supplies, diabetic testing supplies, wound care products, and other items that patients use regularly. These codes often require understanding of both medical conditions and the supplies needed to manage them effectively.

Consider the complexity of ostomy care, which might seem straightforward to those unfamiliar with the medical reality. Ostomy patients need pouching systems that fit properly, skin barriers that protect against irritation, and accessories that allow them to maintain active lifestyles. Different ostomy types require different supplies, and individual patient needs vary based on anatomy, activity level, and personal preferences.

Administrative Services: Some A codes capture administrative services like case management or care coordination that don't involve direct patient care but are essential for effective healthcare delivery. These services recognize that modern healthcare often requires coordination among multiple providers and systems.

E Codes: Durable Medical Equipment Durable medical equipment (DME) represents one of HCPCS Level II's most important and complex areas, covering items from simple canes to sophisticated power wheelchairs and home oxygen systems.

Equipment Hierarchy: E codes are organized to reflect relationships between basic equipment and more sophisticated versions. Understanding these relationships helps you select appropriate codes and understand when upgrades or modifications might be justified.

A basic manual wheelchair might meet some patients' needs, but others might require power wheelchairs with specialized seating systems, tilt-and-recline functions, and environmental control interfaces. The code structure reflects these varying levels of complexity and functionality.

Home vs. Institutional Use: Many DME codes distinguish between equipment intended for home use and that designed for institutional settings. This distinction reflects different durability requirements, maintenance needs, and regulatory standards that apply in different settings.

J Codes: Drugs Administered Other Than Oral Method J codes represent one of HCPCS Level II's most financially significant categories, covering expensive medications that are administered by injection, infusion, or other non-oral routes.

Dosage-Based Coding: Many J codes specify exact dosages, reflecting the fact that drug costs are often directly related to the amount of medication used. Understanding these dosage specifications is crucial for accurate billing and appropriate reimbursement.

Brand vs. Generic Considerations: Some J codes distinguish between brand-name and generic versions of medications, while others cover both. Understanding these distinctions helps ensure appropriate billing and can affect both reimbursement and patient access to medications.

Administration vs. Supply: J codes cover only the medication itself, not the professional service of administering the medication. This separation requires understanding of both HCPCS Level II drug codes and CPT® administration codes to bill complete services.

Temporary Code Categories

C Codes: Hospital Outpatient Prospective Payment System C codes represent temporary codes used in hospital outpatient settings to capture new technologies, procedures, or services that don't have permanent CPT® codes. These codes often transition to permanent CPT® codes as technologies become established.

Understanding C codes requires appreciating the rapid pace of medical technology development and the need for coding systems that can adapt quickly to new innovations. A new medical device might receive a temporary C code within months of FDA approval, allowing hospitals to be reimbursed for using the device while permanent coding is developed.

G Codes: Procedures and Services Temporarily Assigned G codes serve various temporary purposes, including quality reporting, demonstration projects, and services under development. These codes often support healthcare initiatives that extend beyond simple fee-for-service payment.

Many G codes support quality improvement initiatives by capturing data about processes, outcomes, or patient characteristics that help healthcare systems demonstrate their performance. Understanding these codes helps you appreciate healthcare's evolution toward value-based payment and quality measurement.

Q Codes: Temporary National Codes Q codes cover a variety of temporary services and supplies that don't fit into other categories. These codes often address unique situations or specialized programs that serve specific patient populations or geographic areas.

The temporary nature of these codes means they can change quickly as programs evolve or as permanent coding solutions are developed. Staying current with Q code changes requires ongoing attention to updates and policy changes.

Durable Medical Equipment (DME): Independence Through Technology

Durable medical equipment represents healthcare technology that extends beyond the clinical setting into patients' daily lives, enabling independence, functionality, and quality of life that might not be possible otherwise. Understanding DME coding requires appreciating both the technology involved and the profound impact these devices have on patients' lives.

The Philosophy and Impact of DME

Independence and Quality of Life: DME serves a fundamental principle of modern healthcare: maintaining patient independence and dignity while managing illness or disability. A wheelchair doesn't just provide mobility—it enables employment, social interaction, and personal autonomy that define quality of life.

Consider the transformation that occurs when a patient with severe mobility limitations receives appropriate DME. What might begin as a simple need for mobility support can evolve into a comprehensive technology solution that includes power mobility, environmental controls, communication devices, and home modification equipment that enables nearly complete independence.

This transformative potential explains why DME coding can be complex—the equipment often represents life-changing interventions that require careful assessment, proper fitting, and ongoing maintenance to achieve optimal outcomes.

Medical Necessity and Functional Assessment: DME coverage depends heavily on demonstrating medical necessity through functional assessment rather than simply diagnosing medical conditions. A patient might have a condition that could benefit from DME, but coverage requires demonstrating that the equipment will meaningfully improve function in the patient's specific circumstances.

This functional focus means that DME coding often requires understanding not just medical conditions but also patients' living situations, activity goals, and long-term care plans. The same medical condition might justify different DME solutions for different patients based on their individual needs and circumstances.

Technology Evolution and Adaptation: DME technology evolves rapidly, incorporating advances in materials science, electronics, and software that create new possibilities for patient care. Modern DME can include smartphone connectivity, artificial intelligence features, and integration with home monitoring systems that weren't imaginable just years ago.

This rapid evolution means that DME coding must adapt frequently to accommodate new technologies and capabilities. Understanding this evolution helps explain why HCPCS Level II updates are so frequent and why staying current with changes is essential for accurate coding.

Mobility Equipment and Coding

Manual Wheelchairs (K0001-K0109): Manual wheelchairs range from basic transport chairs to sophisticated lightweight models with specialized seating systems and customization options. Understanding the coding requires appreciating the functional differences between various wheelchair types and how these differences affect patient outcomes.

Basic vs. Lightweight Wheelchairs: The distinction between basic and lightweight wheelchairs isn't just about convenience—it can significantly affect a user's ability to propel the chair independently, transfer safely, and participate in activities. Lightweight wheelchairs reduce energy expenditure and can mean the difference between independence and dependence on others.

Customization and Modifications: Many wheelchair users require customizations like specialized seating, positioning equipment, or functional accessories. Understanding how these modifications are coded requires knowledge of both the base wheelchair codes and the additional codes for modifications and accessories.

The complexity of wheelchair customization reflects the diversity of user needs. A young athlete might need a lightweight sports wheelchair with specialized wheels and positioning, while an elderly patient might need a wheelchair with enhanced stability features and comfortable cushioning for extended sitting.

Power Wheelchairs (K0813-K0898): Power wheelchairs represent sophisticated medical devices that can provide mobility for patients who cannot propel manual wheelchairs effectively. These devices often include complex seating systems, environmental controls, and specialized driving interfaces that accommodate various disabilities.

Power Wheelchair Categories: Power wheelchairs are categorized based on their intended use environment and functionality. Group 1 power wheelchairs are designed for basic indoor use, while Group 5 wheelchairs can handle outdoor terrain and extended daily use. Understanding these categories helps ensure that patients receive appropriate equipment for their lifestyle needs.

Seating and Positioning Systems: Many power wheelchair users require specialized seating systems that provide pressure relief, positioning support, and accommodation for orthopedic needs. These seating systems can be as important as the wheelchair base for patient health and comfort.

Complex seating systems might include multiple components like specialized cushions, back supports, lateral supports, and positioning devices that work together to maintain proper body alignment and prevent complications like pressure sores or contractures.

Home Oxygen Systems (E0424-E0486): Home oxygen therapy allows patients with chronic respiratory conditions to maintain independence while receiving life-sustaining treatment. Understanding oxygen equipment coding requires knowledge of different delivery methods, flow requirements, and mobility considerations.

Oxygen Concentrators vs. Cylinders: Oxygen concentrators extract oxygen from room air, providing an unlimited supply without requiring tank replacements. Portable oxygen concentrators allow patients to maintain mobility while receiving continuous oxygen therapy. Understanding when each system is appropriate requires knowledge of patient lifestyle needs and oxygen requirements.

Flow Rate and Delivery Methods: Different patients require different oxygen flow rates and delivery methods. Some patients need continuous oxygen, while others need it only during sleep or exertion. These varying needs affect equipment selection and coding requirements.

The impact of portable oxygen therapy on quality of life can be dramatic. Patients who were previously homebound due to oxygen requirements can return to work, travel, and participate in family activities when appropriate portable equipment is available.

Home Medical Equipment and Monitoring

CPAP and BiPAP Equipment (E0601-E0619): Sleep apnea affects millions of Americans and can have serious cardiovascular and neurological consequences if untreated. CPAP (Continuous Positive Airway Pressure) and BiPAP (Bilevel Positive Airway Pressure) equipment provide effective treatment that can dramatically improve both sleep quality and overall health.

Equipment Complexity: Modern CPAP systems include sophisticated monitoring capabilities, automatic pressure adjustments, and data recording features that help healthcare providers optimize treatment. Understanding these capabilities helps explain why different CPAP codes exist and why equipment selection should match patient needs.

Compliance Monitoring: Insurance coverage for CPAP equipment often includes compliance requirements that patients must meet to continue coverage. Understanding these requirements helps explain the importance of patient education and follow-up care in CPAP therapy.

Successful CPAP therapy requires more than just equipment—it requires proper fitting, patient education, ongoing support, and regular follow-up to ensure continued effectiveness. The coding system recognizes these various components of comprehensive sleep apnea management.

Diabetic Equipment and Supplies (A4233-A4259): Diabetes management requires continuous monitoring and medication administration that depends heavily on accurate, reliable equipment. Understanding diabetic supply coding requires appreciating both the medical complexity of diabetes management and the technology that makes effective self-management possible.

Blood Glucose Monitoring: Modern glucose meters provide sophisticated features like data storage, trend analysis, and smartphone connectivity that help patients and healthcare providers optimize diabetes management. Different patients might need different meter features based on their management goals and technical capabilities.

Continuous Glucose Monitoring (CGM): CGM systems provide real-time glucose readings and trend information that can dramatically improve diabetes management outcomes. These systems represent sophisticated medical devices that require proper training and ongoing support for optimal effectiveness.

The evolution from simple glucose meters to continuous monitoring systems demonstrates how technology can transform chronic disease management. Patients who once managed diabetes with occasional glucose checks can now have continuous awareness of their glucose levels and trends.

Insulin Pumps and Supplies (A4230-A4232): Insulin pumps provide continuous subcutaneous insulin delivery that can improve glucose control while providing lifestyle flexibility for diabetes patients. Understanding pump coding requires knowledge of the technology involved and the comprehensive support systems needed for successful pump therapy.

Pump Technology: Modern insulin pumps include features like programmable delivery rates, meal bolus calculations, and integration with continuous glucose monitors. Some systems can automatically adjust insulin delivery based on glucose readings, representing a significant step toward automated diabetes management.

Training and Support Requirements: Successful insulin pump therapy requires extensive patient education, ongoing technical support, and regular follow-up care. The complexity of pump therapy means that coding must capture not just the equipment but also the professional services needed to support successful outcomes.

Transportation Services: Access to Care

Healthcare transportation represents a critical link in the healthcare delivery system, ensuring that patients can access necessary care regardless of their mobility limitations, geographic location, or economic circumstances. Understanding transportation coding requires appreciating both the medical aspects of patient transport and the logistical challenges of providing safe, appropriate transportation services.

Emergency Medical Transportation

Advanced Life Support (ALS) Ambulance Services (A0426-A0433): ALS ambulance services provide sophisticated emergency medical care during transport, essentially bringing emergency room capabilities to patients wherever they are located. Understanding these codes requires appreciating the medical complexity and resource requirements of advanced prehospital care.

Paramedic-Level Care: ALS ambulances are staffed with paramedics who can provide advanced interventions including cardiac monitoring, defibrillation, advanced airway management, medication administration, and other life-saving treatments. These capabilities can mean the difference between life and death for critically ill patients.

The training and certification requirements for paramedics are extensive, often requiring thousands of hours of education and ongoing continuing education to maintain certification. This expertise justifies the higher reimbursement rates for ALS transport compared to basic life support.

Equipment and Technology: Modern ALS ambulances carry sophisticated medical equipment including cardiac monitors, defibrillators, ventilators, medication pumps, and communication systems that allow real-time consultation with hospital physicians. This equipment represents significant investment and ongoing maintenance costs.

Clinical Decision-Making: ALS providers must make rapid clinical assessments and treatment decisions in challenging environments with limited information. These decisions can significantly affect patient outcomes and require specialized training and experience that goes far beyond basic transportation services.

Basic Life Support (BLS) Ambulance Services (A0428-A0429): BLS ambulance services provide essential medical transportation with basic emergency medical capabilities. While less sophisticated than ALS services, BLS transport serves essential functions in the healthcare system and requires trained personnel and appropriate equipment.

Emergency Medical Technician (EMT) Care: BLS ambulances are staffed with EMTs who can provide basic life support interventions including oxygen administration, basic airway management, bleeding control, and other fundamental emergency care measures.

Appropriate Utilization: Understanding when BLS transport is appropriate versus when ALS transport is necessary requires knowledge of both patient conditions and available treatment capabilities. Appropriate level selection ensures that patients receive necessary care while controlling costs.

Many non-emergency medical conditions require ambulance transportation due to patient mobility limitations or medical monitoring needs, but don't require advanced life support interventions. BLS transport serves these needs effectively while being more cost-efficient than ALS services.

Non-Emergency Medical Transportation

Wheelchair Van Transportation (A0130): Wheelchair van transportation serves patients who use wheelchairs but don't require medical monitoring during transport. This service enables access to healthcare for patients whose mobility equipment makes standard vehicle transportation impossible.

Vehicle Specifications: Wheelchair vans require specialized equipment including wheelchair lifts or ramps, wheelchair securement systems, and modified seating arrangements. These modifications represent significant vehicle costs and ongoing maintenance requirements.

Driver Training and Certification: Wheelchair van drivers often require specialized training in wheelchair securement, patient assistance, and emergency procedures. This training ensures passenger safety and regulatory compliance.

The availability of wheelchair van transportation can significantly affect healthcare access for wheelchair users. Without appropriate transportation options, routine medical appointments can become major logistical challenges that might result in delayed or foregone care.

Stretcher Transportation (A0382-A0384): Some patients require transportation on stretchers due to medical conditions that prevent sitting upright, but don't need continuous medical monitoring during transport. Stretcher transportation provides a middle ground between wheelchair transport and ambulance services.

Medical Necessity Requirements: Stretcher transportation typically requires documentation of medical necessity explaining why the patient cannot be transported in a wheelchair or standard vehicle. These requirements ensure appropriate utilization while providing necessary access to care.

Vehicle and Equipment Requirements: Stretcher transport vehicles must include appropriate stretcher securement systems, patient monitoring capabilities, and emergency equipment. These requirements ensure patient safety during transport.

Geographic and Access Considerations

Rural Transportation Challenges: Rural areas often face unique transportation challenges due to long distances, limited provider availability, and sparse population density that makes specialized transportation services difficult to sustain economically.

Mileage and Distance Factors: Transportation coding often includes mileage components that recognize the significant costs associated with long-distance medical transport. Rural patients might need to travel hundreds of miles for specialized care, creating transportation costs that urban patients don't face.

Provider Network Limitations: Rural areas might have limited choices for specialized medical transportation, affecting both service availability and pricing. Understanding these limitations helps explain why transportation policy often includes special provisions for rural areas.

Air Transportation (A0430-A0436): Medical helicopter and fixed-wing aircraft transportation serves patients who need rapid transport over long distances or access to specialized care that's not available locally. These services represent the most sophisticated and expensive forms of medical transportation.

Clinical Capabilities: Medical aircraft often carry advanced medical equipment and specialized flight crews who can provide intensive care during transport. These capabilities enable inter-facility transfers of critically ill patients who might not survive ground transportation.

Geographic Coverage: Air medical services can reach remote areas that might be hours away from definitive care by ground transportation. This capability can be life-saving for patients in rural or wilderness areas who experience medical emergencies.

Cost and Utilization: Air medical transportation represents one of the most expensive forms of medical care, with costs often exceeding tens of thousands of dollars per transport. Understanding appropriate utilization criteria helps ensure that this resource is used effectively while controlling costs.

Drugs and Biologicals: Precision Medicine and Therapeutic Innovation

The pharmaceutical landscape has undergone revolutionary changes in recent decades, evolving from primarily small-molecule drugs to sophisticated biologicals, personalized medicines, and targeted therapies that can dramatically alter disease courses. Understanding HCPCS Level II drug coding requires appreciating both the science behind modern pharmaceuticals and the economic considerations that affect patient access to these life-changing treatments.

The Revolution in Pharmaceutical Medicine

From One-Size-Fits-All to Precision Medicine: Traditional pharmaceutical development focused on creating drugs that would work for most patients with a particular condition. Modern medicine increasingly recognizes that individual patients respond differently to medications based on their genetic makeup, disease characteristics, and other factors that require personalized treatment approaches.

This shift toward precision medicine is reflected in HCPCS Level II coding through increasingly specific drug codes that distinguish between different formulations, dosages, and even genetic variants of similar medications. Understanding this evolution helps explain why drug coding has become more complex and why accurate coding is so important for ensuring patients receive appropriate treatments.

Biologic vs. Traditional Pharmaceuticals: Biologic medications represent one of the most significant advances in modern medicine, offering treatment options for conditions that were previously considered untreatable or poorly manageable. These medications are derived from living organisms rather than synthesized chemically, creating unique manufacturing, storage, and administration challenges.

Biologics often require special handling, including refrigeration, protection from light, and specialized preparation techniques. They may also require specialized administration methods, extended infusion times, and intensive monitoring for adverse reactions. These complexities are reflected in both coding requirements and coverage policies that recognize the additional resources needed for biologic therapy.

Cost and Access Considerations: Many modern medications, particularly biologics and specialty pharmaceuticals, carry enormous costs that can exceed hundreds of thousands of dollars per year for individual patients. These costs create significant challenges for healthcare systems and require careful management to ensure patient access while maintaining financial sustainability.

Understanding these cost considerations helps explain why drug coding often requires detailed documentation of medical necessity, prior authorization processes, and ongoing monitoring requirements that demonstrate continued therapeutic benefit. Accurate coding ensures that patients can access necessary medications while helping healthcare systems manage these significant expenses responsibly.

Injectable and Infusion Medications

Chemotherapy Agents (J9000-J9999): Chemotherapy represents one of medicine's most sophisticated pharmaceutical applications, using highly toxic medications in carefully calculated doses to destroy cancer cells while minimizing damage to healthy tissues. Understanding chemotherapy coding requires appreciating both the precision required for safe administration and the complexity of modern cancer treatment protocols.

Dosage Precision: Chemotherapy dosing often requires calculations based on patient body surface area, kidney function, liver function, and other factors that affect drug metabolism and toxicity. Small errors in dosing can result in either treatment failure or life-threatening toxicity, making accurate coding essential for patient safety.

Combination Therapy: Modern cancer treatment often involves multiple chemotherapy agents given in specific sequences and combinations that have been proven effective through clinical research. Understanding these treatment protocols helps explain why multiple drug codes might be used for single patients and why timing and sequencing are important factors in treatment success.

Administration Complexity: Chemotherapy administration requires specialized facilities, trained personnel, emergency equipment, and extensive safety protocols to protect both patients and healthcare workers. The complexity of safe chemotherapy administration justifies the professional fees associated with these services and explains why specialized oncology practices often provide these treatments.

Biologic Response Modifiers (J0100-J3590): Biologic response modifiers represent a revolutionary approach to treating autoimmune diseases, cancers, and other conditions by modifying immune system function rather than simply suppressing symptoms. These medications can provide dramatic improvements for patients with conditions like rheumatoid arthritis, inflammatory bowel disease, and multiple sclerosis.

Mechanism of Action: Unlike traditional medications that affect broad physiological processes, many biologics target specific immune system components or cellular processes that are involved in disease development. This targeted approach can provide superior effectiveness with fewer side effects compared to traditional treatments.

Administration Requirements: Many biologics require intravenous infusion over extended periods, specialized preparation techniques, and intensive monitoring for infusion reactions. Some newer biologics can be self-administered by patients using prefilled syringes or auto-injectors, providing greater convenience and potentially improved outcomes.

Monitoring and Safety: Biologic therapy often requires ongoing monitoring for effectiveness and side effects, including regular laboratory testing, imaging studies, and clinical assessments. Understanding these monitoring requirements helps explain why biologic therapy involves ongoing professional services in addition to the medication costs.

Oral and Self-Administered Medications

Oral Anticancer Agents (J8500-J9070): The development of oral chemotherapy agents has revolutionized cancer treatment by allowing patients to receive sophisticated cancer therapy at home rather than requiring frequent visits to infusion centers. However, oral chemotherapy requires different management approaches and coding considerations.

Patient Education and Compliance: Oral chemotherapy success depends heavily on patient understanding and compliance with complex dosing schedules, drug interaction precautions, and side effect management. The responsibility for safe medication management shifts from healthcare providers to patients and their families, requiring extensive education and support.

Cost and Access Issues: Oral chemotherapy agents are often extremely expensive, with monthly costs that can exceed traditional chemotherapy regimens. Insurance coverage for oral medications may differ from coverage for infused medications, creating potential access barriers that require careful navigation.

Monitoring and Follow-up: Patients receiving oral chemotherapy require regular monitoring for effectiveness and toxicity, including laboratory testing, imaging studies, and clinical assessments. Understanding these monitoring requirements helps explain why oral chemotherapy involves ongoing professional services despite the medication being self-administered.

Specialty Drug Categories

Blood Products and Derivatives (P9010-P9100): Blood products represent life-saving treatments for patients with various conditions including bleeding disorders, immune deficiencies, and other conditions requiring blood component replacement. Understanding blood product coding requires knowledge of different blood components and their therapeutic applications.

Blood Component Therapy: Different blood components serve different therapeutic purposes. Red blood cells treat anemia and blood loss, platelets prevent bleeding in patients with low platelet counts, and plasma products treat clotting disorders and other conditions. Each component has specific storage, preparation, and administration requirements.

Safety and Testing: Modern blood products undergo extensive testing and processing to ensure safety and effectiveness. These safety measures have dramatically reduced the risk of blood-borne disease transmission but require significant resources and specialized facilities.

Immunoglobulins and Vaccines: Some blood-derived products like immunoglobulins provide passive immunity for patients with immune deficiencies or specific infection risks. Understanding these products requires knowledge of immune system function and the conditions that benefit from passive immunization.

Diagnostic Agents (A9500-A9700): Diagnostic pharmaceuticals enable sophisticated imaging and testing procedures that provide critical information for medical decision-making. Understanding these agents requires knowledge of diagnostic imaging and laboratory testing procedures.

Contrast Agents: Different imaging procedures require different contrast agents that enhance visualization of specific organs or tissues. These agents must be selected based on the imaging modality, anatomical area of interest, and patient factors like kidney function and allergy history.

Radiopharmaceuticals: Nuclear medicine procedures use radioactive pharmaceuticals that concentrate in specific organs or tissues, allowing functional imaging that provides information not available through other imaging modalities. These agents require special handling and safety precautions due to their radioactive properties.

Temporary Codes: Navigating the Ever-Changing Landscape

Temporary codes represent one of HCPCS Level II's most dynamic and challenging aspects. These codes serve as placeholders for new technologies, emerging treatments, and evolving healthcare services that don't yet have permanent codes assigned. Understanding temporary codes requires both technical knowledge and the flexibility to adapt as healthcare continues its rapid evolution.

Understanding the Purpose of Temporary Codes

Why Temporary Codes Exist: Healthcare innovation moves faster than the formal code development process. New medical devices, medications, and treatment approaches emerge constantly, driven by research breakthroughs, technological advances, and clinical innovation. Without temporary codes, there would be no mechanism to bill for these new services while permanent codes are being developed and approved.

Think of temporary codes as healthcare's beta testing phase. They allow new treatments to be tried in real-world settings, reimbursement data to be collected, and clinical effectiveness to be evaluated—all while providers can still bill for their services. This system supports innovation by ensuring that cutting-edge treatments don't languish unbillable while waiting for the slow wheels of code development to turn.

The Temporary Code Lifecycle: Temporary codes typically follow a predictable lifecycle. When a new technology or service emerges, a temporary code is assigned to allow billing while usage patterns and clinical effectiveness are established. If the technology proves valuable and usage becomes widespread, the temporary code may transition to a permanent HCPCS or

CPT® code. If the technology doesn't gain traction or proves ineffective, the temporary code may simply be discontinued.

This lifecycle means that temporary codes require constant monitoring. What's coded correctly today might change tomorrow as codes transition, are discontinued, or have their definitions refined based on real-world usage data.

C Codes: Hospital Outpatient Prospective Payment System

The C Code Category: C codes (C1000-C9999) represent one of the most clinically significant temporary code categories, covering drugs, biologicals, and devices used in hospital outpatient settings. These codes play a crucial role in hospital billing and often involve expensive, innovative treatments that significantly impact both patient care and hospital finances.

Understanding C Code Applications: C codes frequently cover cutting-edge medical technologies that would otherwise have no billing mechanism. Imagine a hospital acquiring a new type of heart valve that hasn't been available long enough to receive a permanent code. The C code system allows the hospital to use this innovative device while still receiving appropriate reimbursement, supporting the adoption of medical advances that benefit patients.

Drug and Biological C Codes: Many C codes represent new medications or biological products that haven't yet been assigned permanent J codes. These might include newly approved chemotherapy agents, innovative biologic treatments for autoimmune diseases, or gene therapies that represent entirely new treatment paradigms.

Clinical Example: A new monoclonal antibody for treating a rare form of cancer receives FDA approval. Before permanent codes are established, a C code allows hospitals to administer this life-saving treatment while documenting usage patterns and outcomes that will inform permanent code development.

Device C Codes: Medical devices ranging from sophisticated cardiac implants to innovative surgical tools often start with C codes. These temporary codes recognize that device technology evolves rapidly, with improvements and innovations emerging faster than the permanent coding system can accommodate.

Clinical Example: A new type of drug-eluting stent with innovative coating technology that reduces restenosis rates receives a temporary C code. Hospitals can begin using this improved technology immediately, with the C code ensuring appropriate reimbursement while permanent coding pathways are established.

C Code Documentation Requirements: Proper C code usage requires meticulous documentation including the specific device or drug name, manufacturer information, lot numbers when applicable, and clinical indication for use. This documentation serves multiple purposes: supporting medical necessity, tracking device performance and safety, and providing data that informs permanent code development.

Remember that C codes often involve expensive items. Documentation must clearly justify the medical necessity of using these specific products rather than less expensive alternatives. Without this justification, claims may be denied, leaving hospitals absorbing significant costs.

G Codes: Temporary Procedures and Professional Services

The G Code Universe: G codes (G0001-G9999) represent an enormous category covering temporary procedure codes, professional services, and quality reporting measures. These codes fill gaps in the CPT® system, providing billing mechanisms for services that don't fit neatly into established categories.

Medicare-Specific Services: Many G codes specifically address services covered by Medicare but lacking CPT® codes. These might include preventive services mandated by legislation, demonstration projects testing new care delivery models, or services unique to Medicare's coverage policies.

Clinical Example: When legislation mandated Medicare coverage for certain preventive services like cardiovascular disease screening, G codes were created to allow billing while permanent codes were developed. These temporary codes enabled immediate implementation of important preventive care benefits.

Quality Reporting G Codes: Some G codes support quality reporting initiatives, documenting specific clinical actions, patient characteristics, or treatment outcomes that inform healthcare quality assessment. While not always separately reimbursed, these codes serve crucial functions in demonstrating quality care and meeting reporting requirements.

Understanding that these G codes support quality initiatives rather than direct reimbursement helps explain why they're used even when no payment is attached. They document quality of care and help practices meet performance requirements that affect other aspects of reimbursement.

Demonstration Project Codes: G codes often support demonstration projects testing innovative care delivery models. These might include telemedicine services, care coordination programs, or new approaches to managing chronic diseases. The temporary codes allow data collection during the demonstration phase, informing decisions about permanent implementation.

Clinical Example: A Medicare demonstration project testing remote monitoring for heart failure patients uses G codes to track services and outcomes. If the demonstration proves successful, permanent codes may be established, making remote monitoring a standard covered benefit.

K Codes: Durable Medical Equipment

DME Temporary Codes: K codes (K0001-K9999) focus on durable medical equipment, orthotics, prosthetics, and supplies that don't yet have permanent codes. These codes are particularly important for assistive technology and medical equipment that helps patients maintain independence and quality of life.

Wheelchairs and Mobility Devices: Many K codes cover specialized wheelchairs and mobility devices with features or technologies that don't fit existing code definitions. As wheelchair technology advances—incorporating improved seating systems, power controls, or specialized functionality—K codes provide billing mechanisms for these innovations.

Clinical Example: A new wheelchair design incorporating advanced pressure-relieving cushioning and customizable seating that prevents pressure ulcers receives a K code. This allows patients to access this technology that could prevent serious complications, while usage data informs whether permanent codes are warranted.

Orthotics and Prosthetics: Prosthetic and orthotic technology continues advancing rapidly, with new materials, designs, and functionalities emerging regularly. K codes ensure that patients can access these advances without waiting years for permanent code development.

Clinical Example: A new prosthetic knee joint using microprocessor technology that adjusts to different walking speeds and terrains receives a K code. Amputees can benefit from this advanced technology that dramatically improves mobility and quality of life, with the K code ensuring providers are reimbursed for this expensive, sophisticated device.

Q Codes: Temporary and Miscellaneous Services

The Q Code Catch-All: Q codes (Q0001-Q9999) represent perhaps the most diverse temporary code category, covering everything from drugs and biologicals to vision services, laboratory tests, and specialized procedures. This diversity makes Q codes particularly challenging—you must understand not just coding rules but also the wide range of clinical situations they address.

Drug and Biological Q Codes: Many Q codes cover drugs administered in specific settings or circumstances that don't fit standard J code categories. These might include drugs used in clinical trials, medications with unique administration requirements, or pharmaceuticals in special FDA programs.

Clinical Example: An oral chemotherapy drug covered under Medicare Part B (which usually covers only injected or infused drugs) receives a Q code recognizing its special coverage status. This allows cancer patients to receive needed oral therapy with appropriate Medicare coverage.

Vision and Hearing Services: Some Q codes cover specialized vision and hearing services, particularly those related to prosthetic devices or rehabilitative services. These codes fill gaps in coverage for services that improve quality of life but don't fit traditional medical service categories.

Clinical Example: Specialized low vision rehabilitation services that teach adaptive techniques for daily living activities use Q codes. These services can dramatically improve independence for patients with vision loss, with Q codes ensuring access while permanent coding pathways are explored.

Casting and Splinting Supplies: Q codes include various casting and splinting supplies, particularly those with specialized features or applications. These codes ensure that orthopedic care can use the most appropriate materials for individual patient needs.

S Codes: Private Payer and State-Specific Services

Understanding S Code Limitations: S codes (S0001-S9999) occupy a unique position—they're created by commercial payers and state Medicaid programs but are NOT recognized by Medicare. This creates an important distinction: S codes may be perfectly appropriate for commercial insurance claims but should never appear on Medicare claims.

Why S Codes Exist: Commercial insurance companies and state Medicaid programs sometimes cover services that Medicare doesn't, or they may define services differently than Medicare does. S codes provide a standardized mechanism for billing these payer-specific services without cluttering the Medicare coding system with codes that aren't relevant to the federal program.

Clinical Example: A commercial insurance company covers acupuncture services for chronic pain management. While Medicare doesn't cover most acupuncture, the commercial payer uses S codes to process these claims consistently across their network. Using S codes prevents confusion with Medicare-approved services while ensuring standardized billing for commercial coverage.

Common S Code Applications: S codes frequently cover services like home infusion therapy, medical foods for inborn errors of metabolism, investigational procedures, and certain preventive services. Understanding which payers accept S codes and for what services is crucial for successful claims processing.

Payer-Specific Policies: Before using S codes, always verify the specific payer's policies. Some commercial payers use S codes extensively, while others prefer different coding approaches. State Medicaid programs vary widely in their S code usage, making payer-specific research essential.

Temporary Code Management Strategies

Staying Current with Code Changes: Temporary codes change more frequently than permanent codes, with updates occurring quarterly or even more often. Successful temporary code management requires systematic monitoring of code updates, including new codes, deleted codes, and redefined code descriptions.

Develop a systematic approach: Set calendar reminders for checking quarterly HCPCS updates. Subscribe to official CMS notifications and professional coding organization updates. Create a simple tracking system noting which temporary codes your organization uses and monitoring their status.

Documentation Excellence: Temporary codes often require more detailed documentation than permanent codes because they're newer, less familiar to reviewers, and may cover innovative or unusual treatments. Your documentation must clearly establish medical necessity and explain why the temporary code-described service is appropriate.

Include specific details: Document the exact device model number and manufacturer for C codes. Explain the clinical rationale for G code services. Describe why standard treatments weren't appropriate, necessitating the temporary code service. This comprehensive documentation prevents denials and supports your coding decisions if questioned.

Payer Policy Verification: Don't assume payers cover temporary codes simply because they exist. Many payers have specific policies about which temporary codes they recognize and under what circumstances they provide coverage. Always verify coverage before providing services when possible, or ensure patients understand potential financial responsibility.

Prior Authorization Management: Many services requiring temporary codes also trigger prior authorization requirements. Build prior authorization processes into your workflow for temporary codes, recognizing that the authorization process itself helps clarify whether the payer covers the service and under what circumstances.

Transition Planning: When temporary codes transition to permanent codes, implement the change promptly to avoid claim denials. Monitor announcements about code transitions and update your charge capture systems, superbills, and billing software before the effective date of changes.

Modifiers in HCPCS Level II: Adding Precision to Your Coding

HCPCS Level II modifiers provide crucial information about how services were performed, who performed them, or what special circumstances apply. While similar in concept to CPT® modifiers, HCPCS modifiers address unique situations related to DME, supplies, and services not covered by CPT® codes. Mastering HCPCS modifiers transforms you from someone who simply finds codes to a professional who communicates precise clinical and billing information.

Understanding HCPCS Modifier Categories

Anatomical Modifiers: Precision in Location Several HCPCS modifiers specify exact anatomical locations with precision impossible using only CPT® codes. These modifiers ensure payers understand exactly where services were provided or supplies were used, preventing confusion and supporting appropriate reimbursement.

Digit-Specific Modifiers (FA, F1-F9, TA, T1-T9): These modifiers specify exactly which finger or toe was involved in treatment, providing detail essential for proper claims processing and medical record documentation.

FA: Left hand, thumb	**TA:** Left foot, great toe
F1: Left hand, second digit	**T1:** Left foot, second digit
F2: Left hand, third digit	**T2:** Left foot, third digit
F3: Left hand, fourth digit	**T3:** Left foot, fourth digit
F4: Left hand, fifth digit	**T4:** Left foot, fifth digit
F5: Right hand, thumb	**T5:** Right foot, great toe
F6: Right hand, second digit	**T6:** Right foot, second digit
F7: Right hand, third digit	**T7:** Right foot, third digit
F8: Right hand, fourth digit	**T8:** Right foot, fourth digit
F9: Right hand, fifth digit	**T9:** Right foot, fifth digit

Clinical Application: A patient with diabetes develops infected ingrown toenails on both great toes. The provider treats each toe separately during the same visit. Using modifiers TA (left great toe) and T5 (right great toe) clearly documents that two separate sites required treatment, supporting separate billing for each service.

Why These Modifiers Matter: Without digit-specific modifiers, payers might assume duplicate billing when multiple digits are treated. The modifiers clarify that legitimate separate services were provided, preventing inappropriate denials while ensuring accurate medical documentation.

Eyelid Modifiers (E1-E4): These modifiers specify which eyelid received treatment, crucial for ophthalmologic and oculoplastic procedures.

E1: Upper left eyelid
E2: Lower left eyelid
E3: Upper right eyelid
E4: Lower right eyelid

Clinical Application: A patient has chalazion lesions on both upper eyelids requiring incision and drainage. Using modifiers E1 (upper left) and E3 (upper right) documents that two separate procedures were performed on different anatomical sites, supporting appropriate reimbursement for both services.

Left/Right Modifiers (LT, RT): These fundamental modifiers specify left or right side for procedures that could be performed on either side of the body. While simple, these modifiers prevent billing confusion and claims processing delays.

LT: Left side
RT: Right side

Clinical Application: A patient receives a knee injection for osteoarthritis in the right knee. Modifier RT clarifies which knee received treatment, ensuring accurate medical records and appropriate claims processing.

Service Delivery Modifiers: How and Where Services Were Provided

Location-Specific Modifiers: Several HCPCS modifiers specify where services were provided, information that can affect reimbursement rates and coverage decisions.

Modifier 77: Repeat service by another physician or other qualified healthcare professional
Modifier 76: Repeat procedure or service by same physician or other qualified healthcare professional
Modifier 95: Synchronous telemedicine service rendered via a real-time interactive audio and video telecommunications system

Telemedicine Modifier 95: The COVID-19 pandemic dramatically expanded telemedicine usage, making modifier 95 increasingly important. This modifier indicates services provided through interactive audio-video technology rather than in-person visits.

Clinical Application: A patient with diabetes receives follow-up care through a video visit, discussing blood sugar control, medication adjustments, and lifestyle modifications. Modifier 95 appended to the E/M code indicates the telemedicine delivery method, ensuring proper claims processing according to payer telemedicine policies.

Remember: Telemedicine policies vary significantly among payers. Some accept modifier 95 for many service types, while others have strict limitations. Always verify specific payer policies before billing telemedicine services.

Service Level Modifiers: Some HCPCS modifiers describe the level or intensity of services provided, helping payers understand service complexity and supporting appropriate reimbursement.

Modifier KX: Requirements specified in the medical policy have been met This modifier indicates that specific coverage criteria were met, often used with services requiring documentation of medical necessity or prior authorization.

Clinical Application: Power wheelchair coding requires extensive documentation of mobility limitations and trial of less expensive equipment. Modifier KX indicates all required documentation has been obtained and coverage criteria have been met, preventing delays in wheelchair approval.

Supplier-Related Modifiers: Clarifying Equipment and Supply Situations

Rental vs. Purchase Modifiers: DME can be rented or purchased, with different reimbursement rules applying to each scenario. Modifiers clarify the billing arrangement, ensuring correct payment processing.

Modifier RR: Rental
Modifier NU: New equipment
Modifier UE: Used equipment

Clinical Application: A patient requires a hospital bed for home use. The DME supplier provides a rental unit initially (modifier RR) to ensure the equipment meets the patient's needs. After three months, if the rental payments would exceed purchase price, the equipment converts to a purchase, requiring modifier NU on subsequent claims.

Understanding DME Payment Rules: DME payment rules are complex, with rental periods, rental caps, and maintenance payments that vary by equipment type. The modifiers you use must align with these payment rules to ensure correct reimbursement.

Modifier Combinations: When Multiple Modifiers Are Necessary

Modifier Sequencing: Sometimes services require multiple HCPCS modifiers to accurately describe all relevant circumstances. Understanding proper modifier sequencing ensures clear communication and appropriate reimbursement.

General Sequencing Principles:

- Pricing modifiers (those affecting reimbursement) typically come first
- Informational modifiers (providing additional detail) follow
- Anatomical modifiers usually appear last

Example: A patient receives bilateral knee injections during a telemedicine encounter. The coding might include modifier 95 (telemedicine), modifier 50 (bilateral procedure), or separate services with modifiers RT and LT depending on payer requirements and coding guidelines.

Payer-Specific Modifier Requirements: Different payers have different modifier preferences and requirements. Medicare might require specific modifiers that commercial payers don't recognize, or commercial payers might require modifiers Medicare doesn't use.

Research Requirements: Before implementing modifier usage, research specific payer requirements. Create payer-specific reference guides noting which modifiers each payer requires, prefers, or prohibits. This research prevents claim denials and resubmission delays.

Practice Questions with Comprehensive Explanations

Now test your HCPCS Level II mastery with these challenging scenarios that mirror real-world coding situations:

Question 1: A patient receives a new lightweight manual wheelchair with specialized seating system. The wheelchair is coded with K0009. Which modifier indicates this is new equipment?

A) RR (rental)
B) NU (new equipment)
C) UE (used equipment)
D) KX (requirements met)

Answer: B
Explanation: Modifier NU indicates new durable medical equipment, distinguishing it from used equipment (UE) or rental equipment (RR). This distinction affects reimbursement rates and documentation requirements. New equipment typically receives higher reimbursement than used equipment, and different documentation may be required to support the medical necessity of new rather than used equipment. The modifier KX relates to meeting coverage requirements but doesn't specify whether equipment is new or used.

Question 2: A patient with diabetes receives treatment for an ingrown toenail on the left great toe and right second toe during the same visit. How should these services be coded?

A) Single code with no modifiers
B) Single code with modifier 50 (bilateral)
C) Separate codes with modifiers TA (left great toe) and T6 (right second digit)
D) Separate codes with modifiers LT and RT

Answer: C
Explanation: Different toes require digit-specific modifiers that precisely identify the anatomical location of each service. Modifier TA identifies the left foot great toe, while T6 identifies the right foot second digit. This precision prevents confusion about which toes were treated and supports billing for two separate services. Modifier 50 (bilateral) would be inappropriate because it indicates identical procedures on both sides of the body, which isn't the case here since different toes on different feet were treated. General left/right modifiers (LT, RT) lack the specificity needed for digit identification.

Question 3: A physician provides a follow-up visit for hypertension management via real-time audio-video telemedicine. Which modifier indicates the telemedicine delivery method?

A) 77 (repeat service by another physician)
B) 95 (synchronous telemedicine service)
C) GT (via interactive audio-video)
D) No modifier needed for telemedicine

Answer: B
Explanation: Modifier 95 indicates services provided through synchronous (real-time) interactive audio-video telecommunications systems. This modifier became crucial during the COVID-19 pandemic as telemedicine usage expanded dramatically. While modifier GT was previously used for some telemedicine services, modifier 95 is now the standard modifier for most telemedicine services under current coding guidelines. The distinction between synchronous (real-time) and asynchronous (store-and-forward) telemedicine is important—modifier 95 specifically indicates real-time interactive communication, not simple review of transmitted information.

Question 4: A patient receives a hospital bed rental for home use after hip surgery. The initial claim should include which modifier?

A) NU (new equipment)
B) RR (rental)
C) UE (used equipment)
D) KX (requirements met)

Answer: B
Explanation: Modifier RR indicates rental equipment, which is the appropriate modifier for the initial rental period of DME. Many types of expensive DME start as rentals, allowing patients to ensure the equipment meets their needs before committing to purchase. DME rental rules are complex—rental payments may continue for specified periods, after which the equipment may convert to purchase or require different billing approaches. Using the correct modifier from the start ensures proper payment processing and prevents billing errors. Modifier KX might also be used if specific coverage requirements have been met, but RR is the primary modifier indicating the rental status.

Question 5: A power wheelchair prescription requires documenting that all Medicare coverage criteria have been met. Which modifier indicates this documentation is complete?

A) NU (new equipment)
B) RR (rental)
C) KX (requirements specified in medical policy have been met)
D) 59 (distinct procedural service)

Answer: C
Explanation: Modifier KX indicates that all requirements specified in the medical policy have been met. For power wheelchairs, this includes extensive documentation of mobility limitations, failure of less expensive alternatives, and compliance with specific coverage criteria defined in Medicare's Local Coverage Determinations (LCDs). Without this modifier, power wheelchair claims may be denied even if coverage criteria were actually met, because the modifier serves as the supplier's certification that required documentation has been obtained. This modifier is particularly important for high-cost DME items subject to stringent coverage criteria.

Question 6: A patient receives orthotic treatment on three fingers of the right hand (thumb, index, and middle fingers) during the same visit. How should this be coded?

A) Single code with no modifiers
B) Single code with modifier 50 (bilateral)
C) Three separate line items with modifiers F5, F6, and F7
D) Single code with modifier 22 (increased procedural services)

Answer: C
Explanation: When multiple digits are treated, each digit requires separate billing with the appropriate digit-specific modifier. F5 identifies the right thumb, F6 the right index finger (second digit), and F7 the right middle finger (third digit). This detailed coding documents exactly which digits received treatment, supports medical necessity for treating multiple digits, and enables appropriate reimbursement for each service. Billing a single code would significantly undervalue the services provided, while modifier 50 (bilateral) would be incorrect because it indicates treatment of corresponding structures on opposite sides of the body.

Question 7: Temporary code G0101 is used for which type of service?

A) New durable medical equipment
B) Cervical or vaginal cancer screening; pelvic and clinical breast examination
C) Outpatient hospital device
D) Vision services

Answer: B
Explanation: G0101 is a specific Medicare temporary code for preventive services—cervical or vaginal cancer screening that includes pelvic and clinical breast examination. This G code illustrates how temporary codes address services covered by Medicare but lacking CPT® codes. The code ensures appropriate billing for these important preventive services while providing data about utilization patterns. Remember that G codes are often Medicare-specific and may not be recognized by commercial payers, which might require different coding approaches for the same services.

Question 8: A patient receives both upper eyelid procedures—right upper lid lesion removal and left upper lid ptosis repair. The coding should include:

A) Single code with modifier 50 (bilateral)
B) Two codes with modifiers E3 (right upper) and E1 (left upper)
C) Two codes with modifiers RT and LT
D) Single code with no modifiers

Answer: B
Explanation: Different procedures on different eyelids require separate coding with specific eyelid modifiers. E3 identifies the right upper eyelid, while E1 identifies the left upper eyelid. Even though both services involve upper eyelids, the procedures are different (lesion removal vs. ptosis repair), so modifier 50 (identical bilateral procedures) would be inappropriate. The eyelid-specific modifiers provide more precise anatomical detail than general left/right modifiers and are required for proper eyelid procedure coding. This precision ensures accurate medical documentation and appropriate reimbursement for distinctly different procedures.

Question 9: An ambulance transports a patient from home to hospital. The appropriate coding requires which type of HCPCS code?

A) C code (outpatient hospital device)
B) A code (transportation services)
C) E code (durable medical equipment)
D) Q code (temporary service)

Answer: B
Explanation: A codes include transportation services, with specific codes for different types of ambulance transport (basic life support, advanced life support, specialty care transport) and different transport scenarios (emergency vs. non-emergency, mileage-based charges). Ambulance coding is highly specific, with separate codes for the base rate and additional mileage, and modifiers indicating origin and destination. Understanding ambulance coding requires knowledge of both the specific HCPCS codes and the complex rules governing medical necessity documentation for non-emergency ambulance transport.

Question 10: A patient uses a hospital bed at home for three months as a rental, then converts to purchase. What coding changes occur?

A) Continue using modifier RR (rental) indefinitely
B) Change from modifier RR (rental) to modifier NU (new) after rental cap reached
C) No modifier changes needed
D) Add modifier KX after purchase conversion

Answer: B
Explanation: When DME rental payments reach the rental cap (typically after 13 months for capped rental items, or sooner for items with shorter rental periods), the equipment converts from rental to purchase. This conversion requires changing the billing modifier from RR (rental) to NU (new equipment purchase). The modifier change reflects the fundamental change in the financial transaction—from temporary equipment use to permanent ownership.

After purchase, different billing rules apply for maintenance, repairs, and replacement, making the correct modifier essential for proper claims processing. Understanding DME rental-to-purchase rules prevents billing errors and ensures appropriate reimbursement throughout the equipment lifecycle.

Chapter 16 Summary: Your HCPCS Level II Mastery

Congratulations! You've now mastered HCPCS Level II coding, adding a crucial dimension to your comprehensive coding expertise. This achievement completes your understanding of the three major coding systems that drive healthcare billing and documentation.

What You've Accomplished

Complete Code System Mastery: You now understand and can confidently use all three major coding systems—ICD-10-CM for diagnoses, CPT® for procedures and professional services, and HCPCS Level II for supplies, equipment, and services not covered by CPT®. This comprehensive expertise makes you invaluable to any healthcare organization.

Temporary Code Navigation: You've mastered the challenging world of temporary codes, understanding how they support healthcare innovation while creating coding complexity. You know how to monitor code changes, apply temporary codes appropriately, and transition smoothly when temporary codes become permanent or are discontinued.

Modifier Precision: Your command of HCPCS modifiers enables you to communicate precise clinical and billing information that affects reimbursement and supports accurate medical documentation. You understand when modifiers are required, how to sequence multiple modifiers, and how to adapt modifier usage to different payer requirements.

DME Expertise: You've developed specialized knowledge of durable medical equipment coding, including complex rental-to-purchase rules, supplier modifiers, and documentation requirements that ensure appropriate reimbursement while preventing fraud and abuse.

Payer Variations: You appreciate how different payers use HCPCS codes differently, with Medicare, Medicaid, and commercial insurance having distinct policies about code acceptance, modifier requirements, and documentation expectations.

Integration with Your Complete Coding Knowledge

Your HCPCS Level II expertise now integrates seamlessly with your other coding skills, creating a complete picture of healthcare coding:

Diagnosis Coding Foundation: Your ICD-10-CM knowledge ensures you can support HCPCS coding with appropriate diagnosis codes that establish medical necessity for equipment, supplies, and services.

Procedure Coding Complement: Your CPT® expertise helps you understand when to use CPT® codes and when HCPCS Level II codes are more appropriate, preventing coding errors that could affect reimbursement.

Complete Claim Preparation: You can now prepare complete, accurate claims that include all necessary diagnoses, procedures, supplies, equipment, and modifiers—nothing missing, nothing incorrect, everything properly documented.

Your Professional Future

This comprehensive coding education positions you for success in any healthcare setting. You're ready to:

Excel in Any Specialty: Your broad knowledge base allows you to work confidently in primary care, specialized medicine, hospital settings, or any other healthcare environment.

Lead Coding Teams: Your comprehensive expertise qualifies you to train others, supervise coding departments, and ensure organizational coding compliance.

Adapt to Changes: Healthcare coding continues evolving, but your systematic understanding of coding principles allows you to adapt quickly to new codes, regulations, and technologies.

Support Quality Care: Most importantly, your accurate coding directly supports quality patient care by ensuring appropriate reimbursement for necessary services, supplies, and equipment.

Remember that coding mastery isn't just about knowing codes—it's about understanding healthcare, appreciating clinical care, and contributing meaningfully to the complex system that delivers medical services to millions of people.

You've built a strong foundation. Now take that knowledge into the world and make a difference through coding excellence!

PART VI: COMPLIANCE AND REGULATORY ISSUES

Chapter 17: Medical Coding Compliance

"In matters of style, swim with the current; in matters of principle, stand like a rock." - Thomas Jefferson

Medical coding compliance represents the intersection of technical accuracy, legal requirements, and ethical responsibility. Every code you assign carries weight far beyond its numerical value—it affects patient care, provider reimbursement, healthcare statistics, and legal liability. Understanding compliance isn't just about avoiding penalties; it's about upholding the integrity of the entire healthcare system.

The landscape of healthcare compliance has evolved dramatically over the past two decades. What once consisted of relatively simple billing rules has transformed into a complex regulatory environment where violations can result in massive fines, criminal prosecution, and career-ending consequences. Yet despite this complexity, the core principle remains simple: code accurately what's documented, document completely what's provided, and always prioritize truthfulness over financial gain.

This chapter transforms compliance from an abstract concept into practical, applicable knowledge that protects you, your employer, and your patients. You'll learn to recognize compliance risks before they become problems, understand the regulatory framework that governs medical coding, and develop the ethical foundation that guides decisions in ambiguous situations.

Your technical coding skills mean nothing if compliance failures undermine your work. The most accurate coder in the world becomes a liability if they don't understand fraud and abuse laws, documentation requirements, and audit processes. This chapter ensures your technical expertise is matched by compliance knowledge that makes you a trusted, valuable professional.

By the end of this chapter, you'll approach coding decisions with a compliance-first mindset that protects everyone involved while maintaining the accuracy and integrity the healthcare system demands. You'll understand not just what the rules are, but why they exist and how to apply them in real-world situations where the right answer isn't always obvious.

HIPAA Privacy and Security Rules

The Health Insurance Portability and Accountability Act of 1996 fundamentally changed how healthcare information is protected, creating a national standard for privacy and security that affects every person who works with medical records. Understanding HIPAA isn't optional for medical coders—it's an essential responsibility that protects patients and keeps you out of legal trouble.

Understanding Protected Health Information (PHI)

Protected Health Information forms the foundation of HIPAA regulations. Before you can protect information properly, you must understand exactly what qualifies as PHI and why it requires special handling.

Defining Protected Health Information: PHI encompasses any individually identifiable health information transmitted or maintained in any form or medium by a covered entity or its business associates. This definition is deliberately broad, capturing virtually all information that could identify a patient and relates to their health, healthcare, or payment for healthcare.

The key phrase is "individually identifiable." Information becomes PHI when it includes or could reasonably be used to identify a specific individual. This goes beyond obvious identifiers like names and social security numbers to include dates, geographic information, and even unique characteristics that might identify someone in a small population.

Examples of Protected Health Information:

Consider a simple scenario: A patient named Maria Rodriguez visits Dr. Smith for diabetes management on March 15, 2025. The following information all constitutes PHI:

Direct Identifiers: Maria Rodriguez's name, her address at 123 Main Street, her phone number (555-1234), her social security number, and her medical record number (MRN: 456789) all directly identify her. These are obvious PHI elements that clearly require protection.

Dates Related to the Individual: The appointment date (March 15, 2025), Maria's date of birth (June 12, 1975), and even the date her diabetes was diagnosed (August 3, 2018) all constitute PHI. Any date related to an individual's health or healthcare qualifies for protection.

Healthcare Information: The diagnosis of diabetes mellitus, her hemoglobin A1c result of 7.2%, her current medications including metformin 1000mg twice daily, and her blood pressure reading of 138/82 all represent health information that, when connected to Maria's identity, becomes PHI.

Payment Information: Maria's insurance company name (Blue Cross Blue Shield), her member ID number, the $30 copay she paid, and the claim submitted for $185 all constitute PHI because they relate to payment for Maria's healthcare.

Photographic Images: If Dr. Smith photographs Maria's diabetic foot ulcer for medical records, that image contains her face and health information, making it PHI requiring the same protections as other medical data.

The 18 HIPAA Identifiers: HIPAA specifically identifies 18 categories of information that must be removed to de-identify health information:

1. Names of patients, relatives, employers
2. Geographic subdivisions smaller than state (except first three digits of ZIP code if area contains more than 20,000 people)
3. Dates directly related to an individual (birth, admission, discharge, death)
4. Telephone numbers
5. Fax numbers
6. Email addresses
7. Social Security numbers
8. Medical record numbers
9. Health plan beneficiary numbers
10. Account numbers
11. Certificate/license numbers
12. Vehicle identifiers and serial numbers
13. Device identifiers and serial numbers
14. Web URLs
15. Internet Protocol (IP) addresses
16. Biometric identifiers (fingerprints, voiceprints)
17. Full-face photographs and comparable images
18. Any other unique identifying number, characteristic, or code

Why This Matters for Coders: As a medical coder, you work with PHI constantly. Every chart you review, every code you assign, and every claim you submit contains PHI that must be protected. Understanding what constitutes PHI helps you recognize when special precautions are needed and avoid inadvertent disclosures.

The Privacy Rule: Patient Rights and Responsibilities

The HIPAA Privacy Rule establishes national standards for protecting PHI, balancing the need for information exchange in healthcare delivery with individuals' rights to privacy. Understanding these rules helps you respect patient rights while performing your coding duties.

Patient Rights Under HIPAA:

Right to Access Medical Records: Patients have the right to inspect and obtain copies of their medical records within 30 days of requesting them. This includes billing records, diagnostic reports, treatment notes, and any other PHI maintained by their healthcare provider. As a coder, you might encounter access requests that require coordination with medical records departments.

When Linda Chen requests copies of her records from the past five years to take to a new physician, the healthcare facility must provide them within 30 days. If records are maintained off-site or in archival storage, an additional 30-day extension may be granted. The facility can charge reasonable, cost-based fees for copying and mailing, but cannot deny access due to inability to pay.

Right to Request Amendments: Patients who believe their medical records contain errors or incomplete information can request amendments. While providers aren't required to make all requested changes, they must have a process for reviewing and responding to amendment requests.

Michael Thompson reviews his medical records and discovers a note stating he's allergic to penicillin, which he's not. He submits an amendment request explaining that he's never had a penicillin allergy and believes this was confused with another patient. The provider must respond within 60 days, either making the amendment or explaining why the request is denied. If denied, Michael has the right to submit a statement of disagreement that becomes part of his permanent record.

Right to an Accounting of Disclosures: Patients can request a list of certain disclosures of their PHI made by the healthcare provider. This accounting includes disclosures for purposes other than treatment, payment, or healthcare operations, helping patients track who has accessed their information.

Sarah Martinez suspects her medical information was inappropriately shared with her employer. She requests an accounting of disclosures for the past six years. The healthcare provider must provide a list showing: date of disclosure, name and address of recipient, brief description of information disclosed, and purpose of disclosure. This accounting doesn't include routine disclosures for treatment, payment, or operations, but does include disclosures to public health authorities, legal proceedings, or other non-routine purposes.

Right to Request Restrictions: Patients can request that healthcare providers limit how PHI is used or disclosed. While providers aren't required to agree to all requests, they must agree to certain restrictions, particularly regarding disclosures to health plans when patients pay out-of-pocket in full.

David Williams undergoes treatment for a minor cosmetic procedure and pays the $500 fee completely out-of-pocket. He requests that the provider not disclose any information about this treatment to his health insurance company. Under HIPAA, the provider must honor this request because David paid for the service in full and the disclosure isn't required by law.

Right to Receive Privacy Notices: Patients must receive a Notice of Privacy Practices (NPP) that explains how their PHI may be used and disclosed, their rights under HIPAA, and the provider's legal duties regarding PHI protection. This notice must be provided at the first service delivery and must be available for review at any time.

Permitted Uses and Disclosures:

HIPAA permits PHI use and disclosure without patient authorization for specific purposes essential to healthcare delivery and operations:

Treatment, Payment, and Healthcare Operations (TPO): This represents the core exception allowing healthcare to function. Treatment includes providing, coordinating, or managing healthcare services. Payment encompasses billing, collection, and reimbursement activities. Healthcare operations include quality assessment, credentialing, training, and business planning.

As a medical coder, most of your PHI access falls under TPO exceptions. When you review a chart to assign diagnosis and procedure codes, you're engaging in payment activities. When you query a physician for clarification, you're supporting both treatment documentation and payment accuracy. When you participate in coding education or quality reviews, you're involved in healthcare operations.

Consider a typical day in a coding department: You review Dr. Johnson's operative report to code a laparoscopic cholecystectomy. This review for coding purposes constitutes payment activity—permitted under TPO. You notice the report mentions complications not reflected in the discharge summary and send a query to Dr. Johnson requesting clarification. This communication supports accurate documentation for treatment continuity and proper coding for payment—both permitted under TPO. Later, you participate in a team meeting reviewing coding accuracy rates, which constitutes healthcare operations—also permitted under TPO.

Required by Law: Certain situations mandate PHI disclosure regardless of patient preference. These include court orders, subpoenas in certain circumstances, mandatory public health reporting, and law enforcement requests meeting specific criteria.

When the local health department contacts the hospital requesting information about a patient diagnosed with tuberculosis, the hospital must provide the information without patient authorization. Tuberculosis is a reportable disease, and public health reporting represents a required disclosure. Similarly, if a court issues a properly executed subpoena for medical records in a personal injury lawsuit, the hospital must comply with the legal order.

Public Health Activities: Healthcare providers must disclose PHI to public health authorities for disease prevention, injury reporting, vital statistics, and public health investigations. These disclosures protect community health even when they involve patient information.

Abuse, Neglect, or Domestic Violence: Providers may disclose PHI when they believe a patient is a victim of abuse, neglect, or domestic violence, particularly when reporting is mandated by state law or when necessary to prevent serious harm.

The Security Rule: Protecting Electronic PHI

The HIPAA Security Rule establishes national standards for protecting electronic protected health information (ePHI), recognizing that electronic data requires specialized safeguards beyond traditional paper record protections. Understanding these requirements helps you work safely in electronic health record systems.

Administrative Safeguards:

Administrative safeguards represent the policies, procedures, and processes that govern information security within healthcare organizations. These create the management framework supporting technical and physical security measures.

Security Management Process: Every covered entity must implement policies and procedures to prevent, detect, contain, and correct security violations. This includes conducting regular risk assessments, implementing risk management strategies, establishing sanction policies for employees who violate security rules, and maintaining information system activity review processes.

At Memorial Hospital, the compliance department conducts annual risk assessments examining potential threats to ePHI security. They evaluate risks ranging from malware and hacking attempts to internal breaches and natural disasters. Based on these assessments, they prioritize security improvements, allocate resources to address high-risk areas, and update security policies to reflect emerging threats. When the assessment reveals that mobile device security is inadequate, the hospital implements new policies requiring encryption on all devices accessing ePHI and establishes procedures for remote wiping of lost or stolen devices.

Workforce Security: Organizations must implement procedures ensuring workforce members have appropriate access to ePHI and preventing unauthorized access. This includes authorization processes, workforce clearance procedures, and termination procedures that ensure departing employees lose system access immediately.

When Maria Rodriguez joins the coding department at Memorial Hospital, her manager submits an access request specifying exactly which systems Maria needs for her job duties. Information technology reviews the request, verifies Maria's employment and role, and grants access to coding software, electronic health records for her assigned patient types, and billing systems—but not to payroll, email archives, or administrative systems she doesn't need for her job. This principle of "minimum necessary access" ensures Maria can perform her duties while limiting potential exposure if her credentials are compromised.

Information Access Management: Policies must govern access to ePHI, including authorization processes, access establishment procedures, and access modification protocols. These policies ensure only appropriate individuals can access patient information and that access levels match job responsibilities.

Security Awareness and Training: All workforce members must receive security awareness training covering security reminders, malware protection, password management, and security incident reporting. This training must occur regularly and be updated to reflect new threats and technologies.

At quarterly staff meetings, Memorial Hospital's security officer presents brief training modules covering current security threats. Recent sessions have addressed phishing emails (with examples of actual attempts targeting the hospital), social engineering tactics used by hackers, proper password management (including why password reuse across accounts is dangerous), and how to recognize and report suspicious activity. These regular reminders keep security awareness high and reduce risk of successful attacks.

Security Incident Procedures: Organizations must establish procedures for identifying and responding to security incidents, including documentation requirements, investigation protocols, and mitigation strategies. These procedures ensure incidents are handled consistently and lessons learned prevent future occurrences.

Physical Safeguards:

Physical safeguards protect the physical computer systems, buildings, and equipment that house ePHI. These measures prevent unauthorized physical access to information systems and the facilities that house them.

Facility Access Controls: Covered entities must implement policies limiting physical access to electronic information systems and the facilities where they're housed. This includes establishing visitor control procedures, maintaining access logs, and implementing emergency access procedures for situations requiring immediate system access.

Memorial Hospital's data center, which houses servers containing all patient records, requires badge access, and all entries are logged electronically. A security guard monitors the entrance 24/7, and visitors must sign in, provide identification, and be escorted at all times. The facility has fire suppression systems, emergency power generators, and environmental controls maintaining optimal temperature and humidity. After discovering that a former employee's badge still granted access weeks after termination, the hospital implemented automated access revocation tied to HR termination processes, preventing future unauthorized access.

Workstation Use: Organizations must specify proper functions for workstations accessing ePHI and the manner in which those functions should be performed. This includes policies on screen positioning, automatic logoff periods, and appropriate use of portable devices.

Memorial Hospital's coding department arranges workstations so screens aren't visible from hallways or public areas. Computer screens automatically lock after five minutes of inactivity, requiring password re-entry to resume work. Coders are trained never to leave workstations unattended while logged into patient records and to position themselves to prevent shoulder-surfing by visitors or colleagues passing by.

Workstation Security: Physical safeguards must protect workstations and electronic media from unauthorized access. This includes securing computers, limiting device movement, and protecting portable devices.

Device and Media Controls: Policies must govern receipt and removal of hardware and electronic media containing ePHI, as well as movement within facilities and disposal/reuse of devices. This prevents ePHI exposure through discarded or reassigned equipment.

When Memorial Hospital replaces aging computer equipment, the IT department follows strict disposal procedures. Hard drives are removed from retired computers and destroyed using industrial shredders that render data unrecoverable. The hospital maintains logs documenting each device's disposal, including date, method, and personnel involved. When selling surplus equipment, the hospital ensures complete data erasure before transfer, and purchasers sign acknowledgments that they understand devices previously contained ePHI.

Technical Safeguards:

Technical safeguards involve the technology and policies protecting ePHI and controlling access to it. These represent the front line of defense against electronic security breaches.

Access Control: Technical safeguards must ensure only authorized individuals can access ePHI. This includes unique user identification, emergency access procedures, automatic logoff, and encryption when appropriate.

Each Memorial Hospital employee receives unique login credentials that identify them individually in all system logs. The hospital implements role-based access control, granting access based on job function rather than individually configured for each user. When Sarah Chen transfers from the emergency department coding team to surgical coding, her access automatically updates to reflect her new role's requirements. If the hospital experiences a mass casualty event requiring emergency department activation, predetermined emergency access procedures grant temporary elevated privileges to responding staff, with all access logged for later review.

Audit Controls: Systems must implement hardware, software, and procedural mechanisms recording and examining access to and activity in information systems containing ePHI. These audit trails enable detection of unauthorized access and investigation of suspected breaches.

Memorial Hospital's EHR system logs every access to patient records, recording user identity, date and time, patient accessed, and actions taken. The compliance department runs regular reports identifying unusual access patterns—employees accessing records of family members, friends, or celebrities; excessive record access; or access outside normal work hours. When these reports flag potential inappropriate access, investigators review the activity and take appropriate action ranging from counseling to termination and, in serious cases, referral to law enforcement.

Integrity: Policies and procedures must protect ePHI from improper alteration or destruction, ensuring information accuracy and completeness.

Person or Entity Authentication: Procedures must verify that persons or entities seeking access to ePHI are who they claim to be. This includes password policies, biometric authentication, and multi-factor authentication for high-risk access.

Memorial Hospital implements multi-factor authentication for remote access to patient records. Employees working from home must enter their password and then confirm identity using a code sent to their registered mobile device. This two-factor authentication significantly reduces risk of unauthorized access even if passwords are compromised through phishing or other attacks.

Transmission Security: Technical safeguards must protect ePHI transmitted over electronic networks from unauthorized access. This includes encryption for transmissions over open networks and careful monitoring of all transmission methods.

HIPAA Violations and Penalties

Understanding potential consequences of HIPAA violations helps you appreciate the seriousness of compliance requirements and motivates careful adherence to security and privacy rules.

Violation Tiers and Penalty Structure:

HIPAA violations are categorized into four tiers based on level of culpability, with penalties increasing based on knowledge and intent:

Tier 1: Lack of Knowledge The covered entity or business associate was unaware and could not have realistically known about the violation. This represents the lowest level of culpability and carries minimum penalties.

Minimum Penalty: $100 per violation **Maximum Penalty:** $50,000 per violation **Annual Cap:** $1.5 million for identical violations

Example: A small medical practice with limited IT expertise unknowingly fails to encrypt laptops used by traveling physicians. Despite reasonable security efforts, the practice wasn't aware of the specific encryption requirement. When discovered during a routine audit, the practice faces Tier 1 penalties but receives credit for good faith efforts and implements corrections immediately.

Tier 2: Reasonable Cause The violation resulted from circumstances that would make it unreasonable to comply, despite reasonable diligence. The entity knew or should have known about the risk but couldn't prevent the violation.

Minimum Penalty: $1,000 per violation **Maximum Penalty:** $50,000 per violation **Annual Cap:** $1.5 million for identical violations

Example: A hospital implements strong security measures, but a sophisticated hacking attack exploits a previously unknown software vulnerability. The hospital had exercised reasonable diligence with firewalls, intrusion detection, and regular security updates, but the zero-day exploit couldn't have been prevented with available technology. The breach qualifies as reasonable cause because the hospital couldn't have prevented it despite due diligence.

Tier 3: Willful Neglect, Corrected The violation involved willful neglect but was corrected within 30 days of discovery. This reflects serious non-compliance but gives credit for prompt correction.

Minimum Penalty: $10,000 per violation **Maximum Penalty:** $50,000 per violation **Annual Cap:** $1.5 million for identical violations

Example: A medical practice ignores repeated warnings from its IT vendor about needed security updates, reasoning that they haven't had problems and updates might disrupt operations. When a breach occurs exploiting these known vulnerabilities, regulators determine the practice demonstrated willful neglect. However, because the practice immediately implements all updates and strengthens security procedures within 30 days of the breach, penalties apply at Tier 3 rather than Tier 4.

Tier 4: Willful Neglect, Uncorrected The violation involved willful neglect and was not corrected. This represents the most serious category with maximum penalties.

Minimum Penalty: $50,000 per violation **Maximum Penalty:** $1.5 million per violation **Annual Cap:** $1.5 million for identical violations

Example: A physician's practice repeatedly violates HIPAA security requirements despite multiple warnings from regulators. Employees routinely email unencrypted patient information to personal email accounts, share passwords, and access records without authorization. Even after receiving notice of violations and specific corrective action requirements, the practice makes no meaningful changes. This willful neglect without correction results in maximum penalties and potential criminal prosecution.

Criminal Penalties:

Beyond civil monetary penalties, certain HIPAA violations can result in criminal prosecution with potential imprisonment:

Tier 1 Criminal Penalties: Knowingly obtaining or disclosing PHI without authorization:

- Fine up to $50,000
- Imprisonment up to 1 year
- Or both

Tier 2 Criminal Penalties: Obtaining PHI under false pretenses:

- Fine up to $100,000
- Imprisonment up to 5 years
- Or both

Tier 3 Criminal Penalties:
Obtaining or disclosing PHI with intent to sell, transfer, or use for commercial advantage, personal gain, or malicious harm:

- Fine up to $250,000
- Imprisonment up to 10 years
- Or both

Real-World HIPAA Violation Examples:

Understanding actual cases helps you recognize risky behaviors and avoid similar violations:

Case Study: The Curious Employee A hospital employee with legitimate system access repeatedly accessed medical records of friends, family members, and local celebrities out of curiosity rather than for any work-related purpose. Audit logs detected the inappropriate access pattern, triggering an investigation. The employee was immediately terminated, and the hospital reported the breach to affected patients and regulatory authorities.

Outcome: The employee faced criminal charges for unauthorized PHI access. The hospital faced civil penalties for inadequate access monitoring and delayed breach detection but received reduced penalties for prompt reporting and implementing enhanced monitoring systems. This case demonstrates that even authorized users commit HIPAA violations when accessing records without legitimate work-related reasons.

Case Study: The Unencrypted Laptop A physician's laptop containing unencrypted patient records was stolen from a locked vehicle. The laptop contained demographic information, diagnoses, and treatment details for approximately 2,000 patients. The theft occurred despite the practice having a policy requiring encryption, but enforcement was lax.

Outcome: The practice faced Tier 3 penalties for willful neglect (failure to enforce its own encryption policy) but received credit for reporting the breach promptly and immediately implementing laptop encryption and tracking software. Affected patients received notification and credit monitoring services. This case illustrates that good policies mean nothing without enforcement and that physical security measures (locked car) don't substitute for technical safeguards (encryption).

Case Study: The Gossiping Staff Clinic staff members routinely discussed patient conditions and treatments in public areas including the waiting room, cafeteria, and parking lot. Complaints from patients who overheard conversations about their own or others' conditions triggered an investigation revealing widespread privacy lapses.

Outcome: The clinic faced penalties for inadequate privacy training and failure to maintain minimum necessary standards for PHI discussions. The investigation revealed no formal privacy training had occurred in over five years, and staff weren't aware of proper communication protocols. The clinic implemented mandatory privacy training, established designated private areas for clinical discussions, and retrained all staff on appropriate communication practices.

Fraud and Abuse Prevention

Healthcare fraud and abuse represent serious crimes that damage the entire healthcare system, increasing costs, undermining trust, and compromising patient care. Understanding the difference between honest coding errors and fraud is essential for protecting yourself and maintaining industry integrity.

Defining Fraud and Abuse

The distinction between fraud, abuse, and honest mistakes determines whether actions result in simple corrections, civil penalties, or criminal prosecution. Understanding these definitions helps you recognize the line between acceptable practice and illegal activity.

Healthcare Fraud: Fraud involves knowingly and willfully executing or attempting to execute a scheme to defraud any healthcare benefit program or obtain, by means of false or fraudulent pretenses, any money or property owned by a healthcare benefit program. The key elements are knowledge and intent—the person committing fraud knows the conduct is wrong and does it anyway.

Consider Dr. Mitchell, who routinely bills office visits as hospital visits because hospital visits reimburse at higher rates. Dr. Mitchell knows the services are provided in the office, knows hospital codes should only be used for hospital locations, and deliberately misrepresents service location to increase reimbursement. This knowing and willful misrepresentation constitutes fraud, not an honest mistake. If investigators demonstrate Dr. Mitchell understands the rules, recognizes the code misapplication, but does it anyway for financial gain, criminal prosecution becomes likely.

Healthcare Abuse: Abuse describes practices inconsistent with sound fiscal, business, or medical practices that result in unnecessary costs or improper payment. Unlike fraud, abuse doesn't require intent to deceive but involves practices that directly or indirectly result in overpayment.

Consider Dr. Roberts, who routinely performs and bills for comprehensive metabolic panels when basic metabolic panels would provide all medically necessary information. Dr. Roberts isn't intentionally defrauding anyone but has developed a habit of ordering more extensive testing than clinically justified. This pattern of excessive testing without medical necessity constitutes abuse—it results in unnecessary costs and inappropriate reimbursement even though Dr. Roberts didn't intend to commit fraud.

Honest Mistakes: Not every coding error represents fraud or abuse. Honest mistakes occur despite reasonable efforts at accuracy and don't involve intent to deceive or patterns of careless disregard for rules. The difference lies in circumstances, patterns, and response to identification.

Consider a coder who accidentally assigns a code for right-sided procedure when documentation clearly indicates left-sided procedure. The coder was working quickly, transposed the laterality, but had no intent to deceive and the error doesn't benefit anyone financially. When quality review identifies the error, the coder immediately corrects it and implements a process to prevent similar mistakes. This represents an honest error, not fraud or abuse.

Key Distinctions:

Intent and Knowledge: Fraud requires knowing and willful conduct. The person must understand they're doing something wrong and choose to do it anyway. Abuse doesn't require intent but involves careless or excessive practices. Honest mistakes occur despite good faith efforts at compliance.

Pattern vs. Isolated Occurrence: Single errors rarely constitute fraud or abuse, though egregious cases might. Patterns of similar errors, especially after correction attempts, suggest something beyond honest mistakes. Courts and regulators look for patterns indicating systemic problems or intentional conduct rather than simple human error.

Response to Identification: How organizations and individuals respond to identified errors helps distinguish between categories. Immediate correction and process improvements suggest honest mistakes. Continued errors despite awareness and correction attempts suggest abuse. Concealment or resistance to correction indicates potential fraud.

Financial Impact: The financial benefit derived from errors matters. Random coding errors that sometimes favor and sometimes disadvantage the provider suggest honest mistakes. Errors that consistently result in higher reimbursement suggest abuse or fraud, depending on intent and knowledge.

Common Fraud and Abuse Schemes

Understanding common fraudulent schemes helps you recognize red flags and avoid practices that might inadvertently involve you in illegal activity. These examples represent real-world cases that have resulted in criminal prosecution and massive penalties.

Upcoding: Upcoding involves billing for services at a higher level than actually provided or documented. This artificially inflates reimbursement by claiming more complex or extensive services than actually occurred.

Example: Evaluation and Management Upcoding Dr. Anderson routinely codes all established patient office visits as 99214 (moderate complexity) or 99215 (high complexity) regardless of actual service provided. A patient presenting for simple blood pressure medication refill receives minimal evaluation and medication adjustment but is billed at 99214 ($150 reimbursement). Another patient with multiple chronic conditions requiring extensive evaluation and medication management also receives 99214 coding. The pattern shows Dr. Anderson billing for complexity not supported by documentation or medical necessity.

Red Flags:

- Billing distributions don't match typical practice patterns
- Disproportionate use of highest-level codes compared to specialty peers
- Documentation doesn't support code level assigned
- All patients coded at same level regardless of actual service complexity

Real-World Consequence: A family practice physician was convicted of healthcare fraud for routinely upcoding office visits over a five-year period. Prosecutors demonstrated through statistical analysis that the physician's coding patterns were statistically impossible given patient demographics and visit types. The physician's average E/M code level was 4.8 out of 5, while specialty peers averaged 3.2. This pattern, combined with documentation reviews showing services didn't support high-level codes, resulted in conviction, $2.3 million in restitution, and 3 years imprisonment.

Unbundling: Unbundling (also called fragmentation) involves separating procedure components normally billed together and billing them separately to increase reimbursement. This violates NCCI edits and coding guidelines requiring comprehensive codes when available.

Example: Surgical Unbundling Dr. Kim performs a colonoscopy with biopsy and polyp removal. Rather than coding the procedure with a single comprehensive code (45385: colonoscopy with removal of tumor, polyp, or lesion), Dr. Kim's billing department codes three separate procedures: diagnostic colonoscopy (45378), biopsy (45380), and polyp removal (45385). This unbundling results in total reimbursement of approximately $900 instead of the appropriate $550 for the comprehensive code.

Red Flags:

- Billing multiple codes when comprehensive code exists
- Coding separate components of procedures typically performed together
- Ignoring NCCI edit

OIG Compliance Program Guidelines

The Office of Inspector General (OIG) provides the roadmap for healthcare compliance programs, offering guidance that has become the industry standard for preventing fraud and abuse. Understanding OIG expectations isn't just about avoiding penalties—it's about building organizational cultures that prioritize integrity and patient care over financial gain.

The OIG's compliance program guidance emerged from decades of healthcare fraud investigations that revealed common vulnerabilities in healthcare organizations. Rather than simply prosecuting fraud after it occurs, the OIG recognized that proactive compliance programs could prevent violations while protecting organizations from catastrophic legal consequences. These guidelines represent lessons learned from thousands of fraud cases and billions of dollars in penalties.

The Seven Elements of an Effective Compliance Program

Every effective healthcare compliance program, regardless of organization size or type, should incorporate seven fundamental elements. These elements work together to create a culture of compliance that permeates every aspect of operations.

Element 1: Written Policies and Procedures

Compliance begins with clear, written standards that define expected behaviors and prohibited practices. These policies must be more than bureaucratic documents collecting dust on shelves—they should be living guidelines that employees understand, reference regularly, and incorporate into daily decision-making.

Developing Comprehensive Policies: Effective compliance policies address specific risks your organization faces while providing practical guidance for common situations. A coding department policy manual should cover topics ranging from query processes and documentation requirements to relationships with pharmaceutical representatives and handling of compliance concerns.

Consider Memorial Hospital's coding compliance policy manual, which spans 150 pages and addresses every aspect of coding operations. The manual begins with a clear statement of the organization's commitment to coding accuracy and compliance, signed by both the CEO and chief compliance officer. It then provides specific guidance on dozens of topics that coding staff encounter regularly.

The section on physician queries demonstrates effective policy development. Rather than simply stating "query when documentation is unclear," the policy provides detailed guidance on when queries are appropriate, how to word them without leading physicians toward specific answers, acceptable query methods (written vs. verbal), documentation requirements for query responses, and what to do when physicians don't respond or provide unclear answers. The policy includes examples of appropriate and inappropriate queries, helping staff understand practical application.

Another section addresses the common challenge of coding incomplete procedures. When a colonoscopy is terminated early due to poor preparation, inadequate sedation, or patient discomfort, coders face questions about appropriate code selection. The policy provides decision trees helping coders determine whether to code the intended procedure with modifier -52 (reduced services) or code based on actual extent of service. It references official coding guidelines, payer-specific policies, and includes examples from actual cases the compliance committee reviewed.

Policy Implementation and Accessibility: Even excellent policies fail if employees don't know they exist or can't access them when needed. Memorial Hospital makes its compliance manual available through multiple channels: printed copies in every department, electronic version on the hospital intranet, mobile-optimized version accessible from smartphones, and searchable PDF allowing quick reference to specific topics.

New employees receive compliance training that walks through key policies during orientation. Department supervisors reference relevant policies during staff meetings. When questions arise, managers encourage staff to consult written policies rather than relying on informal practices or assumptions. This consistent emphasis on written standards creates a culture where employees expect clear guidance and feel comfortable seeking clarification.

Policy Review and Updates: Healthcare regulations, coding guidelines, and organizational practices evolve constantly. Policies must be reviewed and updated regularly to remain relevant and effective. Memorial Hospital's compliance committee reviews all policies annually, with interim updates when regulations change or new risks emerge.

When CPT® releases new codes or modifies existing ones each year, the compliance officer works with coding leadership to assess policy implications. Do new codes require additional training? Do they create fraud risks the organization should address proactively? Should query processes be modified? These questions drive policy updates that keep the organization current with evolving standards.

Element 2: Compliance Officer and Committee

Every healthcare organization needs designated individuals responsible for overseeing compliance efforts. The compliance officer serves as the organization's conscience—the person who raises uncomfortable questions, challenges questionable practices, and ensures compliance considerations influence business decisions.

The Compliance Officer's Role: An effective compliance officer must balance multiple responsibilities: educator, investigator, advisor, and enforcer. They must understand healthcare operations deeply enough to identify compliance risks while maintaining sufficient independence to challenge executives and physicians when necessary.

Sarah Martinez serves as compliance officer for Metropolitan Medical Center, a 400-bed hospital with multiple outpatient clinics. Her background as a registered nurse and certified coder gives her credibility with clinical staff, while her law degree helps her understand regulatory requirements and legal implications of compliance decisions.

Sarah's typical week demonstrates the breadth of compliance officer responsibilities. Monday morning starts with reviewing overnight incident reports for potential compliance issues. A nurse reported administering medication to the wrong patient—a serious error requiring investigation to determine if documentation was falsified or if reporting requirements were met. Sarah coordinates with risk management, quality improvement, and nursing leadership to investigate the incident and implement corrective measures.

Tuesday brings a meeting with the billing department to review recent claim denials. One pattern particularly concerns Sarah: multiple denials for medical necessity involving a specific physician. The denials suggest the physician may be performing procedures without adequate documentation of medical necessity or inappropriately coding routine services as more complex procedures. Sarah schedules a meeting with the physician to discuss documentation expectations and offers coding education to prevent future issues.

Wednesday includes compliance committee meetings where Sarah presents investigation findings, proposes policy updates, and discusses emerging compliance risks. The committee reviews a situation where several employees accessed a celebrity patient's medical record without legitimate work-related reasons. While existing policies prohibit inappropriate access, enforcement has been inconsistent. The committee approves Sarah's recommendation to implement automated monitoring that flags unusual access patterns and requires employees to document their reason for accessing records of VIP patients.

Thursday brings external auditor visits reviewing the organization's compliance with conditions of participation for Medicare certification. Sarah coordinates the audit, provides requested documentation, and addresses auditor questions. The audit identifies minor deficiencies in medical record documentation that Sarah immediately begins addressing through physician education and documentation improvement initiatives.

Friday involves strategic planning for next year's compliance priorities. Sarah analyzes data on coding denials, billing errors, and compliance incidents to identify trends requiring attention. She works with finance to develop the compliance budget, with human resources to plan employee training, and with IT to implement technical solutions supporting compliance objectives.

The Compliance Committee: No single person can oversee all compliance activities in a complex healthcare organization. Effective compliance requires a multidisciplinary committee bringing together perspectives from across the organization.

Memorial Hospital's compliance committee meets monthly and includes representatives from medical staff, nursing, coding and billing, health information management, quality improvement, legal, finance, and administration. This diverse membership ensures compliance initiatives consider clinical, operational, financial, and legal perspectives.

Committee meetings follow a structured agenda addressing standing items and emerging issues. Each meeting begins with reviewing compliance metrics: coding error rates, billing denials, documentation deficiencies, employee hotline calls, and investigation outcomes. These metrics help the committee identify trends and assess whether compliance initiatives are working.

Recent meetings addressed several significant issues. The committee reviewed findings from an external audit that identified systematic upcoding of evaluation and management services by hospitalists. Investigation revealed the problem stemmed from inadequate training rather than intentional fraud, but correction required comprehensive education, revised documentation templates, and enhanced monitoring. The committee approved a corrective action plan including mandatory coding education for all hospitalists, revision of admission and progress note templates to prompt appropriate documentation, and random chart audits for six months to verify improvement.

Another discussion addressed relationships with pharmaceutical representatives who provide meals, conference sponsorships, and other benefits to physicians and staff. While federal anti-kickback laws allow certain interactions, the committee concluded that current practices created compliance risks and appearance problems. They approved new policies limiting pharmaceutical representative access, prohibiting meals except in educational contexts, and requiring disclosure of all industry relationships. These changes required careful communication to physicians who valued relationships with representatives, but the committee determined compliance risks outweighed relationship benefits.

Element 3: Effective Training and Education

Compliance programs succeed or fail based on whether employees understand expectations and know how to apply them in real situations. Training can't be a once-yearly box-checking exercise—it must be ongoing, relevant, and engaging enough to actually change behavior.

Comprehensive New Employee Orientation: Compliance education begins during new employee orientation, before bad habits form. Memorial Hospital dedicates four hours of orientation to compliance topics, recognizing that foundation-setting pays dividends throughout employment.

New employee compliance training covers the organization's mission and values, emphasizing that financial success never justifies compromising integrity. It introduces the code of conduct, explaining expectations for ethical behavior and decision-making. It teaches employees about fraud and abuse laws, using real cases to illustrate consequences of violations. It explains how to use compliance resources including the compliance officer, hotline, and policy manual. It emphasizes that reporting concerns is not just permitted but expected, with clear explanations of non-retaliation policies.

The training uses interactive methods rather than lecture. Small group discussions explore ethical dilemmas employees might encounter. Case studies present situations requiring judgment calls about appropriate behavior. Videos featuring the CEO and compliance officer emphasize that leadership takes compliance seriously and expects the same from every employee.

Role-Specific Training: General compliance training provides foundation, but employees need specialized training addressing risks they encounter in their specific roles. Coding staff require different training than nurses, physicians, or billing specialists.

Memorial Hospital provides specialized compliance training for coders covering topics directly relevant to their daily work. The training addresses proper use of coding guidelines, including the difference between coding rules and billing policies. It teaches appropriate query processes, with extensive practice writing queries that request clarification without leading physicians toward specific responses. It covers common fraud schemes in coding, using de-identified real cases from OIG settlements to illustrate risks. It explains how to handle pressure from administration or physicians to code in ways that maximize reimbursement but violate coding accuracy.

One particularly valuable session uses actual documentation from the hospital to practice coding decision-making. Participants review operative reports, clinic notes, and diagnostic studies to assign codes, then discuss their choices. Experienced coders share how they approach ambiguous documentation, handle conflicting information, and determine when queries are necessary. This peer learning reinforces that coding often requires judgment and that seeking guidance when uncertain is expected, not a sign of weakness.

Ongoing Education and Updates: Initial training provides foundation, but ongoing education keeps compliance top-of-mind and addresses emerging issues. Memorial Hospital uses multiple methods for ongoing compliance education:

Monthly compliance newsletters highlighting recent regulatory changes, addressing common compliance questions, and sharing lessons from investigations keep compliance visible. The newsletters feature real scenarios (anonymized and generalized) that staff might encounter, with discussion of appropriate responses.

Quarterly department meetings include compliance segments addressing recent issues and upcoming changes. When OIG releases new guidance or regulatory agencies announce enforcement priorities, these meetings ensure staff understand implications for their work.

Annual mandatory training reinforces core compliance concepts while addressing new topics. Recent annual training focused on updated evaluation and management coding guidelines, requiring all coders to complete modules explaining changes and testing understanding through scenario-based questions.

Just-in-time training addresses immediate needs when changes occur. When ICD-10 codes updated mid-year with significant changes affecting frequently-used diagnoses, the compliance and coding departments developed brief training modules explaining changes and providing coding examples. Staff completed these modules within one week of the effective date, ensuring accurate coding from day one.

Element 4: Effective Lines of Communication

Compliance programs fail when employees don't feel safe raising concerns or don't know how to report suspected violations. Organizations must create multiple pathways for communication while ensuring those who report concerns face no retaliation.

The Compliance Hotline: Anonymous reporting mechanisms enable employees to raise concerns without fear of identification or retaliation. Memorial Hospital contracts with an external hotline vendor providing 24/7 reporting through multiple methods: toll-free phone number, secure website, text messaging, and postal mail.

The hotline accepts reports on any compliance concern: fraud, abuse, harassment, discrimination, safety issues, or other misconduct. Trained operators collect detailed information about reported concerns while maintaining caller anonymity. Operators ask clarifying questions, record relevant details, and assign case numbers allowing anonymous follow-up.

Hotline effectiveness depends on employee awareness and trust. Memorial Hospital promotes hotline availability through posters in break rooms, information cards included with paychecks, mentions in employee newsletters, and reminders during training. The organization tracks hotline usage as a compliance metric, concerned if call volume seems suspiciously low (suggesting employees don't feel safe reporting) or unusually high (suggesting systemic compliance problems).

Recent hotline data reveals typical patterns. Annual call volume averages 150 reports, with about 60% involving human resources issues (harassment, discrimination), 25% involving compliance matters (billing concerns, documentation issues), and 15% involving operational issues (safety concerns, policy violations). Investigations substantiate about 40% of reports, with others involving misunderstandings, insufficient evidence, or situations not actually violating policies.

Investigation and Follow-Up: Reports mean nothing without thorough investigation and appropriate response. Every hotline report triggers an investigation proportional to allegation seriousness. The compliance officer reviews each report, assigns an investigator, and establishes investigation timelines.

Consider a recent hotline report alleging that a physician was billing for services provided by nurse practitioners without appropriate supervision or billing protocols. The anonymous caller provided specific dates and patient names for review.

The compliance officer assigned a senior auditor to investigate. The auditor reviewed medical records for identified patients, examining who actually provided services, whether documentation supported billed codes, and whether supervision requirements were met. The investigation expanded to review a larger sample of the physician's billing to determine if the pattern extended beyond reported cases.

Investigation revealed the physician was billing for nurse practitioner services under his name and provider number, which is permissible under "incident-to" billing rules if strict requirements are met. However, the physician wasn't consistently meeting supervision requirements, wasn't in the office during some billed services, and wasn't maintaining documentation demonstrating his involvement. This created both compliance and fraud risks.

The compliance officer met with the physician, explained findings, and outlined required corrections. The physician agreed to modify his practice, refund inappropriate payments, and complete education on incident-to billing requirements. The compliance department implemented quarterly audits of the physician's billing for one year to verify sustained compliance.

The organization reported investigation findings to the hotline caller through their anonymous case number, explaining what actions were taken without disclosing confidential personnel information. This feedback loop demonstrates that reports are taken seriously and investigated thoroughly, encouraging future reporting.

Non-Retaliation Policies: Fear of retaliation prevents many employees from reporting concerns. Organizations must not only prohibit retaliation but actively demonstrate that reporting concerns enhances rather than harms careers.

Memorial Hospital's non-retaliation policy explicitly protects employees who report compliance concerns in good faith, even if investigation reveals no violation occurred. The policy defines retaliation broadly, including termination, demotion, reduced hours, negative performance reviews, social ostracism, or any adverse action motivated by reporting.

When a coder reported concerns about pressure from her supervisor to code cases in ways that maximized reimbursement despite questionable documentation support, she feared career consequences. Investigation revealed the supervisor had indeed made inappropriate comments suggesting coders should "give physicians the benefit of the doubt" when documentation was ambiguous, and questioned why the coder's productivity was lower than peers who "weren't so picky about documentation."

The investigation substantiated the coder's concerns. The supervisor received corrective action including mandatory compliance training and performance improvement plan. The organization took visible steps ensuring the reporting coder faced no retaliation: she received a positive performance review noting her ethical judgment, was invited to participate in compliance training development, and was promoted six months later to a senior coder position.

This visible reinforcement of non-retaliation policies demonstrates that the organization values employees who raise concerns, encouraging future reporting while discouraging managers from pressuring staff to cut compliance corners.

Element 5: Well-Publicized Disciplinary Standards

Effective compliance requires consistent enforcement of policies through appropriate disciplinary measures. Employees must understand that violations have consequences while recognizing that discipline is corrective rather than purely punitive.

Progressive Discipline Framework: Most organizations use progressive discipline, with consequences escalating based on violation severity and whether prior violations occurred. This framework balances accountability with opportunities for correction.

Memorial Hospital's discipline policy establishes escalating responses:

First violation (minor): Verbal warning with documentation, mandatory retraining on relevant policy, and enhanced monitoring for 90 days. This applies to honest mistakes or minor policy violations without intent to deceive.

Example: A coder consistently codes procedures without checking for updated codes, resulting in minor reimbursement errors. The supervisor provides verbal warning, requires the coder to complete coding update training, and reviews her work daily for 90 days to ensure improvement.

Second violation or first violation (moderate): Written warning placed in personnel file, mandatory corrective action plan with specific improvement expectations and timeline, and suspension of bonus eligibility for one year.

Example: The same coder continues making preventable errors despite previous warning and training. She receives written warning outlining specific improvements required (error rate below 5%, completion of advanced coding education, demonstration of appropriate guideline use). Her coding is audited weekly for six months, and she loses annual bonus eligibility.

Third violation or first violation (serious): Suspension without pay (1-5 days depending on severity), final warning status, and mandatory re-certification of training. The employee understands that further violations will result in termination.

Example: Investigation reveals the coder knowingly assigned codes not supported by documentation to increase reimbursement after being warned that such practices constitute fraud. She receives three-day suspension without pay, final warning status, and must complete comprehensive compliance training. All her coding is reviewed for six months, and she understands that any further integrity violations will result in immediate termination.

First violation (severe) or pattern of violations: Immediate termination with possible referral to law enforcement or regulatory agencies.

Example: A coder deliberately upcodes services over an extended period, falsifies documentation to support incorrect codes, or accesses patient records without work-related reasons after multiple warnings.

Consistency in Enforcement: Nothing undermines compliance programs faster than inconsistent discipline. Employees lose faith in the system when connected individuals receive lenient treatment while others face harsh consequences for similar conduct.

Memorial Hospital tracks all disciplinary actions in a centralized database, allowing the compliance officer to review patterns and ensure consistency. When a department manager recommends terminating an employee for a first-time minor violation while similar violations by others resulted in warnings, the compliance officer questions the inconsistency and ensures fair treatment.

Recent review revealed concerning patterns in one department where minority employees received harsher discipline than white employees for similar violations. This prompted comprehensive review of the department's discipline practices, mandatory unconscious bias training for management, and enhanced compliance officer oversight of all disciplinary decisions. The organization recognized that fair enforcement isn't just about compliance—it's about equal treatment and legal protection.

Element 6: Auditing and Monitoring

The only way to know if compliance efforts are working is through systematic auditing and monitoring. Effective programs combine proactive monitoring detecting problems early with targeted audits investigating specific concerns.

Routine Monitoring Systems: Automated monitoring systems flag potential compliance issues for human review, allowing organizations to identify problems before they escalate into serious violations.

Memorial Hospital's coding compliance monitoring system tracks dozens of metrics providing early warning of potential problems:

Code Distribution Analysis: The system tracks each provider's coding patterns and compares them to specialty peers. When a physician's average evaluation and management level is significantly higher than peers seeing similar patients, the system flags the discrepancy for investigation.

Dr. Thompson's E/M coding average is 4.6 on a 5-point scale, while family medicine peers average 3.2. The system flags this pattern, triggering an audit of Dr. Thompson's documentation. Review reveals that Dr. Thompson provides comprehensive care warranting high-level coding, but his documentation doesn't consistently support code selection. This isn't fraud—it's a documentation problem. The compliance department provides education on documentation requirements and works with Dr. Thompson to improve medical record details supporting his coding.

Diagnosis-Procedure Matching: The system identifies claims where diagnoses don't typically support reported procedures, suggesting possible coding errors or insufficient documentation.

Claims review flags multiple cases where Dr. Rodriguez performed nerve conduction studies (CPT 95907-95913) for patients whose only diagnosis was general "pain in limb" without specific neurological complaints. While nerve studies are sometimes appropriate for limb pain, the pattern suggests either documentation doesn't capture medical necessity justification or studies are being performed without adequate indications. Investigation reveals Dr. Rodriguez routinely performs comprehensive nerve studies but documents only chief complaints without detailed examination findings or clinical reasoning. The compliance department works with Dr. Rodriguez to improve documentation explaining why studies are medically necessary.

Modifier Use Patterns: Unusual modifier use often indicates coding confusion or deliberate manipulation. The system tracks modifier frequency and flags unusual patterns.

One coder's use of modifier -22 (increased procedural services) is three times higher than peer coders. Modifier -22 should be rare, used only when procedures require significantly more work than typical. The high usage suggests the coder either doesn't understand appropriate modifier use or is inappropriately trying to increase reimbursement. Audit reveals the coder applies modifier -22 to any slightly longer procedure without determining if additional work meets "significantly greater" threshold. The compliance department provides education on modifier use and implements pre-submission review of all modifier -22 claims for 90 days.

Focused Audits: While routine monitoring identifies broad patterns, focused audits examine specific areas in detail, often prompted by monitoring alerts, hotline reports, or external concerns.

Memorial Hospital conducts several types of focused audits:

Pre-payment audits review claims before submission, catching errors that would result in overpayment. These audits focus on high-risk areas like evaluation and management coding, modifier use, and new procedures where coding guidance is limited.

Post-payment audits review previously paid claims to identify errors requiring refunds. These audits often focus on specific providers, services, or time periods where monitoring systems flagged concerns.

Educational audits provide feedback to physicians and staff about coding accuracy without direct financial consequences. These audits emphasize improvement rather than blame, though patterns of errors trigger formal compliance reviews.

External audits conducted by contracted specialists provide independent assessment of compliance program effectiveness and identify risks internal reviewers might miss.

Element 7: Response to Detected Offenses

How organizations respond when problems are discovered determines whether compliance programs truly protect against fraud or merely create illusion of compliance. Effective response requires thorough investigation, appropriate correction, and genuine efforts preventing recurrence.

Investigation Protocols: Every potential compliance violation triggers investigation proportional to its seriousness. Minor issues might be addressed through supervisor discussion and immediate correction. Serious allegations require formal investigation with documentation, witness interviews, and detailed analysis.

Consider a recent investigation at Memorial Hospital triggered by medical record audit. Review of several cases billed by Dr. Phillips revealed procedures billed as "moderate complexity" that documentation suggested were actually "low complexity," resulting in overpayment of approximately $150 per case. The auditor identified similar patterns across multiple dates of service.

The compliance officer initiated formal investigation. The investigator reviewed 30 randomly selected cases from Dr. Phillips's recent billing, coding each based on actual documentation without reference to submitted codes. The analysis revealed that 18 of 30 cases were overcoded, with excess payments totaling approximately $2,400.

The investigator interviewed Dr. Phillips's coder to understand her code selection process. The coder explained that Dr. Phillips had told her he performed "moderate complexity" procedures, so she coded accordingly without independently reviewing documentation. She thought physicians determined code levels and coders just translated physician determinations into proper codes. This revealed a fundamental misunderstanding of coding roles—coders must assign codes based on documented services, not physician opinions about appropriate codes.

The investigator interviewed Dr. Phillips, who was surprised to learn his procedures had been overcoded. He hadn't intentionally committed fraud but had misunderstood coding rules and delegated responsibility inappropriately. This represented abuse through inadequate oversight rather than intentional fraud.

Correction and Remediation: Once investigations determine that violations occurred, organizations must correct past errors and prevent future occurrences. This often requires multiple intervention types.

Memorial Hospital's response to Dr. Phillips's overcoding included:

Financial correction: The organization refunded overpayments totaling $2,400 to affected payers, with interest as required by regulations. This demonstrated good faith and compliance with self-disclosure obligations.

Education: Both Dr. Phillips and his coder completed comprehensive training on proper coding procedures, documentation requirements, and their respective responsibilities. They learned that physicians provide clinical services and document thoroughly, while coders assign codes based on documentation.

Process changes: The practice implemented pre-submission review of all Dr. Phillips's coding for six months to verify accuracy. The compliance department created standardized templates for the procedure types Dr. Phillips performs, prompting documentation of elements needed for accurate coding.

Monitoring: Random audits of Dr. Phillips's billing continued quarterly for 18 months to verify sustained improvement. Results showed significant improvement, with error rates dropping from 60% to less than 5%.

Systemic assessment: The compliance department recognized that if Dr. Phillips misunderstood coding procedures, other physicians probably did too. They implemented organization-wide physician education on documentation and coding responsibilities, clarifying that physicians document clinical services while coders translate documentation into codes following official guidelines.

Documentation Requirements

Medical record documentation serves multiple critical functions: communicating patient care between providers, supporting medical necessity of services, defending against liability claims, and justifying codes assigned for billing. Understanding documentation requirements protects both coding accuracy and legal defensibility.

The Link Between Documentation and Coding

Every code assignment must be supported by documentation in the medical record. This fundamental principle of coding creates an unbreakable link between what's written and what's billed. Understanding this relationship helps coders recognize when documentation is insufficient and when queries are necessary.

Documentation Must Support Every Code Element: Consider a simple example: coding an evaluation and management service requires documentation supporting the code level assigned. For 99214 (office visit, established patient, moderate complexity), documentation must demonstrate either moderate medical decision-making or 30-39 minutes of total time on the date of service.

When reviewing Dr. Chen's progress note for established patient Maria Santos, you find: "Patient here for blood pressure follow-up. Reports feeling well. Blood pressure 128/78. Continue current medications. Return in 3 months." This documentation supports 99212 or possibly 99213 at most. It doesn't demonstrate the multiple problem management, data review, or moderate risk required for 99214. If Dr. Chen's billing shows 99214, either the documentation is incomplete or the code is wrong.

Appropriate response requires understanding the actual service provided. If Dr. Chen spent 35 minutes with Maria discussing medication side effects, reviewing recent lab results, and adjusting treatment plans, the documentation should reflect this work. A query to Dr. Chen might elicit additional information: "Please document the specific issues discussed, lab results reviewed, and treatment changes made during this 35-minute visit. Current documentation doesn't support the 99214 code billed."

If Dr. Chen's response indicates the visit actually was routine blood pressure check taking 10 minutes, the 99214 code is wrong and must be corrected to 99212. This protects the organization from fraud allegations while ensuring Dr. Chen receives appropriate credit for work actually performed.

Linking Diagnoses to Services: Medical necessity requires that services provided are appropriate for the patient's condition. Documentation must establish this link clearly.

Dr. Patel performs nerve conduction studies (expensive tests) for patient James Wilson. The only diagnosis documented is "shoulder pain." While shoulder pain might result from nerve problems justifying nerve studies, it's not specific enough to demonstrate medical necessity. The documentation needs more detail: examination findings suggesting nerve involvement, previous conservative treatments that failed, or specific symptoms indicating possible nerve damage.

A query might request: "Please document examination findings suggesting nerve involvement and clinical reasoning supporting medical necessity for nerve conduction studies in this patient with shoulder pain." Dr. Patel's response might explain: "Patient has radiating pain down arm, weakness in grip strength, abnormal reflexes, and findings consistent with possible nerve root compression. Previous physical therapy and medication trials provided no relief. Nerve studies ordered to localize nerve dysfunction and guide treatment planning."

This additional documentation establishes medical necessity, supporting code assignment and protecting against denial or fraud allegations. Without such documentation, the service appears unnecessary and might trigger audit or investigation.

Documentation Integrity and Requirements

Medical records must be complete, accurate, timely, and authenticated. These quality characteristics protect patients, providers, and organizations while supporting appropriate reimbursement.

Completeness: Complete documentation includes all elements necessary for continuity of care, code assignment, and legal protection. Incomplete documentation creates patient safety risks, billing vulnerabilities, and legal exposure.

Essential documentation elements include:

Patient identification: Every page must identify the patient (name, date of birth, medical record number) to prevent mixing records between patients.

Date and time of service: When was care provided? This basic information supports medical necessity, distinguishes between services, and establishes provider responsibility.

Provider identification: Who provided care? Clear identification of treating providers is essential for continuity of care and liability purposes.

Chief complaint: Why did the patient seek care? This explains medical necessity and provides context for services.

History: What symptoms, previous conditions, and relevant background affect current care? Adequate history supports clinical decision-making and coding.

Physical examination: What objective findings were discovered? Examination documentation demonstrates provider assessment and supports medical necessity.

Medical decision-making: What was assessed, what diagnostic testing or treatment was ordered, and why? This demonstrates clinical reasoning and justifies services.

Plan of care: What treatment was provided or recommended? Clear care plans support continuity and document provider instructions.

Signature and credentials: Who is attesting to documentation accuracy? Authenticated records have legal weight while unsigned notes don't.

Accuracy: Documentation must reflect actual care provided without exaggeration, omission, or misrepresentation. Inaccurate documentation creates patient safety risks when providers rely on false information, exposes organizations to fraud liability, and undermines medical record integrity.

Common accuracy problems include:

Copy-forward errors: Electronic health records make copying previous documentation easy, but copying can perpetuate inaccuracies. When providers copy yesterday's examination findings into today's note without actually performing today's examination, the record doesn't reflect current patient status.

Dr. Wilson's progress notes for patient Sarah Johnson show identical examination findings for six consecutive visits over three months: "Alert and oriented times three. Heart regular rate and rhythm without murmur. Lungs clear bilaterally. Abdomen soft and non-tender." Either Sarah's condition has been remarkably stable or Dr. Wilson is copying examination findings without performing examinations. Quality review suggests the latter—office visit times don't allow for documented comprehensive examinations, and other evidence suggests cursory examinations followed by copying previous findings.

This practice creates multiple problems: care quality suffers because Dr. Wilson isn't actually examining patients thoroughly, coding might be inappropriate if billed codes assume examination elements that weren't performed, and medical records don't accurately reflect patient status. When complications arise, the inaccurate documentation creates legal liability.

Up-coding through documentation inflation: Some providers document excessive detail not actually observed or needed to support higher-level coding. This "documentation for coding" rather than "documentation for care" approach violates medical record integrity.

Timeliness: Documentation should occur as soon as possible after care is provided, while memory is fresh and details are accurate. Delayed documentation increases error risk and raises questions about accuracy.

Regulations generally require documentation completion within 24-30 days after service, though best practice suggests same-day completion when possible. Delayed documentation beyond regulatory limits can result in payment denials, compliance violations, and questions about documentation authenticity.

Memorial Hospital monitors documentation timeliness, tracking how long after service provision documentation is completed. Recent analysis revealed concerning patterns for Dr. Martinez, who routinely signs operative reports 15-20 days after surgery. Investigation revealed Dr. Martinez dictates reports promptly, but transcription and review processes are slow. The hospital implemented electronic dictation with faster transcription turnaround, reducing Dr. Martinez's signature delays to 2-3 days.

Authentication: Medical records must be signed (manually or electronically) by the responsible provider. Unsigned documentation has no legal weight and cannot support code assignment or medical necessity.

Authentication requirements include:

Clear identification: Signatures must identify the provider unambiguously, typically through printed name accompanying signature or electronic authentication.

Credentials: Provider credentials (MD, DO, NP, PA) should appear with signature, clarifying provider type and qualifications.

Date and time: When was the documentation authenticated? This distinguishes between when care occurred and when documentation was finalized.

Electronic signature security: Electronic authentication systems must verify signer identity through password, biometric, or other secure means preventing fraudulent signatures.

Query Process and Best Practices

Queries bridge gaps between what's documented and what's needed for accurate coding and complete medical records. Effective queries improve documentation quality without inappropriately influencing provider responses.

When to Query: Queries are appropriate when documentation is unclear, incomplete, or inconsistent. They're not appropriate when documentation is simply inadequate to support desired code selection or when trying to increase reimbursement through leading questions.

Legitimate query situations:

Clinical indicators present but not documented: Examination findings suggest pneumonia, but the assessment lists only "respiratory symptoms." Query: "Based on examination findings of decreased breath sounds, productive cough, and fever, does the patient have pneumonia?"

Conflicting documentation: Progress note says "diabetes well-controlled" but lab shows HbA1c of 9.5%, indicating poor control. Query: "Please clarify diabetes control status given discrepancy between clinical note and lab values."

Specificity needed: Documentation states "infection" without identifying site or causative organism. Query: "Please specify infection site and causative organism if known."

Missing clinical significance: Test results documented without interpretation. Query: "Please provide clinical significance of elevated troponin level. Does this indicate myocardial infarction?"

Inappropriate query situations:

Leading toward specific diagnosis: "Would you say this is acute or chronic respiratory failure?" when documentation doesn't support either diagnosis.

Multiple choice limiting options: "Is this Type 1 or Type 2 diabetes?" when other diabetes types exist.

Queries designed to increase reimbursement: "Can you document additional complications to support higher DRG assignment?"

How to Write Effective Queries: Well-written queries request clarification without leading providers toward specific responses. They're open-ended when possible, provide relevant clinical context, and reference specific documentation prompting the question.

Query template: "Based on [specific clinical indicators or documentation], please clarify [specific information needed]. This information will allow for [explanation of why information is needed]."

Good query example: "Your operative report documents 'significant blood loss requiring transfusion' during the hysterectomy. Please document the estimated blood loss volume and number of units transfused. This information is needed to accurately code the complexity of the procedure and ensure appropriate capture of complications."

This query references specific documentation, requests factual information the provider should know, explains why information is needed, and doesn't suggest a specific response.

Poor query example: "To code this as a complicated procedure, we need you to document blood loss over 500ml. Can you verify blood loss exceeded this amount?"

This query is leading, suggests a minimum threshold for desired response, and makes the coding implication obvious. It's inappropriate because it tells the provider what response supports higher reimbursement.

Query Response and Documentation: Provider responses to queries become part of the medical record. Responses must be authenticated and should directly answer the question posed.

When Dr. Anderson responds to a query about diabetes complications by stating "Patient has diabetic nephropathy and retinopathy," this response can support code assignment for these specific complications. The response should be dated, authenticated, and filed with the original query in the medical record.

If Dr. Anderson doesn't respond or provides an incomplete response, follow-up is required. You might need to rephrase the question, provide additional clinical context, or explain why the information matters. Never accept vague responses or assume information not clearly stated.

Documentation of the query process itself is critical. Maintain records showing what was queried, when it was queried, who responded, and what response was provided. This audit trail demonstrates you sought appropriate clarification rather than making assumptions, protecting you if questions arise later about coding decisions.

Audit Preparation and Response

Audits are inevitable in healthcare coding. Whether conducted internally for quality improvement or externally by payers or government agencies, audits test your organization's coding accuracy, documentation adequacy, and compliance with regulations. Understanding how to prepare for audits and respond to findings can mean the difference between minor corrections and catastrophic penalties.

Types of Audits Coders Face

Different audit types serve different purposes and require different preparation strategies. Knowing what to expect helps you prepare effectively and respond appropriately.

Internal Audits: Your own organization conducts internal audits to assess coding accuracy, identify improvement opportunities, and catch problems before external reviewers find them. These audits should feel collaborative rather than punitive, focused on education and improvement.

Memorial Hospital's coding department conducts regular internal audits using multiple approaches. Prospective audits review claims before submission, catching errors that would result in incorrect payment. Retrospective audits examine previously paid claims, identifying patterns requiring correction or education. Focused audits target high-risk areas like evaluation and management coding, new procedures, or providers showing unusual coding patterns.

Sarah Chen, a senior coder, participates in monthly peer audits where coders review each other's work. This month, she's auditing cases coded by her colleague Marcus Williams. Sarah selects ten random cases from Marcus's work, codes them independently, and compares her results to Marcus's original codes.

When Sarah's codes differ from Marcus's, she reviews the reasoning behind each decision. In one case, Marcus coded a wound repair as complex when Sarah believes simple repair was appropriate. Rather than simply marking this as an error, Sarah meets with Marcus to discuss their different interpretations. They review the operative report together, consult coding guidelines, and ultimately agree that Sarah's interpretation is correct. But the discussion reveals that Marcus misunderstood when extensive undermining qualifies a repair as complex. This identifies an education opportunity rather than just an error.

The collaborative nature of internal audits makes them valuable learning tools. When conducted properly, they improve accuracy, identify systemic issues, and prepare coders for external scrutiny. The key is creating a non-punitive environment where finding errors leads to education rather than discipline.

Payer Audits: Insurance companies conduct audits to verify they've paid claims correctly and to identify potential overpayments requiring refunds. These audits can be routine reviews of random claims or targeted investigations of specific concerns.

Payer audits typically involve requesting medical records for selected claims, reviewing documentation to verify services were provided as billed, and assessing whether medical necessity supported services rendered. When auditors find discrepancies between billing and documentation, they calculate overpayments and request refunds.

Medicare's Recovery Audit Contractor (RAC) program conducts post-payment audits identifying improper payments. RAC auditors review claims using automated systems flagging unusual patterns, then examine medical records to verify appropriateness. When they identify overpayments, they send demand letters requiring refunds within 30 days.

Dr. Martinez's practice recently received a RAC audit notification requesting records for 30 inpatient consultation claims from the previous year. The audit letter explained that national data showed Dr. Martinez billed consultations at much higher rates than specialty peers, suggesting potential upcoding.

The practice's compliance officer coordinated the response, gathering requested medical records, reviewing each case for coding accuracy, and preparing a response letter. Record review revealed that 8 of the 30 cases were indeed overcoded, with documentation not supporting the high consultation levels billed. However, 22 cases were coded correctly, with comprehensive documentation justifying code selection.

The practice's response included:

- Complete medical records for all requested cases
- Explanation of coding rationale for correctly coded cases
- Acknowledgment of errors in 8 cases
- Voluntary refund of overpayments for identified errors ($4,200)
- Explanation of corrective actions taken (education, enhanced auditing)
- Request for reconsideration on the 22 correctly coded cases

This proactive approach demonstrated good faith, showed the practice takes compliance seriously, and positioned them favorably in the audit resolution process. The RAC ultimately agreed that 22 cases were appropriately coded, and the matter was resolved with only the voluntary refund and no additional penalties.

Government Audits: Federal and state government agencies conduct audits ensuring compliance with Medicare, Medicaid, and other public program requirements. These audits carry the highest stakes, potentially resulting in criminal prosecution, massive penalties, and program exclusion.

Office of Inspector General (OIG) audits examine whether healthcare providers are complying with Medicare regulations and identify areas of risk across the industry. These audits might target specific billing practices, provider types, or geographic regions based on data analysis suggesting problems.

Centers for Medicare & Medicaid Services (CMS) conducts various audit programs including Comprehensive Error Rate Testing (CERT), which measures improper payment rates in Medicare, and Medicare Administrative Contractors (MAC) audits examining claims for specific providers or services.

State Medicaid agencies audit providers participating in their programs, often with assistance from contracted audit firms. These audits verify compliance with state-specific Medicaid rules, which may differ from Medicare requirements.

When Memorial Hospital received notice of a CERT audit, the compliance department understood the gravity of the situation. CERT audits examine random Medicare claims across the country to calculate overall improper payment rates. While individual providers aren't penalized based on CERT findings, discovery of improper billing patterns can trigger additional scrutiny.

The hospital received requests for medical records supporting 45 Medicare claims spanning various service types: inpatient admissions, outpatient surgeries, emergency department visits, and diagnostic testing. For each claim, auditors would verify:

- Was the patient eligible for Medicare at time of service?
- Was service actually provided as billed?
- Did documentation support codes assigned?
- Was service medically necessary?
- Were billing rules followed correctly?

The compliance officer assembled a response team including medical records staff, coding professionals, and billing specialists. They gathered all requested records, verified their completeness, and conducted pre-submission review to identify any potential issues.

Internal review revealed several concerns. One inpatient admission was coded based on discharge summary only, without review of complete medical record. When the team examined the full record, they discovered complications not captured in original coding, actually justifying a higher DRG than originally billed. Another case involved outpatient surgery with missing operative report—the service was provided but documentation wasn't in the record as required.

The team corrected identified issues before submitting records, ensuring auditors would see accurate documentation and appropriate coding. They included explanatory letters for cases requiring clarification, demonstrated proactive quality assurance, and showed they take documentation seriously.

Preparing for Audits: Best Practices

Success in audits comes from preparation long before audit notices arrive. Organizations with strong documentation, accurate coding, and comprehensive compliance programs handle audits far better than those scrambling to prepare after receiving audit notifications.

Maintain Excellent Documentation: The single most important audit preparation is ensuring documentation is complete, accurate, timely, and authenticated. When medical records clearly support codes assigned, audits become routine rather than threatening.

Implement Regular Internal Auditing: Organizations conducting frequent internal audits identify and correct problems before external auditors find them. This proactive approach not only improves accuracy but demonstrates commitment to compliance.

Establish Clear Query Processes: Well-documented query processes show you sought clarification when documentation was unclear rather than making assumptions. This protects coding accuracy and demonstrates appropriate care in code assignment.

Track and Trend Coding Metrics: Monitor coding patterns over time, comparing your statistics to national benchmarks and peer practices. Unusual patterns might indicate problems requiring investigation or education.

Memorial Hospital tracks dozens of coding metrics, creating dashboards that managers review monthly:

Case Mix Index (CMI): Average complexity/reimbursement of inpatient cases. When CMI increases without corresponding changes in patient acuity, this might indicate upcoding. When CMI decreases despite sicker patients, this might indicate undercoding or documentation problems.

Recent analysis showed the hospital's CMI increased from 1.45 to 1.62 over six months. This substantial increase raised concerns about potential upcoding. Investigation revealed two factors: (1) the hospital opened a cardiac surgery program, treating more complex patients, and (2) coders received training improving capture of complications and comorbidities. Both factors legitimately explained the increase, but proactive investigation ensured no inappropriate coding was occurring.

Average E/M Level: Tracks evaluation and management service complexity by provider and specialty. Providers coding significantly above or below peers require investigation.

Dr. Thompson's average E/M level was 4.1 while internal medicine peers averaged 3.3. Investigation revealed Dr. Thompson sees more complex patients than typical internists, including many referred for specialty evaluation of difficult cases. His documentation consistently supported high-level coding. This demonstrates the importance of understanding context before assuming high averages indicate problems.

Denial Rates: Track claim denials by reason, payer, and provider. High denial rates suggest coding errors, documentation problems, or medical necessity issues.

Compliance Findings: Track internal audit results, showing trends in error types, rates, and whether issues are improving or worsening.

Education and Training: Regular education ensures coding staff understand current guidelines, documentation requirements, and compliance expectations. Well-trained coders make fewer errors and handle challenging situations more appropriately.

Responding to Audit Findings

How organizations respond to audit findings significantly affects outcomes. Defensive posturing, incomplete responses, or attempts to hide problems typically worsen situations. Transparent, comprehensive, and proactive responses usually result in better outcomes.

Initial Response Strategy: When receiving audit findings, take time to thoroughly understand what auditors identified, why they believe problems exist, and what they're requesting. Rushed responses often overlook important details or fail to address auditor concerns completely.

Assemble Response Team: Complex audits require multidisciplinary response teams including:

- Compliance officer coordinating overall response
- Coding professionals addressing technical coding questions
- Clinical staff clarifying medical necessity and documentation issues
- Legal counsel advising on legal implications
- Finance staff calculating financial impact
- Senior leadership providing strategic direction

Conduct Independent Review: Before responding to auditors, conduct your own thorough review of questioned cases. Sometimes auditors make mistakes or misunderstand documentation. Other times they correctly identify problems you hadn't noticed. Independent review helps you understand ground truth before formulating responses.

Formulate Comprehensive Response: Effective audit responses typically include:

Acknowledgment of valid findings: When auditors correctly identify errors, acknowledge them clearly and take responsibility. Attempting to defend indefensible positions damages credibility.

Explanation of disagreements: When you believe auditors are wrong, explain your position clearly with supporting references to coding guidelines, medical literature, or other authoritative sources.

Documentation of corrective actions: Show what you've done to prevent similar problems in the future. This might include education, policy changes, enhanced monitoring, or personnel actions.

Voluntary refunds when appropriate: Proactively refunding identified overpayments demonstrates good faith and often results in reduced penalties.

Request for reconsideration: When you disagree with findings, follow payer-specific processes for appealing determinations.

Real-World Example: Responding to Audit Findings

Regional Medical Center received audit findings from Medicare identifying $125,000 in alleged overpayments across 50 inpatient admissions. The audit claimed inadequate documentation of medical necessity for inpatient status, suggesting patients could have been treated in observation or outpatient settings.

The compliance officer assembled a response team and conducted detailed review of all 50 cases. Their analysis found:

- 15 cases: Auditors were correct; documentation didn't adequately support inpatient necessity
- 25 cases: Additional documentation existed supporting inpatient status but wasn't provided to auditors
- 10 cases: Clinical judgment differences; physicians believed inpatient status was appropriate even though auditors disagreed

The organization's response strategy addressed each category differently:

For the 15 cases with inadequate documentation:

- Acknowledged the findings were correct
- Immediately refunded overpayments totaling $42,000
- Implemented physician education on inpatient vs. observation criteria
- Created admission documentation templates prompting appropriate medical necessity justification
- Established prospective utilization review to catch inappropriate admissions before they occur

For the 25 cases with additional documentation:

- Provided the missing documentation to auditors
- Explained why documentation wasn't initially provided (records request was unclear about which specific documents were needed)
- Requested reconsideration based on complete records
- Ultimately, auditors agreed 22 of these 25 cases were appropriately billed, reducing disputed amount by $60,000

For the 10 clinical judgment cases:

- Provided detailed explanation of clinical factors supporting inpatient admission
- Referenced medical literature supporting admission decisions
- Obtained letters from treating physicians explaining their clinical reasoning
- Requested independent medical review
- Ultimately settled these cases by refunding payment for 3 cases while maintaining that 7 were appropriate

The total financial impact was $53,000 in refunds rather than the initially claimed $125,000, and the organization avoided penalties because they demonstrated good faith, implemented meaningful corrective actions, and showed commitment to compliance.

Ethical Coding Practices

Ethics in medical coding extends beyond simply avoiding fraud. Ethical coders balance competing pressures—accuracy, productivity, employer expectations, physician preferences, and payer requirements—while maintaining integrity and professionalism. Understanding ethical principles that guide coding decisions helps you navigate these complex situations.

Core Ethical Principles for Coders

Several fundamental ethical principles should guide every coding decision you make:

Accuracy Above All: The coder's primary obligation is assigning the most accurate codes supported by documentation, regardless of financial or political pressure to do otherwise. When accuracy conflicts with productivity expectations, revenue goals, or relationships, accuracy must prevail.

You're reviewing a complex surgical case where documentation is ambiguous about whether the procedure meets criteria for a more extensive code paying $2,000 additional reimbursement. Your supervisor pressures you to "give the surgeon the benefit of the doubt" and code the higher-paying procedure. The surgeon calls personally, insisting the more complex code is appropriate despite documentation ambiguity.

The ethical response is sending a query requesting documentation clarification rather than making assumptions. If the surgeon provides additional information supporting the higher code, you can code accordingly with clear conscience. If clarification reveals the lower code is appropriate, you assign it regardless of disappointed expectations. Your obligation is to documentation and coding guidelines, not to making people happy or maximizing revenue.

Independence and Objectivity: Coders must maintain independence from financial pressures, personal relationships, and organizational politics that might compromise coding accuracy. This doesn't mean being adversarial, but it does mean making coding decisions based on documentation and guidelines rather than external pressures.

Memorial Hospital recently implemented a new compensation structure linking coding manager bonuses to departmental productivity and revenue accuracy. While the intention was encouraging efficiency and accuracy, it created an ethical concern. If the coding manager's compensation increases when coders assign higher-paying codes, this creates pressure—whether explicit or implicit—toward upcoding.

The compliance officer raised concerns about this compensation structure, noting it created conflicts between the manager's financial interests and the organization's compliance obligations. Leadership modified the structure to base bonuses on coding accuracy metrics, turnaround time, and employee development rather than revenue generated. This change aligned incentives with compliance rather than creating conflicts.

Professional Integrity: Ethical coders maintain professional standards even when facing personal consequences. This might mean reporting concerns about inappropriate pressure to upcode, refusing to participate in fraudulent schemes, or accepting lower productivity ratings rather than cutting accuracy corners.

Marcus, a hospital coder, discovered that his department manager regularly changes codes after coders submit them, consistently changing to higher-paying codes without reviewing documentation or consulting coders. When Marcus questioned this practice, the manager told him to "mind his own business" and implied his job might be at risk if he complained.

Marcus faces a difficult ethical decision. Reporting the manager's behavior might result in retaliation despite non-retaliation policies. But remaining silent makes him complicit in fraudulent coding. The ethical choice is clear even though the personal consequences are uncertain.

Marcus reports the situation to the compliance officer, providing specific examples and explaining the manager's response to his concerns. The compliance officer investigates, discovers the manager has been systematically upcoding claims for months, and terminates the manager for fraud. Marcus receives protection under non-retaliation policies and ultimately earns respect for his integrity.

This case illustrates that ethical choices sometimes involve personal risk. But compromise of integrity creates far greater long-term risks—to your career, your organization, and your profession.

Continuous Learning: Medical coding changes constantly with new procedures, coding guideline updates, and regulatory modifications. Ethical coders maintain competency through continuous learning, recognizing that yesterday's knowledge might not support today's coding decisions.

You've coded orthopedic procedures for fifteen years and feel confident in your expertise. But CPT® releases significant changes to musculoskeletal coding, consolidating some codes, splitting others, and modifying guidelines substantially. Rather than assuming your experience makes education unnecessary, you recognize your obligation to learn new guidelines before coding affected procedures.

Ethical practice requires humbling yourself to acknowledge knowledge gaps and investing time to stay current. Coding based on outdated knowledge isn't just technically incorrect—it's ethically problematic because you're claiming expertise you no longer possess.

Handling Ethical Dilemmas

Real-world coding involves situations where the right answer isn't obvious and competing values create difficult choices. Understanding how to analyze ethical dilemmas helps you navigate these challenges systematically rather than reacting emotionally or impulsively.

The Ethical Decision-Making Framework:

When facing ethical dilemmas, work through a systematic decision-making process:

Step 1: Identify the ethical issue clearly What specific ethical principle or value is at stake? Is this about accuracy, independence, integrity, or some other ethical concern?

Step 2: Gather relevant information What facts do you need to understand the situation completely? What documentation exists? What coding guidelines apply? What organizational policies are relevant?

Step 3: Identify stakeholders and their interests Who will be affected by your decision and how? Consider patients, providers, your organization, payers, and yourself.

Step 4: Consider alternative courses of action What different actions could you take? What would be the consequences of each alternative?

Step 5: Apply ethical principles to alternatives How does each alternative align with ethical principles of accuracy, independence, integrity, and professional responsibility?

Step 6: Make and implement your decision Choose the course of action that best upholds ethical principles while considering practical consequences.

Step 7: Reflect on the outcome After implementing your decision, consider what happened and what you learned for future situations.

Scenario: Productivity Pressure vs. Accuracy

Your coding manager calls you into her office and expresses concern about your productivity. You're coding 15 charts per day while department standards are 25 charts daily. The manager explains that low productivity affects the department's financial performance and suggests you need to "work smarter, not harder" to meet expectations.

You explain that you take time to thoroughly review documentation, formulate appropriate queries when needed, research coding guidelines for unusual cases, and ensure accuracy before submitting codes. The manager responds that other coders meet productivity standards while maintaining acceptable accuracy rates, suggesting you're being "too cautious."

Applying the ethical framework:

Ethical issue: Productivity pressure potentially compromising coding accuracy

Relevant information:

- Your accuracy rate is 98% based on recent audits (significantly above department average of 93%)
- Your query rate is 12% (department average 4%)
- Cases assigned to you are complex cases requiring more time
- Other coders achieving higher productivity have lower accuracy rates and rarely query

Stakeholders:

- You: Concerned about maintaining quality and integrity
- Manager: Responsible for department efficiency and financial performance
- Organization: Needs both productivity and accuracy
- Patients: Deserve accurate coding for proper care documentation
- Payers: Entitled to accurate billing

Alternatives:

1. Increase speed by reducing review thoroughness (compromises accuracy)
2. Maintain current practices while accepting productivity criticism (personally costly)
3. Request case complexity review to adjust productivity expectations (addresses underlying issue)
4. Propose different productivity metrics valuing accuracy over speed (systemic solution)

Ethical analysis: Alternative 1 violates accuracy principles but satisfies manager Alternative 2 maintains ethical standards but creates career problems Alternative 3 addresses legitimate concern about case complexity Alternative 4 proposes systemic change benefiting entire department

Decision: Request meeting with manager and compliance officer to discuss case complexity and productivity measurement. Propose adjusting productivity expectations based on case mix complexity and accuracy rates. Suggest department-wide shift toward quality metrics rather than pure speed metrics.

Implementation: Present data showing your assigned cases are more complex, document the relationship between your thorough review process and high accuracy rates, and propose alternative productivity measurement considering both speed and quality.

Outcome: After reviewing data, management agrees your case mix is more complex and adjusts productivity expectations accordingly. They also implement department-wide quality metrics balancing speed with accuracy, ultimately improving overall coding quality.

This scenario demonstrates that ethical dilemmas often have solutions addressing underlying systemic issues rather than requiring you to choose between your values and your career.

Common Ethical Challenges Coders Face

Understanding common ethical challenges helps you recognize them when they arise and respond appropriately:

Pressure to Upcode: Physicians, administrators, or managers may pressure coders to assign higher-level codes than documentation supports, explicitly or implicitly suggesting financial considerations should influence coding decisions.

Appropriate response: Explain that codes must reflect documented services, offer to educate providers on documentation requirements supporting higher-level codes, and involve compliance officer if pressure continues.

Inadequate Documentation: Documentation doesn't clearly support services provided, leaving you uncertain about appropriate code assignment.

Appropriate response: Query for clarification rather than making assumptions. If queries aren't answered, code based on available documentation even if this results in lower reimbursement.

Productivity Demands: Expected coding volume requires cutting corners on review, query processes, or guideline research.

Appropriate response: Discuss concerns with management, document that productivity demands compromise accuracy, and involve compliance if productivity expectations create compliance risks.

Relationships Influencing Coding: Personal relationships with physicians or colleagues create pressure to code favorably regardless of documentation support.

Appropriate response: Maintain professional boundaries, apply the same standards to everyone regardless of relationships, and recuse yourself from coding cases where relationships might compromise objectivity.

Knowledge Gaps: You encounter procedures or situations you're unsure how to code correctly.

Appropriate response: Research coding guidelines, consult experienced colleagues, seek compliance guidance, and never guess when uncertain. Hold claims rather than submitting codes you're not confident about.

Building and Maintaining Professional Ethics

Ethical practice isn't just about individual decisions—it's about developing character and habits that make ethical choices natural rather than difficult.

Cultivate Ethical Awareness: Stay alert to situations creating ethical risks. Recognize when financial pressures, relationships, or organizational cultures might compromise your independence or objectivity.

Seek Ethics Education: Participate in ethics training, case discussions, and professional development addressing ethical challenges coders face. Learning from others' experiences prepares you for similar situations.

Build Support Networks: Develop relationships with colleagues who share your commitment to ethical practice. Having people you can consult when facing difficult situations provides both practical guidance and moral support.

Document Ethical Concerns: When you encounter ethically problematic situations, document what happened, what you observed, and what actions you took. This documentation protects you if questions arise later and demonstrates your commitment to appropriate practice.

Report Concerns Appropriately: When you observe unethical behavior by others, report concerns through appropriate channels—compliance officers, hotlines, or management. While reporting takes courage, silence makes you complicit.

Maintain Professional Boundaries: Keep professional relationships professional. Don't let personal friendships, romantic relationships, or family connections influence your coding decisions.

Stay Current: Maintain and enhance your professional knowledge through continuing education, certification maintenance, and regular guideline review. Competence is an ethical obligation.

Chapter 17 Summary and Practice Questions

You've now mastered the critical compliance and ethical concepts that protect you, your organization, and your patients. Your achievements include:

HIPAA Understanding: You know how to protect patient information, recognize PHI, and comply with privacy and security requirements in your daily work.

Fraud Prevention: You can distinguish between honest errors, abuse, and fraud, recognizing common schemes and understanding the serious consequences of violations.

OIG Guidelines: You understand the seven elements of effective compliance programs and can contribute to your organization's compliance efforts.

Documentation: You recognize the critical link between documentation and coding, know when queries are appropriate, and can write effective queries that improve documentation quality.

Audit Preparation: You understand different audit types, know how to prepare for audits proactively, and can respond effectively when findings are issued.

Ethical Practice: You've developed a framework for ethical decision-making and understand how to handle common ethical challenges that coders face.

These compliance and ethical principles aren't separate from your technical coding skills—they're integral to being a complete, professional coder. The most technically skilled coder becomes a liability if they don't understand compliance obligations and ethical responsibilities.

Chapter 17 Practice Questions

Test your understanding of compliance and ethical concepts:

Question 1: Which of the following represents Protected Health Information (PHI) under HIPAA?

A) Statistical data about hospital readmission rates B) A patient's medical record number and diagnosis C) De-identified research data D) Aggregate billing data without patient identifiers

Answer: B Explanation: A patient's medical record number combined with diagnosis information constitutes PHI because it contains individually identifiable health information. The other options either lack individual identifiers (statistical and aggregate data) or have been properly de-identified (research data).

Question 2: The difference between fraud and abuse is:

A) Fraud involves small amounts of money; abuse involves large amounts B) Fraud requires intent and knowledge; abuse does not require intent C) Fraud is a civil matter; abuse is criminal D) There is no difference between fraud and abuse

Answer: B Explanation: Fraud requires knowing and willful conduct—the person understands they're doing something wrong and does it anyway. Abuse involves practices that result in improper payments but doesn't require proof of intent to deceive.

Question 3: According to OIG compliance guidelines, an effective compliance program must include:

A) At least 50 employees dedicated to compliance B) Annual compliance audits by external consultants C) Written policies and procedures addressing compliance risks D) Bonuses for employees who report compliance concerns

Answer: C Explanation: One of the seven essential elements of an effective compliance program is written policies and procedures. The other options aren't requirements—the necessary number of compliance staff depends on organization size, external audits aren't required (though internal auditing is), and bonus programs for reporting aren't mandated.

Question 4: When should you query a physician about documentation?

A) Whenever you want to assign a higher-paying code B) When documentation is unclear, incomplete, or inconsistent C) Every time you code a complex case D) Only when explicitly instructed by your supervisor

Answer: B Explanation: Queries are appropriate when documentation is unclear, incomplete, or inconsistent—situations where clarification is needed for accurate coding. Queries should never be used simply to obtain higher reimbursement or when documentation is clear and complete.

Question 5: During an audit, you discover that your organization has been systematically overcoding services. The most appropriate response is:

A) Ignore the findings and hope auditors don't discover the problem B) Immediately report the findings to the compliance officer C) Correct future coding but don't address past errors D) Blame physicians for inadequate documentation

Answer: B Explanation: Ethical and legal obligations require reporting compliance concerns to appropriate authorities within your organization. The compliance officer can investigate, implement corrections, and determine whether self-disclosure to payers or government agencies is necessary.

Question 6: You're pressured by your supervisor to code all E/M services at the highest level to maximize revenue. The ethically appropriate response is:

A) Follow the supervisor's instructions to keep your job B) Code accurately and report the pressure to the compliance officer C) Agree to upcode but document that you were pressured D) Quit immediately without reporting the problem

Answer: B Explanation: Ethical coders maintain accuracy despite pressure and report inappropriate demands through proper channels. Following instructions to upcode would make you complicit in fraud. Documenting the pressure doesn't excuse participation in fraudulent billing. Quitting without reporting allows the fraudulent practice to continue.

Question 7: HIPAA's Security Rule specifically addresses:

A) All patient information regardless of format B) Only paper medical records C) Electronic protected health information (ePHI) D) Financial records but not medical information

Answer: C Explanation: The HIPAA Security Rule establishes safeguards specifically for electronic protected health information (ePHI), recognizing that electronic data requires specialized technical protections. The Privacy Rule addresses all PHI regardless of format.

Question 8: When documentation doesn't support the code a physician wants to bill, you should:

A) Code what the physician requests since they provided the care B) Query the physician for additional documentation supporting the desired code C) Assign a code supported by existing documentation D) Code based on what you think probably happened

Answer: C Explanation: Codes must be supported by documentation in the medical record. If documentation doesn't support a desired code, you should code based on what is documented. You may query for additional information, but if clarification isn't provided or doesn't support the higher code, you must code accurately based on available documentation.

Question 9: The primary purpose of the OIG Work Plan is:

A) Providing a list of all healthcare regulations B) Identifying areas the OIG plans to investigate in the coming year C) Teaching coders how to assign codes correctly D) Establishing Medicare reimbursement rates

Answer: B Explanation: The OIG Work Plan identifies specific areas the OIG plans to investigate in the coming year, helping healthcare organizations anticipate compliance risks and focus their internal auditing on high-risk areas.

Question 10: You accidentally access a coworker's medical record without a work-related reason. The appropriate response is:

A) Don't say anything since it was an accident B) Delete your access logs to hide the mistake C) Report the accidental access to your supervisor or compliance officer D) Access other records to make your access look routine

Answer: C Explanation: Even accidental PHI access should be reported. Organizations need to know about all access incidents to determine if they require breach notification. Self-reporting demonstrates integrity and allows appropriate response. Attempting to hide or cover up access would compound the problem.

Your Compliance Foundation Is Complete

You now possess comprehensive knowledge of the regulatory framework governing medical coding, the ethical principles guiding professional practice, and the practical skills needed to navigate complex compliance situations. This foundation protects you throughout your coding career, ensuring that your technical expertise is matched by compliance wisdom and ethical judgment.

Chapter 18: Reimbursement and Revenue Cycle

"The intersection of medicine and money requires coders who understand both the clinical and the financial." - Anonymous Healthcare CFO

Welcome to the chapter where your coding expertise meets the business reality of healthcare. Every code you assign triggers a financial transaction that ripples through the entire healthcare system. Understanding how reimbursement works, how claims are processed, and how denials are managed transforms you from a technical coder into a strategic partner who directly impacts your organization's financial health.

Many coders think their job ends when they submit a claim. But the truth is, that's just the beginning. Your codes start a journey through complex payment systems, payer edits, medical necessity reviews, and appeals processes. When you understand this entire revenue cycle, you code smarter—anticipating payer requirements, preventing denials before they happen, and supporting successful appeals when denials do occur.

This chapter reveals the financial machinery underlying every healthcare encounter. You'll discover how different payers calculate payments, why some claims sail through while others get rejected, and how to navigate the appeals process when payers disagree with your coding. More importantly, you'll learn to think strategically about coding decisions, balancing accuracy with payer requirements and documentation realities.

The revenue cycle knowledge you gain here makes you invaluable to any healthcare organization. While many coders can assign technically correct codes, few understand how those codes translate into revenue, why certain documentation elements protect payment, and how to prevent the denials that cost organizations millions of dollars annually. This strategic understanding elevates your career from routine coding to revenue cycle expertise that commands premium compensation and leadership opportunities.

By the end of this chapter, you'll see every coding decision through a dual lens: clinical accuracy and financial impact. You'll understand that your role isn't just documenting what happened—it's ensuring your organization gets paid appropriately for the care provided while maintaining absolute compliance with regulations and ethical standards.

Understanding Payment Systems

Healthcare reimbursement operates through multiple payment methodologies, each with unique logic, incentives, and challenges. Understanding these systems helps you code in ways that ensure appropriate payment while maintaining accuracy and compliance.

Fee-for-Service: Paying for Each Service

Fee-for-service remains the most intuitive payment model: providers get paid for each service they perform, with payment rates varying by service complexity, geographic location, and payer contracts. This system dominated healthcare for decades and still governs much of outpatient care.

How Fee-for-Service Works:

Every procedure code has an assigned relative value reflecting the resources required to provide that service. Medicare's Physician Fee Schedule exemplifies this approach, using the Resource-Based Relative Value Scale (RBRVS) to determine payment rates.

Consider Dr. Sarah Martinez, a family physician seeing patients in her San Diego office. When she performs a level 4 office visit for an established patient (CPT 99214), Medicare doesn't just pull a random payment number. Instead, the system calculates payment using three components:

Work Relative Value Units (RVUs): Measures the physician effort, skill, and time required. For 99214, this is 1.50 work RVUs, reflecting moderate complexity care requiring significant clinical judgment and time.

Practice Expense RVUs: Captures overhead costs like staff salaries, equipment, supplies, and rent. For 99214 in a non-facility setting (like Dr. Martinez's office), this is 1.43 practice expense RVUs.

Malpractice RVUs: Accounts for professional liability insurance costs, which vary by specialty and procedure risk. For 99214, this is 0.07 malpractice RVUs.

Medicare adds these components (1.50 + 1.43 + 0.07 = 3.00 total RVUs) and multiplies by the geographic adjustment factor for San Diego, then by the conversion factor (approximately $33.00 in 2025). Dr. Martinez receives about $99 for this visit from Medicare.

The Fee-for-Service Incentive Structure:

Fee-for-service creates clear financial incentives that profoundly affect healthcare delivery. Since providers get paid for each service, more services generate more revenue. This can align well with quality when treating complex patients requiring extensive care, but it can also incentivize overutilization—providing services that may not add meaningful value to patient care.

Dr. Martinez faces these tensions daily. When a patient with diabetes comes for routine follow-up, comprehensive care might include foot examination, retinal screening, kidney function testing, and medication review. Fee-for-service compensates all these services appropriately, supporting thorough care. But the system also compensates unnecessary testing, creating temptation to over-order without clinical justification.

As a coder, you navigate this landscape carefully. Your job isn't policing medical necessity—that's the physician's responsibility. But you must code accurately based on documentation, avoiding both undercoding (failing to capture legitimate services) and upcoding (billing for services not provided or documented). Understanding fee-for-service incentives helps you recognize patterns suggesting documentation or medical necessity concerns that might warrant compliance review.

Geographic Variations in Payment:

Medicare recognizes that practicing medicine in Manhattan costs more than in rural Montana. Geographic Practice Cost Indices (GPCIs) adjust RVUs based on local wage rates, practice costs, and malpractice insurance premiums.

The same 99214 office visit that pays Dr. Martinez $99 in San Diego might pay $121 in Manhattan (higher practice costs) or $91 in rural Mississippi (lower overhead). These adjustments ensure payment reasonably reflects local economic realities, though whether adjustments adequately capture true cost differences remains debated.

For you as a coder, geographic variations matter when comparing your facility's payments to national benchmarks or peer institutions. Low reimbursement might reflect geographic adjustment rather than coding problems, while unusually high payments might warrant investigation to ensure codes aren't inflated.

Prospective Payment Systems: Getting Paid Per Episode

While fee-for-service pays for individual services, prospective payment systems provide a predetermined amount for an entire episode of care regardless of specific services provided. These systems shift financial risk from payers to providers, creating incentives for efficiency.

Inpatient Prospective Payment System (IPPS):

When Memorial Hospital admits Margaret Thompson for pneumonia treatment, Medicare doesn't pay separately for each medication dose, nursing hour, or lab test. Instead, the hospital receives a single payment based on the Diagnosis Related Group (DRG) assigned at discharge.

DRG assignment depends critically on accurate diagnosis and procedure coding. Margaret's case might be assigned to DRG 177 (Respiratory Infections & Inflammations with MCC) if she has major complications like respiratory failure, paying the hospital approximately $8,500. Without those complications, she'd be assigned DRG 195 (Simple Pneumonia & Pleurisy with CC), paying only $5,800. That $2,700 difference hinges entirely on documentation and coding accuracy.

Understanding DRG Logic:

DRGs group patients with similar clinical characteristics and expected resource consumption. The system considers:

Principal Diagnosis: The condition determined after study to be chiefly responsible for admission. This drives DRG assignment more than any other factor. Coding Margaret's principal diagnosis as "pneumonia due to Pseudomonas" versus generic "bacterial pneumonia" might not change the DRG, but coding "respiratory failure" instead would dramatically shift payment.

Secondary Diagnoses: Complications and comorbidities (CCs) and major complications and comorbidities (MCCs) increase expected resource use. Margaret's diabetes with complications qualifies as a CC, while her respiratory failure would be an MCC. Accurate capture of these conditions directly impacts payment.

Procedures Performed: Certain procedures change DRG assignment, particularly when they represent significantly different treatment approaches. If Margaret requires mechanical ventilation, this procedure dramatically changes both the DRG and the payment.

Patient Demographics: Age and discharge status affect some DRG assignments and payment adjustments.

The Coding Imperative in Prospective Payment:

Under fee-for-service, missing a diagnosis or procedure code means missing payment for that specific service. Under prospective payment, incomplete coding can misrepresent case complexity, resulting in payment that doesn't reflect actual resource consumption.

Consider what happens if you code Margaret's case incompletely. You document pneumonia (principal diagnosis) but miss her respiratory failure, chronic kidney disease, and diabetes complications. The hospital gets paid for simple pneumonia when they actually treated a much sicker patient requiring intensive monitoring, aggressive treatment, and extended stay. The hospital loses thousands of dollars not because they didn't provide the care, but because coding didn't capture the complexity.

This creates enormous pressure on hospital coders to "capture everything." But there's a critical line between thorough, accurate coding and inflating case complexity through inappropriate code assignment. You must code all documented, clinically significant conditions affecting care, resource use, or patient outcomes. You must not code conditions not clearly documented, not affecting current care, or included simply to inflate payment.

Case Mix Index: Measuring Your Impact:

Hospitals track their average DRG weight (Case Mix Index or CMI) as a key performance metric. CMI reflects average patient complexity and directly affects revenue. A hospital with CMI of 1.5 gets paid 50% more per case than a hospital with CMI of 1.0, assuming similar patient volumes.

Your coding accuracy directly influences CMI. When you accurately capture complications, properly sequence diagnoses, and thoroughly document secondary conditions, CMI rises appropriately. When you miss documented conditions or code conservatively to avoid scrutiny, CMI falls and your hospital loses legitimate revenue.

But CMI can also rise inappropriately through upcoding—coding conditions not truly present or inflating severity beyond documentation support. This creates compliance risks far exceeding any revenue benefits. Your challenge is maximizing legitimate CMI through excellent documentation and thorough coding while maintaining rigid accuracy standards that prevent inappropriate inflation.

Value-Based Payment: Getting Paid for Quality

Healthcare is transitioning from "volume to value"—from paying providers for services rendered to paying for outcomes achieved. Value-based payment models tie reimbursement to quality metrics, patient outcomes, and cost efficiency rather than just service quantity.

How Value-Based Payment Works:

Under traditional Medicare, Dr. James Wilson gets paid the same whether his diabetic patients achieve excellent glucose control or suffer repeated hospitalizations for complications. Value-based models change this calculus, adjusting payments based on quality performance.

Dr. Wilson participates in Medicare's Merit-based Incentive Payment System (MIPS), which evaluates physician performance across four categories:

Quality (45% of score): Did Dr. Wilson's diabetic patients receive appropriate screenings? What percentage achieved target glucose levels? How many suffered preventable complications?

Cost (15% of score): Did Dr. Wilson's care cost more or less than expected given patient complexity? Did he avoid unnecessary testing and treatment?

Improvement Activities (15% of score): Did Dr. Wilson participate in quality improvement initiatives, care coordination programs, or practice transformation activities?

Promoting Interoperability (25% of score): Did Dr. Wilson effectively use electronic health records for patient care coordination, information exchange, and quality reporting?

Based on overall performance, Dr. Wilson receives payment adjustments ranging from -9% to +9% of his Medicare payments. Poor performance costs him tens of thousands of dollars annually, while excellent performance generates substantial bonuses.

The Coding Connection to Value-Based Payment:

You might wonder how coding affects value-based payments since they're based on quality rather than code assignment. The connection is profound but sometimes subtle.

Accurate Risk Adjustment: Many value-based models "risk adjust" performance expectations based on patient complexity. If Dr. Wilson's diabetic patients are elderly with multiple complications, he's held to different standards than physicians treating young, otherwise healthy diabetics.

Risk adjustment depends entirely on coding. When you accurately code all of Dr. Wilson's patients' conditions, the risk adjustment recognizes he treats complex patients. When you undercode, the system assumes he treats simple cases, and holds him to unrealistic performance standards given his actual patient population.

Quality Measure Denominator Definition: Many quality measures apply only to patients with specific conditions identified through diagnosis codes. Incomplete coding can exclude patients from quality measures, skewing performance metrics.

Cost Attribution: Value-based models attribute costs to physicians based on patients they treat. Accurate coding ensures costs are attributed appropriately, preventing unfair cost assessments.

Documentation Supporting Quality: Quality measures often require specific documentation elements beyond codes. But coding reviews frequently identify documentation gaps that also affect quality reporting.

Bundled Payments: Getting Paid for Complete Episodes

Bundled payment models provide a single payment covering all services related to a treatment episode, regardless of how many providers are involved or what specific services are rendered. This approach creates strong incentives for care coordination and efficiency.

Understanding Bundled Payment Episodes:

When Robert Chen needs hip replacement surgery, traditional fee-for-service involves separate payments to the surgeon, hospital, anesthesiologist, physical therapist, and any physicians managing complications. Each provider maximizes their own revenue without particular incentive to coordinate care or minimize overall costs.

Under bundled payment, all providers share a single payment covering the entire episode from pre-surgical evaluation through 90-day post-operative recovery. If the episode costs less than the bundled payment, providers share savings. If costs exceed the payment, providers share losses.

This fundamentally changes incentives. Now all providers benefit from smooth, efficient care that avoids complications and unnecessary services. The surgeon cares whether Robert gets appropriate pre-surgical optimization (reducing complication risk), whether the hospital uses cost-effective implants, and whether physical therapy proceeds efficiently.

Coding Implications for Bundled Payments:

Bundled payments might seem to reduce coding's importance since the payment is predetermined rather than calculated from individual codes. Actually, accurate coding becomes more critical, just in different ways.

Episode Definition: Bundled payment episodes are identified through specific procedure codes. Coding Robert's surgery as revision hip replacement versus primary hip replacement puts him in completely different bundles with different payment amounts.

Risk Adjustment: Like value-based payments, many bundles risk-adjust for patient complexity. Robert's diabetes, obesity, and heart disease all legitimately increase expected episode costs. Accurate coding of these conditions ensures the bundled payment reflects his complexity.

Exclusion Identification: Many conditions or circumstances exclude patients from bundles or adjust payments. Accurately coding these situations protects appropriate payment.

Quality and Outcome Tracking: Bundles often include quality incentives or penalties based on outcomes. Accurate coding of complications, readmissions, and outcomes enables proper performance assessment.

Medicare and Medicaid Guidelines

Medicare and Medicaid represent the largest payers in American healthcare, covering over 130 million people and accounting for 40% of national healthcare spending. Understanding their unique requirements, coverage policies, and payment methodologies is essential for any medical coder.

Medicare Part A and Part B Coverage

Medicare divides coverage into distinct "parts," each covering different service types with different payment methods and beneficiary cost-sharing.

Medicare Part A: Hospital Insurance

Part A covers inpatient hospital care, skilled nursing facility care, home health services, and hospice care. Most beneficiaries pay no premium for Part A since they (or their spouse) paid Medicare taxes during their working years.

When 72-year-old Dorothy Martinez is admitted to Memorial Hospital with congestive heart failure, Part A covers her hospital stay. But "coverage" doesn't mean Dorothy pays nothing. She's responsible for a substantial deductible ($1,632 in 2025) covering the first 60 days of any benefit period, plus increasing copays for longer stays.

Your Coding Impact on Part A:

Part A payments to hospitals use the IPPS system described earlier, with DRG assignment driving payment. Your accurate diagnosis and procedure coding determines whether the hospital receives appropriate reimbursement for Dorothy's care.

But you're not just affecting hospital payment. Your coding also determines Dorothy's financial responsibility. If coding errors result in DRG assignment suggesting shorter stay expectations,

Dorothy might face pressure for early discharge even though her clinical status requires continued hospitalization. Conversely, if upcoding inflates the DRG beyond her actual severity, the hospital gains revenue at Medicare's expense, creating fraud risk.

Medicare Part B: Medical Insurance

Part B covers physician services, outpatient care, preventive services, durable medical equipment, and other healthcare services not covered by Part A. Unlike Part A, Part B requires monthly premiums ($174.70 standard premium in 2025, though higher earners pay more) plus 20% coinsurance on most services.

When Dorothy visits Dr. Chen for heart failure follow-up two weeks after hospital discharge, Part B covers the office visit. Dr. Chen performs a detailed examination, reviews recent lab results, adjusts medications, and schedules echocardiogram (ultrasound of the heart) to assess heart function. Each of these services is separately coded and billed to Medicare Part B.

Understanding Part B Payment:

Part B uses fee-for-service payment based on the Medicare Physician Fee Schedule. Dr. Chen's level 4 established patient visit (99214) is paid based on RVUs as described earlier. The echocardiogram has both professional (Dr. Chen's interpretation) and technical (equipment and technician) components, each separately coded and paid.

Your coding determines Dr. Chen's payment and Dorothy's cost-sharing. An incorrectly downcoded visit (coding 99213 instead of documented 99214) causes Dr. Chen to lose about $30 in payment while saving Dorothy about $6 in coinsurance. Upcoding the visit (coding 99215 instead of appropriate 99214) inappropriately increases both Dr. Chen's payment and Dorothy's coinsurance.

Medicare Coverage and Medical Necessity

The most frequent denial reason in Medicare coding isn't incorrect code assignment—it's failure to demonstrate medical necessity. Medicare pays only for services that are "reasonable and necessary" for diagnosis or treatment of illness or injury.

What Makes Services Medically Necessary:

Medical necessity is a clinical determination based on accepted standards of medical practice. But demonstrating necessity to Medicare requires clear documentation linking services to patient conditions and showing the services are appropriate for those conditions.

Consider Dr. Chen's decision to order echocardiogram for Dorothy's heart failure follow-up. The test is expensive (about $900 for complete study) and Medicare scrutinizes high-cost diagnostic testing. To support medical necessity, documentation should address:

Clinical indication: Why is the test needed? Dorothy's heart failure symptoms have worsened despite medication adjustments. The echocardiogram assesses whether her heart function has deteriorated, helping guide treatment decisions.

Appropriateness: Is this the right test for the clinical question? Echocardiogram is the standard, non-invasive method for assessing heart function in heart failure patients. Alternative tests (like cardiac catheterization) are more invasive, expensive, and risky without providing better information for this clinical question.

Timing: Is the test needed now? Dorothy's change in clinical status and medication adjustments warrant reassessment. Performing the same test in stable patients without clinical changes would lack medical necessity.

Impact on treatment: How will results change management? If Dorothy's heart function has declined significantly, she may need referral to cardiology, medication intensification, or even consideration for advanced heart failure therapies. The test directly guides treatment decisions.

When documentation addresses these elements, medical necessity is clear and payment is likely. When documentation simply states "order echo," medical necessity is questionable and denial risk is high.

Your Role in Medical Necessity:

You might think medical necessity is the physician's responsibility, not the coder's concern. Actually, coders play a crucial role in protecting medical necessity payments through several mechanisms:

Linking diagnoses to services: Your diagnosis coding must establish medical necessity. If Dr. Chen orders echocardiogram but you code only hypertension (a condition not typically requiring echocardiogram), you've created a medical necessity problem even though the actual indication (heart failure) is documented.

Recognizing documentation gaps: When documentation doesn't clearly establish medical necessity, query the physician. A brief query might result in clarifying statement that protects payment.

Understanding coverage policies: Medicare publishes Local Coverage Determinations (LCDs) and National Coverage Determinations (NCDs) specifying coverage criteria for many services. Familiarity with these policies helps you identify potential coverage issues.

Coding covered alternatives: When Medicare doesn't cover a service for a particular indication, sometimes alternative codes represent covered approaches to the same clinical problem.

Medicaid Variations by State

While Medicare is a federal program with relatively uniform national rules (though local contractors create some variation), Medicaid represents 50+ different programs administered by states within broad federal guidelines. Understanding Medicaid requires knowing both federal requirements and your state's specific policies.

Federal Medicaid Requirements:

Federal law mandates that state Medicaid programs cover certain populations (pregnant women, children, people with disabilities, elderly needing nursing home care) and certain services (hospital care, physician services, lab and X-ray, nursing facility care for adults). Beyond these requirements, states have enormous flexibility in who they cover and what services they provide.

State Medicaid Variations:

California's Medi-Cal program differs substantially from Texas Medicaid, which differs from New York Medicaid. These differences affect:

Eligibility: Some states expanded Medicaid under the Affordable Care Act, covering adults with incomes up to 138% of federal poverty level. Other states didn't expand, leaving significant coverage gaps.

Covered services: While mandatory services must be covered, optional services (dental, vision, prescription drugs, physical therapy, etc.) vary widely by state.

Payment rates: Medicaid notoriously pays providers less than Medicare or commercial insurance. But payment rates vary dramatically by state, affecting provider willingness to accept Medicaid patients.

Prior authorization: States impose varying prior authorization requirements, with some requiring approval for services covered automatically in other states.

Coding and billing rules: States adopt varying coding requirements, sometimes differing from standard Medicare rules.

Managed care penetration: Most states now deliver Medicaid through managed care plans rather than traditional fee-for-service, creating additional complexity.

Coding for Medicaid:

Medicaid coding generally follows standard CPT and ICD-10-CM guidelines, but important variations exist:

State-specific codes: Some states have state-specific code requirements or modifiers not used in Medicare.

Service limitations: States may cover a service but limit frequency (e.g., routine physicals once yearly, mental health visits limited to certain number annually).

Documentation requirements: States may impose documentation requirements beyond Medicare standards, particularly for services they scrutinize carefully.

Prior authorization documentation: When prior authorization is required, claim submission must include authorization numbers and may require specific codes or modifiers indicating authorization was obtained.

Commercial Insurance Processes

Commercial insurance companies—the Blue Cross plans, United Healthcare, Aetna, Cigna, and hundreds of smaller payers—provide coverage for about 160 million Americans, primarily through employer-sponsored health plans. Unlike Medicare's relatively standardized rules, commercial payers create enormous variation in coverage policies, payment methods, and coding requirements.

Understanding Commercial Insurance Contracts

When Memorial Hospital negotiates a contract with Blue Cross, they're not just agreeing on payment rates. They're establishing a complex set of rules governing which services are covered, how they're coded, what documentation is required, and how disputes are resolved.

Provider Contract Essentials:

Commercial insurance contracts typically address:

Payment methodology: Fee-for-service (with fee schedules specifying payment for each CPT code), case rates (paying fixed amounts for specific procedures or diagnoses), capitation (paying per member per month regardless of services provided), or bundled payments.

Fee schedules: For fee-for-service contracts, detailed fee schedules list payment amounts for thousands of CPT codes. These rates are often expressed as percentage of Medicare (e.g., "Medicare plus 40%" means each service pays 140% of Medicare's rate).

Code bundling edits: Contracts specify which code combinations are separately payable versus bundled together.

Medical necessity policies: Payer-specific policies defining coverage criteria for services, often differing from Medicare standards.

Documentation requirements: Some payers require specific documentation elements beyond standard medical record requirements.

Prior authorization: Lists of services requiring approval before performance, with consequences for performing without authorization.

Timely filing limits: Deadlines for claim submission after service dates (typically 90 days to one year, varying by payer and state).

Claims submission requirements: Electronic submission requirements, specific forms, required attachments, etc.

Your Role in Contract Compliance:

As a coder, you're not negotiating contracts or making business decisions. But you implement contractual requirements through daily coding decisions. Understanding these requirements protects both appropriate payment and compliance.

Applying Payer-Specific Edits:

Medicare publishes National Correct Coding Initiative (NCCI) edits that define which codes can be billed together. Commercial payers often apply these edits but also impose additional payer-specific bundling rules.

When you code Dr. Singh's office visit (99214) and same-day EKG (93000), Medicare allows both codes separately. But Aetna's contract with Dr. Singh bundles EKG with same-day E/M services for patients over 65, paying only for the office visit. United Healthcare allows separate payment but requires modifier -25 on the E/M code demonstrating it was significant and separately identifiable from the EKG.

You must know each major payer's requirements to code correctly. This typically requires:

Reference materials: Maintaining payer policy manuals, coding guidelines, and fee schedules for major payers you work with regularly.

Coding edits in billing system: Implementing payer-specific edits in your practice management or billing system to flag violations before claim submission.

Regular updates: Monitoring payer communications for policy changes and updating your processes accordingly.

Prior Authorization Tracking:

Many commercial payers require prior authorization for expensive services, procedures, or medications. Performing services without authorization typically results in complete payment denial, even when the service was medically appropriate.

Your billing system should flag services typically requiring authorization, but ultimately you're responsible for verifying authorization was obtained before submitting claims. When coding cases, check that authorization numbers are documented for services requiring them. If authorization wasn't obtained, alert appropriate staff immediately so they can pursue authorization retroactively if the payer allows.

Negotiating Payment Rates

While you don't negotiate contracts, understanding how payment rates are established helps you recognize when payments seem incorrect and may warrant investigation.

Determining Fee Schedule Rates:

Commercial payers establish payment rates through various methodologies:

Percentage of Medicare: Many contracts pay a percentage above or below Medicare's rates. "Medicare plus 35%" means every CPT code pays 135% of Medicare's allowed amount. This creates predictable payment relationships—if Medicare pays $100 for a service, this payer pays $135.

UCR (Usual, Customary, and Reasonable): Payers analyze what providers typically charge (usual), what most providers in the area charge (customary), and what's reasonable given service complexity. This methodology fell out of favor due to manipulation concerns but some payers still use variations.

Resource-based pricing: Like Medicare's RBRVS system, some payers establish payment rates based on estimated resource consumption, practice costs, and physician work.

Negotiated rates: The most common approach for large provider organizations is negotiating specific rates with payers based on market leverage, quality metrics, and volume expectations.

Understanding Payment Discrepancies:

When expected payment doesn't match actual payment, investigate possible causes:

Wrong fee schedule applied: Payers may have multiple fee schedules (for different plan types, provider types, or service locations) and apply the wrong one.

Outdated fee schedule: Payment rates change periodically (usually annually), and payers sometimes fail to update their systems timely.

Incorrect code: Payment seems wrong because the wrong code was submitted or the payer's system mapped your code to a different one.

Bundling or modifier edit: Payer reduced or denied payment due to bundling rules or missing/inappropriate modifiers.

Contractual adjustment: Payment is correct per contract terms, but contract rates are lower than you expected.

Claims Processing and Denials Management

Every claim you code starts a complex journey through multiple review stages before payment is issued. Understanding this process helps you code in ways that minimize denials and support successful appeals when denials occur.

The Claims Processing Journey

When you submit a claim for Dr. Martinez's patient visit, it enters the payer's claims processing system where it faces multiple scrutiny layers:

Initial Registration:

The claim is received electronically (or occasionally on paper) and undergoes initial validation. This first checkpoint verifies:

Formatting: Is the claim in the required electronic format or does it have critical format errors preventing processing?

Completeness: Are required data elements present (patient demographics, provider identifiers, service dates, diagnosis and procedure codes)?

Eligibility: Was the patient covered by this insurance on the service date? Surprisingly many claims fail here due to coverage terminations, incorrect policy numbers, or patients using insurance they don't actually have.

Provider validation: Is the servicing provider contracted with this payer and properly credentialed?

Claims failing initial registration are rejected immediately (usually within 24-48 hours), never entering the formal claims adjudication process. You receive rejection notices identifying missing information so you can correct and resubmit.

Automated Claims Processing:

Claims passing initial registration enter automated review applying pre-programmed rules checking:

Coding validity: Are the procedure and diagnosis codes valid in the current code sets? Are codes formatted correctly?

Medical necessity: Does automated screening suggest services might not be medically necessary? Claims raising necessity concerns are flagged for manual review.

Billing rules: Do code combinations violate bundling edits? Are modifiers used appropriately? Is service frequency reasonable?

Payment calculation: Based on contracted rates, patient cost-sharing, and applicable adjustments, what payment amount is correct?

Most claims (typically 80-90%) pay automatically within days, never touching human hands. But claims raising any red flags are routed to manual review.

Manual Claims Review:

Claims flagged by automated screening undergo manual review by claims examiners (and sometimes nurse reviewers or physician medical directors). Reviewers assess:

Medical necessity: Does documentation support that the service was appropriate for the patient's condition?

Coding accuracy: Are codes assigned correctly based on documentation?

Policy compliance: Does the service meet payer-specific coverage criteria?

Potential fraud or abuse: Do patterns suggest intentional billing irregularities?

Manual review takes much longer (often weeks) and results in higher denial rates than automated processing. When possible, coding to avoid manual review flags improves cash flow even though you can't always prevent it.

Common Denial Reasons and Prevention

Understanding why claims get denied helps you code in ways that prevent denials before they happen.

Denial Reason #1: Medical Necessity

Medical necessity denials assert that the service, while provided, wasn't "reasonable and necessary" for the patient's condition. These denials are particularly frustrating because you coded correctly—the problem is documentation or clinical decision-making.

Prevention strategies:

Link diagnoses appropriately: Ensure diagnosis codes clearly establish medical necessity for services provided. Don't code just the patient's chronic conditions—code the specific symptoms or acute conditions justifying today's services.

Code to highest specificity: Vague diagnosis codes raise necessity questions. "Chest pain, unspecified" provides less necessity support than "chest pain with exertion, consistent with angina."

Include all relevant conditions: Patients with multiple problems often require more extensive or frequent services. Accurately coding all conditions helps establish why seemingly extensive care was necessary.

Flag potential coverage issues: When you recognize a service that payers frequently deny for necessity, alert clinical staff so they can ensure documentation strongly supports necessity.

Denial Reason #2: Invalid or Incorrect Codes

These denials occur when you've submitted codes the payer doesn't recognize or claims contain code combinations that don't make logical sense.

Prevention strategies:

Verify current codes: Ensure you're using current year code sets. CPT and ICD-10-CM update annually, and submitting deleted codes causes automatic denials.

Check code validity: Some code combinations are logically impossible (e.g., pregnancy complication codes for male patients). Front-end edits catching these issues before submission prevent denials.

Use appropriate specificity: ICD-10-CM codes often require 6-7 characters for full specificity. Submitting truncated codes may cause denials even though "the payer should know what I meant."

Denial Reason #3: Bundling and Unbundling

Bundling denials occur when you've billed separately for services the payer considers included in another service. Unbundling allegations suggest you've deliberately split services to increase payment.

Prevention strategies:

Understand bundling rules: Know NCCI edits and payer-specific bundling policies for services you code frequently.

Use modifiers appropriately: When separate payment is appropriate despite bundling edits, proper modifiers (particularly -59 and X{EPSU} modifiers) prevent denials.

Document separately identifiable services: When billing same-day E/M and procedure, ensure documentation clearly shows the E/M was significant and separately identifiable beyond the procedure's usual pre- and post-work.

Denial Reason #4: Authorization and Referral Issues

Many payers require authorization before performing certain services. Providing services without authorization usually results in payment denial even when medically necessary and appropriately coded.

Prevention strategies:

Verify authorization requirements: Maintain current lists of services requiring authorization for each major payer.

Check authorization status before coding: Don't code and submit claims for services performed without required authorization until authorization is obtained (even retroactively).

Include authorization numbers: When services required authorization, include authorization numbers on claims.

Track authorization specifics: Authorizations often limit approved services (specific procedures, number of visits, date ranges). Claims exceeding authorization scope will be denied.

Appeals and Reconsiderations

Even with perfect coding, some claims will be denied. Understanding the appeals process transforms denials from revenue losses into opportunities to educate payers and secure appropriate payment.

Understanding the Appeals Process

Payers provide multiple levels of appeal when claims are denied, each with specific timelines and requirements.

First-Level Appeal (Reconsideration):

When a claim is denied, you typically have 90-180 days (varying by payer and state) to file first-level appeal. This appeal goes to the payer's internal appeals department and often involves fresh review by someone who didn't process the original claim.

First-level appeals should:

Clearly identify the claim: Include patient name, dates of service, claim number, and all identifying information allowing the payer to locate the original claim.

State what you're appealing: Specify which denied services you're contesting and what payment you believe is correct.

Explain why the denial was incorrect: Provide clear rationale addressing the stated denial reason. If they denied for medical necessity, explain why necessity exists. If they denied for coding errors, explain why your coding was correct.

Provide supporting documentation: Include medical records, operative reports, coding guidelines, payer policy references, or other evidence supporting your position.

Request specific action: Clearly state that you're requesting payment reversal and claim reprocessing.

Second-Level Appeal (External Review):

If first-level appeal is denied, you typically can pursue second-level appeal, often involving review by independent third parties or state insurance departments. Requirements and processes vary significantly by payer and state. These appeals often require more formal documentation and may involve independent medical reviews.

Building Successful Appeals:

Effective appeals share common characteristics that increase success rates dramatically. Understanding these elements transforms you from someone who simply resubmits denied claims to a strategic appeals professional who consistently overturns denials.

Element 1: Address the Specific Denial Reason

The most common appeals mistake is creating generic appeals that don't directly address why the claim was denied. Payers deny claims for specific reasons, and your appeal must directly rebut those reasons.

When Blue Cross denies Dr. Patterson's nerve conduction studies claiming "medical necessity not established," your appeal must specifically demonstrate medical necessity. Explaining that the codes were correct or that the service was performed doesn't address the denial reason. Your appeal needs to show why the patient's symptoms, examination findings, and clinical circumstances warranted nerve studies.

Building the Medical Necessity Appeal:

"Patient presented with three-month history of radiating arm pain, numbness in fingers, and progressive weakness in grip strength. Physical examination revealed positive Spurling's test, decreased sensation in C6 dermatome, and diminished triceps reflex. These findings are consistent with possible cervical radiculopathy affecting C6 nerve root.

Nerve conduction studies were ordered to localize the site and severity of nerve dysfunction, differentiating between cervical radiculopathy, peripheral neuropathy, or carpal tunnel syndrome—conditions requiring different treatment approaches. Studies confirmed C6 radiculopathy, guiding treatment decisions including physical therapy focus and neurosurgical consultation.

American Academy of Neurology guidelines (attached) support nerve conduction studies for evaluating radicular symptoms when clinical examination suggests nerve root compression. Patient's clinical presentation meets these evidence-based criteria."

This appeal directly addresses medical necessity by explaining clinical indications, diagnostic reasoning, and how results guided treatment. It references authoritative clinical guidelines supporting the decision. Most importantly, it tells a clinical story demonstrating why this specific patient needed this specific test at this specific time.

Element 2: Provide Supporting Documentation

Appeals without supporting documentation rarely succeed. Payers need evidence verifying your assertions, not just your word that documentation exists.

Essential Documentation Elements:

Complete medical records: Include all relevant documentation showing medical necessity. For the nerve study appeal, include the initial evaluation note with symptom history and examination findings, any previous treatment records, the nerve study order, and study results with interpretation.

Highlighted key elements: Don't expect reviewers to hunt through lengthy records. Use highlighting, margin notes, or cover letters directing reviewers to specific documentation supporting your appeal.

Clinical guidelines or literature: When appealing medical necessity denials, including relevant clinical guidelines, peer-reviewed literature, or specialty society recommendations strengthens your case by showing the service follows accepted standards of care.

Coding guidelines or policy references: For coding disputes, include relevant coding guidelines from AMA, coding clinic, or other authoritative sources supporting your code selection.

Element 3: Present Professional, Respectful Tone

Frustrated, angry, or accusatory appeals rarely succeed. Even when payers make obvious errors, maintaining professional tone increases your chances of favorable review.

Ineffective appeal language: *"Your denial is absurd and shows complete ignorance of medical practice. Any competent reviewer would recognize this service was medically necessary. Your denial is simply a way to avoid paying legitimate claims."*

This approach antagonizes reviewers, making them defensive rather than receptive to your arguments. Even if factually correct, the tone undermines your case.

Effective appeal language: *"We respectfully disagree with the denial determination. As the attached documentation demonstrates, medical necessity for this service is well-established by patient symptoms, clinical findings, and evidence-based treatment guidelines. We request reconsideration of this claim based on the additional information provided."*

This professional tone invites reconsideration while firmly asserting your position. You're treating reviewers as professional colleagues who will recognize merit when it's clearly presented.

Element 4: Request Specific Action

Vague appeals asking for "review" or "reconsideration" don't clearly communicate what you want. Be specific about the action you're requesting.

Clear request examples:

- "We request payment of the denied claim in the amount of $____"
- "We request the claim be reprocessed with payment for all services at contracted rates"
- "We request the medical necessity denial be overturned and full payment issued"

Clear requests eliminate ambiguity about what constitutes successful appeal resolution.

Maximizing Appeal Success Rates

Not all denied claims warrant appeal efforts. Understanding which denials to appeal and when to accept unfavorable determinations helps you allocate resources effectively.

Denials Worth Appealing:

High-dollar claims: When denied payment exceeds $500-1,000, appeal costs are justified by potential recovery.

Pattern denials: When a payer routinely denies a service you provide frequently, successful appeal may establish precedent preventing future denials.

Clear coding or policy errors: When the payer clearly misapplied coding guidelines or their own policies, appeals often succeed quickly.

Strong clinical documentation: When you have comprehensive documentation clearly supporting medical necessity, success rates are high enough to justify appeal efforts.

Denials Rarely Worth Appealing:

Small-dollar claims: When denied payment is under $100, appeal costs often exceed potential recovery unless it's a pattern issue.

Clear coverage exclusions: When the payer's contract explicitly excludes the service, appeals won't succeed unless you can argue the exclusion doesn't apply.

Weak documentation: When your own record review reveals documentation gaps, appeal efforts rarely succeed. Better to focus on improving future documentation than appealing weak cases.

Timely filing denials: When you missed filing deadlines through your own delays, appeals rarely overturn these denials unless you can demonstrate extenuating circumstances.

Creating Appeals Tracking Systems:

Effective denials management requires systematic tracking of denied claims, appeal status, and outcomes. This tracking helps you:

Identify patterns: Which services, providers, or payers generate the most denials? Pattern recognition guides targeted improvement efforts.

Measure success rates: What percentage of appeals succeed? Which appeal strategies work best? Data-driven approaches optimize resource allocation.

Track financial impact: How much revenue is recovered through appeals? This quantifies the value of your denials management program.

Monitor aging: How long have denied claims been pending? Aging reports ensure appeals are filed timely and prevent write-offs of recoverable revenue.

Memorial Hospital's denials tracking system captures detailed information on every denied claim:

Denial information: Claim number, patient, service date, provider, billed amount, denial reason, denial code, initial denial date

Appeal information: First appeal filed date, appeal level (first, second, third), appeal outcome, payment recovered, time to resolution

Categorization: Denial reason category (medical necessity, coding error, authorization, etc.), service type, payer

Outcome analysis: Final disposition (paid, upheld denial, partial payment), revenue recovered, appeal costs

This comprehensive tracking enables sophisticated analysis revealing that:

- Medical necessity denials have 65% overturn rate on first appeal
- Authorization denials have only 15% overturn rate (usually legitimate)
- Coding error denials have 85% overturn rate (often payer mistakes)
- Dr. Thompson's services have 3x higher denial rate than peer physicians

These insights drive targeted interventions: education for Dr. Thompson on documentation, enhanced authorization verification processes, and systematic coding error appeals that reliably recover revenue.

Quality Measures and Reporting

Healthcare has moved beyond simply paying for services to measuring and rewarding quality performance. Understanding quality measures, how they're calculated, and how your coding affects them is increasingly essential for medical coders.

Understanding Healthcare Quality Measurement

Quality measurement attempts to objectively assess whether healthcare providers deliver appropriate, effective, safe care. But measuring quality is remarkably complex—healthcare involves thousands of conditions, countless interventions, and highly variable patient circumstances that make standardization challenging.

Types of Quality Measures:

Quality measures fall into several categories, each capturing different aspects of healthcare quality:

Structure Measures: Assess whether providers have systems and resources supporting quality care. Examples include having electronic health records, providing after-hours access, or maintaining board certification.

These measures are easiest to evaluate but least directly connected to patient outcomes. Just because a practice has an EHR doesn't mean they use it effectively for patient care.

Process Measures: Evaluate whether providers perform evidence-based processes known to improve outcomes. Examples include screening diabetics for kidney disease, prescribing appropriate medications after heart attacks, or immunizing children on schedule.

Process measures dominate current quality measurement because they're more directly controllable by providers than outcomes while still strongly correlating with better results. Your coding directly impacts many process measures.

Outcome Measures: Assess actual health results achieved. Examples include mortality rates after surgery, hospital readmission rates, or diabetic patients achieving target glucose control.

Outcome measures most directly reflect quality but are heavily influenced by factors beyond provider control, including patient adherence, genetic factors, and social determinants of health.

Patient Experience Measures: Capture patients' perception of care quality through surveys. Examples include communication ratings, care coordination assessments, and overall satisfaction scores.

These measures recognize that quality includes how patients experience care, not just clinical metrics. Your coding doesn't directly affect patient experience measures but documentation quality often correlates with communication quality.

How Coding Affects Quality Measures

You might wonder how coding—a billing function—affects quality measurement focused on clinical care. The connection is profound and often underappreciated.

Risk Adjustment Through Coding:

Most quality measures "risk adjust" to account for patient complexity. Treating sicker patients is harder, so quality expectations adjust accordingly. Risk adjustment depends entirely on diagnosis coding.

The Risk Adjustment Mechanism:

Consider diabetes quality measures evaluating the percentage of diabetic patients achieving target glucose control (HbA1c < 8%). Dr. Martinez's diabetic patients average HbA1c of 8.2%, slightly above target. Is this poor quality care?

Without risk adjustment, the answer seems to be yes—Dr. Martinez's patients aren't achieving target control. But suppose Dr. Martinez specializes in complex diabetes cases—patients with multiple complications, poorly controlled despite multiple medications, and significant comorbidities making control challenging.

Risk adjustment recognizes this complexity through diagnosis coding. When you accurately code all of Dr. Martinez's patients' complications—diabetic nephropathy, retinopathy, neuropathy, cardiovascular disease, depression—the risk adjustment system recognizes he treats unusually complex patients. Quality expectations adjust accordingly, and Dr. Martinez's 8.2% average might actually represent excellent care given his patient population.

Conversely, incomplete coding makes Dr. Martinez's patients appear simpler than they actually are. The system assumes he treats straightforward diabetes cases and expects better outcomes than are reasonably achievable. He's unfairly penalized not because his care quality is poor but because coding didn't capture complexity.

Denominator Definition Through Coding:

Quality measures apply to specific patient populations identified through diagnosis codes. Incomplete coding can exclude patients from quality measures inappropriately, skewing performance assessments.

Example: Breast Cancer Screening Measure

One quality measure evaluates what percentage of women ages 50-74 receive breast cancer screening mammography every two years. This measure applies only to women meeting age criteria without certain exclusions (history of mastectomy, current breast cancer).

When 52-year-old Jennifer Thompson has bilateral mastectomy for breast cancer, she should be excluded from this measure—screening mammography isn't appropriate for someone without breasts. But if you don't code her mastectomy history (Z90.13 for bilateral mastectomy status), she remains in the measure denominator.

Now Dr. Chen, Jennifer's primary care physician, gets "dinged" for not performing screening mammography on a patient who doesn't need it. The quality report shows he's not screening appropriately when actually he's providing exactly appropriate care—not ordering tests patients don't need.

This example illustrates how incomplete coding creates false quality failures, unfairly penalizing physicians who are actually practicing good medicine.

Quality Reporting Programs

Healthcare providers participate in numerous quality reporting programs, each with unique measures, reporting requirements, and financial implications.

Medicare Quality Programs:

Medicare operates several major quality programs affecting physician and hospital payment:

Merit-based Incentive Payment System (MIPS):

MIPS represents Medicare's primary physician quality program, affecting about 200,000 physicians and generating payment adjustments from -9% to +9% of Medicare payments.

MIPS evaluates performance across four categories:

Quality (45% of score): Physicians report on six quality measures relevant to their specialty and patient population. Measures include clinical processes (like screening diabetics for kidney disease), intermediate outcomes (like percentage of patients achieving blood pressure control), and patient safety indicators (like catheter-associated infection rates).

Cost (15% of score): Medicare evaluates total costs of caring for physicians' patients, comparing actual costs to expected costs given patient complexity. Physicians treating patients more efficiently than expected score positively; those with higher-than-expected costs score negatively.

Improvement Activities (15% of score): Physicians attest to participating in activities improving care quality, care coordination, or patient safety. Activities include implementing care management programs, using shared decision-making tools, or participating in quality improvement collaboratives.

Promoting Interoperability (25% of score): Measures meaningful use of electronic health records for care coordination, patient engagement, and health information exchange.

Your Role in MIPS Success:

MIPS might seem like a physician responsibility, but coders significantly influence performance:

Accurate measure denominator definition: As discussed earlier, complete diagnosis coding ensures patients are correctly included or excluded from quality measures.

Risk adjustment coding: Thorough coding of patient complexity ensures fair risk adjustment when calculating quality scores.

Cost attribution: Diagnosis coding affects which costs are attributed to which physicians, impacting cost performance scores.

Supporting documentation: Quality measure reporting often requires specific documentation elements. Your documentation reviews frequently identify gaps affecting both billing and quality reporting.

Hospital Quality Programs:

Hospitals participate in several Medicare quality programs affecting billions in annual payments:

Hospital Value-Based Purchasing:

This program adjusts hospital payments (up or down by 2%) based on quality performance across multiple domains:

Clinical outcomes: Mortality rates, complication rates, healthcare-associated infection rates

Person and community engagement: Patient experience scores from surveys

Safety: Measures of common hospital-acquired conditions and adverse events

Efficiency and cost reduction: Medicare Spending Per Beneficiary, comparing costs to peer hospitals

Accurate coding directly affects several of these domains. Hospital-acquired condition rates depend on Present on Admission (POA) coding distinguishing conditions present at admission from those developing during hospitalization. Mortality rates require accurate case mix coding for appropriate risk adjustment.

Hospital Readmissions Reduction Program:

Medicare penalizes hospitals with higher-than-expected 30-day readmission rates for certain conditions. Penalties can reduce hospital payments by up to 3%.

Coding affects readmission penalties through:

Index admission coding: Accurate coding of the initial hospitalization ensures appropriate risk adjustment when calculating expected readmission rates.

Readmission coding: Proper coding of the readmission determines whether it "counts" as a readmission for the measured condition versus an unrelated readmission.

Complication identification: Thorough coding of complications during index admission helps explain readmissions that occur due to complex clinical circumstances.

Documentation Supporting Quality Reporting

Quality reporting requires documentation beyond traditional medical necessity requirements. Understanding these additional needs helps you recognize documentation gaps and support both billing and quality goals.

Quality-Specific Documentation Elements:

Many quality measures require specific documentation that might not be captured in routine clinical notes:

Counseling and education: Quality measures increasingly evaluate whether providers counsel patients about important health behaviors. Documentation must specifically state that counseling occurred, what topics were discussed, and patient response.

When Dr. Rodriguez counsels diabetic patient Maria Santos about the importance of daily foot inspections, routine documentation might note "discussed diabetes care." But quality reporting requires more specificity: "Counseled patient on importance of daily foot inspections due to diabetic neuropathy risk. Demonstrated proper inspection technique. Patient verbalized understanding and agreed to perform daily inspections."

This enhanced documentation supports both quality reporting and medical necessity justification for future services that might be needed.

Screening and prevention: Process measures evaluating screening rates require clear documentation that screening was offered, completed, or refused.

Insufficient: "Patient declined mammogram" **Adequate:** "Discussed breast cancer screening guidelines with patient. Explained benefits and risks of screening mammography. Patient declined screening, stating personal preference to avoid medical procedures. Will revisit at next annual visit."

The enhanced documentation shows the screening was appropriately offered and patient refusal was informed, protecting the physician's quality scores when patients decline recommended care.

Risk factor assessment: Many measures require documentation of risk factor assessment beyond simply noting conditions exist.

Insufficient: "Patient smokes" **Adequate:** "Patient currently smokes 1 pack per day for 15 years (15 pack-year history). Discussed smoking cessation. Offered counseling resources and pharmacotherapy options. Patient not ready to quit at this time but willing to consider at future visits."

This thorough documentation supports risk adjustment coding, quality measure reporting, and demonstrates appropriate clinical care regardless of patient's readiness to change behaviors.

Chapter 18 Summary and Practice Questions

You've now mastered the business side of medical coding, understanding how your technical coding decisions translate into financial impact for your organization and quality performance for your providers. Your achievements include:

Payment System Expertise: You understand fee-for-service, prospective payment, value-based payment, and bundled payment systems, recognizing how each methodology creates different coding imperatives.

Payer Knowledge: You can navigate Medicare Part A and B, Medicaid state variations, and commercial insurance complexities, understanding unique requirements each payer type imposes.

Claims Processing Insight: You understand the journey claims take from submission through payment, recognizing points where denials occur and strategies for preventing them.

Appeals Mastery: You can build effective appeals that address specific denial reasons, provide supporting documentation, and maximize recovery of denied claims.

Quality Measurement Understanding: You recognize how your coding affects quality measures, risk adjustment, and performance assessment that increasingly drive provider payment.

This revenue cycle knowledge elevates you from a technical coder to a strategic revenue cycle professional. You understand that accurate coding isn't just about correctness—it's about ensuring your organization receives appropriate payment while supporting quality measurement and performance reporting that increasingly determine success in modern healthcare.

Chapter 18 Practice Questions

Test your understanding of reimbursement and revenue cycle concepts:

Question 1: In a fee-for-service payment system, the physician gets paid:

A) A fixed amount per patient per month regardless of services B) For each individual service provided based on relative value units C) A predetermined amount for an entire episode of care D) Based primarily on quality metrics and patient outcomes

Answer: B Explanation: Fee-for-service pays providers for each individual service performed, with payment calculated based on relative value units (RVUs) that measure the work, practice expense, and malpractice risk associated with each service.

Question 2: DRG assignment for inpatient hospital payment is primarily determined by:

A) Length of hospital stay B) Principal diagnosis assigned at discharge C) Total charges billed by the hospital D) Patient's insurance type

Answer: B Explanation: The principal diagnosis (condition determined after study to be chiefly responsible for admission) is the primary driver of DRG assignment. Secondary diagnoses, procedures performed, and patient demographics also affect assignment, but principal diagnosis is the most critical factor.

Question 3: Medical necessity denials can best be prevented by:

A) Coding all services at the highest level possible B) Avoiding complex procedures that are frequently denied C) Linking diagnosis codes that clearly establish need for services provided D) Never querying physicians about clinical indications

Answer: C Explanation: Medical necessity requires clear linkage between patient conditions (diagnoses) and services provided. Accurate diagnosis coding that establishes why services were needed is the best prevention for medical necessity denials.

Question 4: When appealing a denied claim, you should:

A) Argue that the payer is wrong and always denies legitimate claims B) Specifically address the stated denial reason with supporting documentation C) Submit the same claim information again hoping for different outcome D) Wait for the payer to contact you requesting additional information

Answer: B Explanation: Effective appeals directly address the specific reason for denial (medical necessity, coding error, etc.) and provide supporting documentation demonstrating why the denial should be overturned. Generic appeals or resubmissions without addressing the denial reason rarely succeed.

Question 5: Risk adjustment in quality measures:

A) Is not affected by coding since quality is purely clinical B) Depends on thorough diagnosis coding to reflect patient complexity C) Only applies to hospital inpatient quality measures D) Penalizes physicians who treat complex patients

Answer: B Explanation: Risk adjustment attempts to fairly compare quality performance by accounting for patient complexity. This adjustment depends entirely on complete and accurate diagnosis coding that captures all patient conditions affecting expected outcomes.

Question 6: Medicare Part A primarily covers:

A) Physician office visits and outpatient services B) Inpatient hospital care and skilled nursing facilities C) Prescription medications D) Preventive care and annual wellness visits

Answer: B Explanation: Medicare Part A is hospital insurance covering inpatient hospital care, skilled nursing facility care, home health services, and hospice care. Part B covers physician services and outpatient care.

Question 7: Commercial insurance contracts often:

A) Use identical payment methods and policies as Medicare B) Have uniform coverage policies across all payers C) Vary significantly in payment rates, bundling rules, and coverage policies D) Never require prior authorization for any services

Answer: C Explanation: Commercial insurance contracts vary enormously in payment methodologies, bundling rules, coverage policies, and documentation requirements. Coders must understand payer-specific requirements for accurate billing.

Question 8: The primary purpose of Case Mix Index (CMI) is:

A) Measuring average patient complexity and expected resource use B) Tracking physician productivity and efficiency C) Calculating nurse staffing requirements D) Determining patient satisfaction scores

Answer: A Explanation: Case Mix Index measures the average complexity and resource intensity of patients treated by a hospital. It's calculated from DRG weights and directly affects hospital revenue since more complex patients generate higher payments.

Question 9: Which denial type typically has the lowest successful appeal rate?

A) Coding errors by the payer B) Timely filing denials due to provider delays C) Medical necessity denials with strong supporting documentation D) Claims denied for missing modifiers

Answer: B Explanation: Timely filing denials are rarely overturned on appeal unless you can demonstrate extenuating circumstances. These denials typically result from provider delays rather than payer errors, making them difficult to successfully appeal.

Question 10: Present on Admission (POA) coding is important because:

A) It determines whether Medicare pays for hospital services B) It distinguishes conditions present at admission from hospital-acquired conditions C) It's required for all outpatient claims D) It only affects quality measures, not payment

Answer: B Explanation: POA indicators distinguish conditions present when the patient arrived at the hospital from those that developed during hospitalization. This affects both payment (Medicare doesn't pay extra for many hospital-acquired conditions) and quality measures (hospitals are evaluated on rates of hospital-acquired complications).

PART VII: PRACTICE EXAMINATIONS

Chapter 19: Practice Test 1

"Success is the sum of small efforts repeated day in and day out." - Robert Collier

You've spent weeks or months building your coding knowledge, mastering anatomy, learning guidelines, and developing systematic approaches to complex scenarios. Now it's time to put everything together and experience what the actual CPC exam feels like. This practice test isn't just about answering questions—it's about building exam-day confidence, identifying remaining knowledge gaps, and fine-tuning your test-taking strategies.

This practice test replicates the actual CPC exam experience as closely as possible. You'll face 100 multiple-choice questions covering all major content areas in proportions that mirror the real exam. The questions progress from straightforward recall to complex scenario-based problems that require integrating knowledge from multiple areas. Some questions will feel easy, confirming what you know well. Others will challenge you, revealing areas that need additional study.

Approach this practice test seriously. Set aside 4 uninterrupted hours, gather your coding books, and create an environment as similar to test day as possible. Turn off your phone, close unnecessary browser tabs, and commit to finishing the entire test in one sitting. This mental and physical endurance practice is as valuable as the content review itself.

Remember: Your goal isn't perfection—it's progress. Every question you answer, whether correctly or incorrectly, teaches you something valuable. Wrong answers are actually gifts because they show exactly where to focus additional study time. The detailed explanations following each question will transform mistakes into learning opportunities that strengthen your overall understanding.

Take a deep breath. Trust your preparation. You've worked hard to reach this point, and you're ready to demonstrate what you've learned. Let's begin.

Instructions for Taking Practice Test 1

Before You Begin

Gather Your Materials:

- CPT® 2025 code book (properly tabbed and marked)
- ICD-10-CM 2025 code book (tabbed with guidelines marked)
- HCPCS Level II 2025 code book
- Pencils or pens for marking answers
- Scratch paper for calculations
- Timer or clock for time management
- This study guide for checking answers afterward

Create Your Test Environment:

- Find a quiet, comfortable location where you won't be interrupted
- Ensure adequate lighting and comfortable seating
- Turn off phone notifications and close social media
- Have water and necessary comfort items nearby
- Set your timer for 4 hours

Set Your Mindset:

- Approach this as if it's the real exam
- Don't rush, but maintain steady pace
- Skip difficult questions and return to them later
- Mark questions you want to review
- Trust your preparation and instincts

Time Management Strategy

Four-Hour Breakdown:

- First pass (2.5 hours): Answer all questions you can without extensive research
- Second pass (1 hour): Return to skipped questions with focused book research
- Final review (30 minutes): Check marked questions and verify answers

Pacing Guidelines:

- Aim for approximately 2.4 minutes per question
- Don't spend more than 5 minutes on any single question initially
- Easy questions might take 30 seconds; hard ones might need 4-5 minutes
- Save time by bookmarking difficult questions for later review

Answering Strategies

Read Carefully:

- Read each question completely before looking at options
- Identify key words like "not," "except," "most," "least"
- Underline or circle critical information in the question
- Don't assume you know the question before finishing it

Eliminate Wrong Answers:

- Cross out obviously incorrect options first
- Look for options that contradict known guidelines
- Be suspicious of extreme words like "always," "never," "only"
- Choose the best answer among remaining options

Use Your Books Effectively:

- Start with the alphabetic index, then verify in tabular list
- Check all instructional notes and guidelines
- Don't code directly from the index
- Verify code descriptions match documentation

Make Educated Guesses:

- Never leave questions blank
- Use medical terminology knowledge to eliminate options
- Consider which answer makes most clinical sense
- Trust your instincts when you've narrowed to two options

After the Test

Immediate Steps:

- Take a short break before reviewing answers
- Note your overall feeling about difficulty and preparation
- Identify questions you felt most confident about
- List topics that seemed particularly challenging

Scoring and Analysis:

- Check all answers against the answer key
- Read explanations for every question, even those you answered correctly
- Calculate your percentage score
- Use the Performance Analysis Guide to identify weak areas

Creating Your Study Plan:

- Review missed questions in detail
- Identify patterns in errors (specific body systems, coding types)
- Schedule focused review of weak areas
- Plan when to take Practice Test 2

Now, set your timer for 4 hours and begin. Good luck!

Practice Test 1: Questions

Section 1: Medical Terminology and Anatomy (Questions 1-8)

Question 1: Which term means surgical removal of the gallbladder?

A) Cholecystitis B) Cholecystectomy C) Cholelithiasis D) Cholecystostomy

Question 2: The prefix "tachy-" means:

A) Slow B) Fast C) Without D) Difficult

Question 3: Which anatomical structure connects the kidney to the bladder?

A) Urethra B) Ureter C) Renal pelvis D) Collecting duct

Question 4: The myocardium refers to which layer of the heart?

A) Outer protective layer B) Middle muscular layer C) Inner smooth lining D) External covering sac

Question 5: Which term describes the study of disease?

A) Pathology B) Physiology C) Histology D) Cytology

Question 6: The suffix "-ostomy" indicates:

A) Surgical removal B) Inflammation C) Surgical opening D) Disease condition

Question 7: Which structure is NOT part of the respiratory system?

A) Trachea B) Bronchi C) Esophagus D) Alveoli

Question 8: The term "bilateral" means:

A) One side only B) Both sides C) Above D) Below

Section 2: ICD-10-CM Diagnosis Coding (Questions 9-28)

Question 9: What is the correct order for using ICD-10-CM code books?

A) Tabular list first, then alphabetic index B) Alphabetic index first, then tabular list C) Either order is acceptable D) Tabular list only is sufficient

Question 10: An "Excludes1" note in ICD-10-CM means:

A) The condition may be coded with other conditions B) The condition cannot be coded here C) Additional codes are required D) The condition is being deleted

Question 11: For Type 2 diabetes with diabetic nephropathy in a patient using insulin, the correct coding is:

A) E11.21 only B) E11.21 and Z79.4 C) E10.21 and Z79.4 D) E11.9 and Z79.4

Question 12: A patient presents with chest pain to rule out myocardial infarction. EKG and cardiac enzymes are normal. How should this be coded in an outpatient setting?

A) I21.9 (acute myocardial infarction) B) R07.9 (chest pain, unspecified) C) I25.10 (atherosclerotic heart disease) D) No code should be assigned

Question 13: For malignant neoplasm described as "metastatic breast cancer," the correct interpretation is:

A) Primary breast cancer only B) Secondary breast cancer only C) Primary breast cancer with unspecified metastases D) Cannot determine without more information

Question 14: Which ICD-10-CM code represents latent tuberculosis infection?

A) A15.9 (respiratory tuberculosis, unspecified) B) Z87.01 (personal history of tuberculosis) C) Z22.7 (latent tuberculosis) D) A19.9 (miliary tuberculosis, unspecified)

Question 15: A patient with acute exacerbation of COPD due to pneumonia should be coded as:

A) J44.1 only B) J18.9 only C) J44.1 first, then J18.9 D) J18.9 first, then J44.1

Question 16: For a patient with a nonunion of a previously closed femur fracture, the correct 7th character is:

A) A (initial encounter) B) D (routine healing) C) G (delayed healing) D) K (nonunion)

Question 17: A patient develops anaphylactic shock from correctly administered penicillin. The condition should be sequenced:

A) T36.0X5A first, then T78.2XXA B) T78.2XXA first, then T36.0X5A C) T36.0X5A only D) T78.2XXA only

Question 18: Combination codes should be used when:

A) Multiple conditions are present B) A single code describes multiple related conditions C) Documentation is unclear D) Provider requests specific coding

Question 19: A patient with sepsis due to E. coli should be coded as:

A) A41.9 (sepsis, unspecified) B) A41.51 (sepsis due to E. coli) C) R65.20 (severe sepsis) D) A41.51 and B96.20

Question 20: For gestational diabetes in a currently pregnant patient at 28 weeks, use:

A) E11.9 (Type 2 diabetes without complications) B) O24.419 (gestational diabetes, unspecified control) C) O99.810 (abnormal glucose complicating pregnancy) D) Z87.59 (personal history of endocrine disorders)

Question 21: Third-degree burn of the chest measuring 8% body surface should be coded with:

A) T21.31XA only B) T21.31XA and T31.0 C) T21.31XA, T31.0, and external cause code D) T31.0 and external cause code only

Question 22: When coding "Type 2 diabetes with diabetic retinopathy and diabetic nephropathy," you should:

A) Use only the most severe complication code B) Code each complication separately with multiple diabetes codes C) Use the most specific combination code available D) Code diabetes once and list all complications separately

Question 23: A patient admitted for chemotherapy to treat lung cancer should be sequenced:

A) C34.10 first, then Z51.11 B) Z51.11 first, then C34.10 C) Z51.11 only D) C34.10 only

Question 24: For sequela of old stroke with current right-sided weakness, use:

A) I63.9 and G81.91 B) I69.351 only C) G81.91 and I63.9S D) G81.91 only

Question 25: A pregnant woman at 28 weeks with gestational hypertension should be coded with:

A) I10 (essential hypertension) B) O13.3 (gestational hypertension, third trimester) C) O16.3 (unspecified maternal hypertension, third trimester) D) O10.13 (pre-existing essential hypertension complicating pregnancy)

Question 26: Multiple trauma with fractures of right femur and left tibia requires:

A) One code for multiple trauma B) Two separate fracture codes C) S06.9XXA (multiple injuries, unspecified) D) T07 (unspecified multiple injuries)

Question 27: Iron deficiency anemia due to chronic blood loss from gastric ulcer should be coded as:

A) D50.9 only B) D50.0 only C) D50.0 and K25.4 D) K25.4 only

Question 28: For late effects of poliomyelitis with current muscle weakness, code:

A) A80.9 and M62.81 B) B91 only C) B91 and M62.81 D) M62.81 and B91

Section 3: CPT® Evaluation and Management (Questions 29-40)

Question 29: A new patient is seen for 45 minutes with moderate complexity medical decision making. The correct code is:

A) 99203 (30-44 minutes, low complexity MDM) B) 99204 (45-59 minutes, moderate complexity MDM) C) 99205 (60-74 minutes, high complexity MDM) D) Either 99203 or 99204 depending on documentation

Question 30: An established patient is seen for routine blood pressure monitoring by a nurse under physician supervision. The appropriate code is:

A) 99211 B) 99212 C) 99213 D) No E/M code appropriate

Question 31: A consultation requires all of the following EXCEPT:

A) Written request from another physician B) Written report back to requesting physician C) Transfer of care to the consulting physician D) Rendering of an opinion or advice

Question 32: Critical care services require a minimum of how many minutes?

A) 15 minutes B) 20 minutes C) 30 minutes D) 45 minutes

Question 33: For Medicare patients, consultation codes should be:

A) Used as normal for all consultations B) Replaced with new/established patient codes C) Used only for office consultations D) Used only for inpatient consultations

Question 34: An established patient is seen for 25 minutes with low complexity medical decision making. The correct code is:

A) 99212 (10-19 minutes, straightforward MDM) B) 99213 (20-29 minutes, low complexity MDM) C) 99214 (30-39 minutes, moderate complexity MDM) D) Either 99212 or 99213

Question 35: Hospital discharge services are reported with:

A) The same code regardless of time spent B) 99238 for 30 minutes or less, 99239 for more than 30 minutes C) The final subsequent hospital care code D) No separate code—included in final hospital day

Question 36: Emergency department coding differs from office coding because:

A) It uses different code ranges B) It has no new vs. established patient distinction C) It requires different documentation D) All of the above

Question 37: Time-based E/M coding includes:

A) Only face-to-face time with the patient B) Only time spent in the examination room C) Total time on the date of encounter including non-face-to-face activities D) Only time spent documenting the encounter

Question 38: Prolonged services codes (99354-99355) are used when:

A) Any E/M service takes longer than expected B) Face-to-face time significantly exceeds the typical time for the highest level E/M code C) Documentation takes longer than usual D) The patient requires extensive counseling

Question 39: An established patient presents with multiple chronic conditions requiring extensive review. The physician spends 50 minutes total time. The correct code is:

A) 99213 (20-29 minutes) B) 99214 (30-39 minutes) C) 99215 (40-54 minutes) D) 99215 + 99354 (prolonged services)

Question 40: Medical decision making complexity is determined by which three elements?

A) History, examination, and time B) Problems addressed, data reviewed, and risk of management C) Chief complaint, assessment, and plan D) Diagnosis complexity, treatment options, and patient compliance

Section 4: CPT® Surgery Coding (Questions 41-65)

Question 41: A patient has three lacerations repaired: 3 cm on forehead (simple), 2 cm on cheek (simple), and 4 cm on scalp (intermediate). How should this be coded?

A) 12014 only (9 cm total, face) B) 12013 (5 cm face) + 12032 (4 cm scalp) C) 12014 (face) + 12032 (scalp) D) Three separate codes for each laceration

Question 42: Excision of a 1.5 cm malignant lesion from the back with 0.5 cm margins should be coded as:

A) 11402 (1.1 to 2.0 cm, benign) B) 11603 (1.1 to 2.0 cm, malignant) C) 11604 (2.1 to 3.0 cm, malignant) D) Cannot code until pathology results available

Question 43: A partial mastectomy with sentinel lymph node biopsy should be coded as:

A) 19301 only B) 19301 + 38500 C) 19302 + 38525 D) 38525 only

Question 44: Closed treatment of a displaced femur fracture with manipulation should be coded as:

A) 27500 (closed treatment without manipulation) B) 27502 (closed treatment with manipulation) C) 27506 (open treatment) D) 27509 (percutaneous skeletal fixation)

Question 45: Arthroscopic partial meniscectomy of the knee should be coded as:

A) 29870 (arthroscopy, diagnostic) B) 29880 (arthroscopy with meniscectomy) C) 29881 (arthroscopy with meniscectomy including repair) D) 27332 (open meniscectomy)

Question 46: Application of a short arm cast for a fracture treated by the same physician should be:

A) Coded separately with 29075 B) Included in the fracture treatment code C) Coded only if applied later D) Never coded separately

Question 47: A diagnostic nasal endoscopy followed by ethmoidectomy should be coded as:

A) 31231 + 31254 B) 31254 only C) 31231 only D) 31255 only

Question 48: Flexible laryngoscopy performed in the office should be coded as:

A) 31575 (flexible laryngoscopy, diagnostic) B) 31576 (flexible laryngoscopy with biopsy) C) 31540 (direct laryngoscopy with excision) D) 31579 (laryngoscopy with stroboscopy)

Question 49: Thoracentesis with image guidance should be coded as:

A) 32554 only B) 32554 + imaging guidance code C) 32555 only D) 32560 only

Question 50: A colonoscopy with biopsy and polyp removal should be coded as:

A) 45380 (colonoscopy with biopsy) only B) 45385 (colonoscopy with polyp removal) only C) 45380 + 45385 (both procedures) D) 45378 (diagnostic colonoscopy) + 45380 + 45385

Question 51: Laparoscopic repair of recurrent ventral hernia should be coded as:

A) 49560 (ventral hernia repair, initial) B) 49565 (ventral hernia repair, recurrent) C) 49650 (laparoscopic hernia repair) D) 49651 (laparoscopic hernia repair, recurrent)

Question 52: EGD with control of bleeding using injection therapy should be coded as:

A) 43235 (EGD, diagnostic) B) 43255 (EGD with control of bleeding) C) 43236 (EGD with injection) D) 43239 (EGD with biopsy)

Question 53: Cystoscopy with biopsy of bladder tumor and fulguration of small lesion should be coded as:

A) 52000 (cystoscopy, diagnostic) B) 52204 (cystoscopy with biopsy) + 52224 (fulguration) C) 52234 (cystoscopy with fulguration/resection of small tumor) D) 52204 (cystoscopy with biopsy) only

Question 54: Radical nephrectomy for renal cell carcinoma should be coded as:

A) 50220 (nephrectomy, including partial ureterectomy) B) 50225 (nephrectomy, complicated) C) 50230 (nephrectomy, radical) D) 50240 (nephrectomy, partial)

Question 55: TURP (transurethral resection of prostate) should be coded as:

A) 52450 (transurethral incision of prostate) B) 52500 (transurethral balloon dilation of prostate) C) 52601 (transurethral electrosurgical resection of prostate) D) 52700 (drainage of prostatic abscess)

Question 56: Bilateral orchiectomy for prostate cancer treatment should be coded as:

A) 54520 (orchiectomy, simple) × 2 B) 54520 with modifier -50 (bilateral) C) 54522 (orchiectomy, partial bilateral) D) 54535 (orchiectomy, radical)

Question 57: Laparoscopic total hysterectomy with bilateral salpingo-oophorectomy should be coded as:

A) 58570 (laparoscopic total hysterectomy) + 58661 (removal of adnexal structures) B) 58571 (laparoscopic total hysterectomy with removal of tubes and ovaries) C) 58150 (total abdominal hysterectomy) + 58720 (salpingo-oophorectomy) D) 58260 (vaginal hysterectomy) + 58661

Question 58: Vasectomy reversal (vasovasostomy) should be coded as:

A) 55250 (vasectomy) B) 55400 (vasovasostomy, vasoepididymostomy) C) 55450 (ligation of vas deferens) D) 54900 (epididymectomy)

Question 59: Carpal tunnel release should be coded as:

A) 64721 (neuroplasty of median nerve at carpal tunnel) B) 25000 (incision, extensor tendon sheath, wrist) C) 64831 (suture of digital nerve) D) 20526 (injection, carpal tunnel)

Question 60: Epidural steroid injection at L5-S1 level should be coded as:

A) 64483 (transforaminal epidural injection, single level) B) 64484 (transforaminal epidural injection, each additional level) C) 62311 (lumbar epidural injection) D) 20610 (arthrocentesis, major joint)

Question 61: Laminectomy for spinal stenosis at L4-L5 and L5-S1 should be coded as:

A) 63030 (laminectomy, lumbar) × 2 B) 63030 + 63035 (each additional segment) C) 63047 + 63048 (each additional segment) D) 22630 (spinal fusion)

Question 62: Simple repair of a 3.0 cm laceration on the face and a 2.5 cm laceration on the scalp should be coded as:

A) 12013 (face, 2.6-5.0 cm) + 12002 (scalp, 2.6-7.5 cm) B) 12014 (face, 7.6-12.5 cm) for combined length C) 12013 (face, 2.6-5.0 cm) only D) Two separate simple repair codes

Question 63: Arthroscopic meniscectomy with repair of anterior cruciate ligament should be coded as:

A) 29880 (meniscectomy) only B) 29888 (ACL reconstruction) only C) 29880 + 29888 (both procedures) D) 29870 (diagnostic arthroscopy) + 29880 + 29888

Question 64: Emergency tracheostomy for acute airway obstruction should be coded as:

A) 31600 (tracheostomy, planned) B) 31601 (tracheostomy, emergency) C) 31603 (tracheostomy, emergency procedure) D) 31605 (tracheostomy, planned procedure)

Question 65: Laparoscopic cholecystectomy with cholangiography should be coded as:

A) 47562 (laparoscopic cholecystectomy) only B) 47563 (laparoscopic cholecystectomy with cholangiography) C) 47562 + 74300 (cholangiography) D) 47600 (open cholecystectomy)

Section 5: CPT® Anesthesia, Radiology, Pathology, and Medicine (Questions 66-85)

Question 66: Anesthesia for appendectomy (00840, 6 base units) lasting 78 minutes in a healthy 45-year-old patient. Calculate total units:

A) 11 units (6 base + 5 time + 0 physical status) B) 12 units (6 base + 6 time + 0 physical status) C) 13 units (6 base + 5 time + 2 physical status) D) 14 units (6 base + 6 time + 2 physical status)

Question 67: Which qualifying circumstance applies to anesthesia for a 2-month-old infant?

A) +99100 (extreme age) B) +99116 (controlled hypotension) C) +99135 (total body hypothermia) D) +99140 (emergency conditions)

Question 68: A patient with severe, poorly controlled diabetes and heart failure would most likely be assigned which physical status modifier?

A) P1 (normal healthy patient) B) P2 (mild systemic disease) C) P3 (severe systemic disease) D) P4 (severe systemic disease, constant threat to life)

Question 69: Anesthesia time units are calculated by:

A) Total procedure time ÷ 15 minutes B) Anesthesia start to surgery end ÷ 15 minutes C) Anesthesia start to patient discharge ÷ 15 minutes D) Surgery start to surgery end ÷ 15 minutes

Question 70: Emergency surgery adds which qualifying circumstance?

A) +99100 (extreme age) B) +99116 (total body hypothermia) C) +99135 (controlled hypotension) D) +99140 (emergency conditions)

Question 71: A radiologist interprets a chest X-ray performed at a hospital. How should the radiologist bill?

A) 71045 (chest X-ray, global) B) 71045-26 (chest X-ray, professional component) C) 71045-TC (chest X-ray, technical component) D) Cannot bill separately

Question 72: Screening mammography for both breasts should be coded as:

A) 77065 (diagnostic mammography, unilateral) × 2 B) 77066 (diagnostic mammography, bilateral) C) 77067 (screening mammography, bilateral) D) 77065 with modifier -50 (bilateral)

Question 73: CT guidance for needle biopsy should be coded as:

A) 77012 (CT guidance for needle placement) only B) Biopsy code only (guidance included) C) Depends on whether guidance is included in biopsy code description D) Both codes always separately reportable

Question 74: Complete abdominal ultrasound should be coded as:

A) 76700 (ultrasound, abdominal, complete) B) 76705 (ultrasound, abdominal, limited) C) 76770 (ultrasound, retroperitoneal) D) Multiple organ-specific ultrasound codes

Question 75: MRI of the knee without and with contrast should be coded as:

A) 73721 (MRI knee, without contrast) B) 73722 (MRI knee, with contrast) C) 73723 (MRI knee, without and with contrast) D) 73721 + 73722 (both codes)

Question 76: A complete blood count (CBC) with differential should be coded as:

A) 85025 (CBC, automated with differential) B) 85027 (CBC, automated without differential) C) 85004 (blood count, automated differential) D) 85009 (blood count, manual differential)

Question 77: Hepatitis C antibody screening should be coded as:

A) 86803 (Hepatitis C antibody) B) 87520 (Hepatitis C, direct probe) C) 87521 (Hepatitis C, amplified probe) D) 87522 (Hepatitis C, quantification)

Question 78: A comprehensive metabolic panel includes all of the following EXCEPT:

A) Glucose B) Creatinine C) Lipid panel D) Total protein

Question 79: Urinalysis with microscopy should be coded as:

A) 81000 (urinalysis, non-automated) B) 81001 (urinalysis, automated) C) 81002 (urinalysis, non-automated without microscopy) D) 81003 (urinalysis, automated without microscopy)

Question 80: Influenza vaccination administration should be coded with:

A) 90471 (immunization administration, first vaccine) B) 90460 (immunization administration through 18 years, with counseling) C) 90472 (immunization administration, each additional vaccine) D) Depends on patient age and counseling provided

Question 81: An EKG with interpretation and report should be coded as:

A) 93000 (electrocardiogram, complete) B) 93005 (electrocardiogram, tracing only) C) 93010 (electrocardiogram, interpretation and report only) D) 93040 (rhythm EKG)

Question 82: Nebulizer treatment for acute bronchospasm should be coded as:

A) 94640 (pressurized or nonpressurized inhalation treatment) B) 94060 (bronchodilation responsiveness) C) 94620 (pulmonary stress testing) D) 94664 (aerosol or vapor inhalation, initial)

Question 83: Physical therapy evaluation should be coded as:

A) 97110 (therapeutic exercises) B) 97140 (manual therapy) C) 97161 (physical therapy evaluation, low complexity) D) Depends on complexity of evaluation

Question 84: Vitamin B12 injection for pernicious anemia should be coded with:

A) 96372 (therapeutic injection, subcutaneous or intramuscular) B) 96365 (intravenous infusion) C) 90471 (immunization administration) D) J3420 (vitamin B12 injection, HCPCS code) only

Question 85: Psychotherapy, 60 minutes, should be coded as:

A) 90832 (psychotherapy, 30 minutes) B) 90834 (psychotherapy, 45 minutes) C) 90837 (psychotherapy, 60 minutes) D) 90853 (group psychotherapy)

Section 6: HCPCS Level II and Modifiers (Questions 86-95)

Question 86: Durable medical equipment (DME) is typically coded using which HCPCS code range?

A) A codes B) E codes C) J codes D) L codes

Question 87: Injectable drug codes are typically found in which HCPCS section?

A) A codes B) E codes C) J codes D) Q codes

Question 88: Modifier -25 indicates:

A) Bilateral procedure B) Significant, separately identifiable E/M service C) Professional component D) Reduced services

Question 89: Modifier -59 is used to indicate:

A) Distinct procedural service B) Bilateral procedure C) Multiple procedures D) Reduced services

Question 90: Modifier -50 indicates:

A) Bilateral procedure B) Multiple procedures C) Reduced services D) Discontinued procedure

Question 91: Which modifier indicates a reduced service?

A) -22 (increased procedural services) B) -52 (reduced services) C) -53 (discontinued procedure) D) -54 (surgical care only)

Question 92: Modifier -26 represents:

A) Technical component B) Professional component C) Bilateral procedure D) Multiple procedures

Question 93: Ambulance transport to the hospital should be coded with:

A) A0426 (ambulance service, advanced life support, non-emergency) B) A0429 (ambulance service, basic life support, non-emergency) C) Depends on level of service and urgency D) E codes (durable medical equipment)

Question 94: A wheelchair for home use should be coded with:

A) A4556 (wheelchair accessory) B) E1130 (standard wheelchair) C) K0001 (standard wheelchair) D) Depends on specific wheelchair type and features

Question 95: Modifier -76 indicates:

A) Repeat procedure by same physician B) Repeat procedure by different physician C) Bilateral procedure D) Multiple procedures

Section 7: Compliance and Regulatory (Questions 96-100)

Question 96: HIPAA Privacy Rule primarily protects:

A) Healthcare provider financial information B) Protected Health Information (PHI) C) Insurance company proprietary data D) Hospital operational procedures

Question 97: Which is NOT considered Protected Health Information under HIPAA?

A) Patient name B) Medical record number C) Date of birth D) Hospital's tax identification number

Question 98: Upcoding is defined as:

A) Billing for services at a lower level than provided B) Billing for services at a higher level than provided or documented C) Billing for services not provided D) Unbundling services

Question 99: The False Claims Act addresses:

A) Knowingly submitting false claims for payment B) HIPAA privacy violations C) Medical malpractice D) Medication errors

Question 100: Medical necessity means:

A) Any service ordered by a physician B) Services reasonable and necessary for diagnosis or treatment C) All preventive care services D) Services covered by insurance

Answer Key with Detailed Explanations

Section 1: Medical Terminology and Anatomy (Questions 1-8)

Question 1: Answer: B) Cholecystectomy

Explanation: The suffix "-ectomy" means surgical removal. Cholecystectomy combines "chole" (bile), "cyst" (bladder/sac), and "-ectomy" (removal), meaning surgical removal of the gallbladder. Cholecystitis is inflammation of the gallbladder, cholelithiasis means gallstones, and cholecystostomy is creating a surgical opening into the gallbladder.

Study Tip: Remember that "-ectomy" always indicates removal. When you see this suffix on the exam, you know the procedure involves taking something out of the body. Create a mental list of common -ectomy procedures: appendectomy, tonsillectomy, hysterectomy.

Question 2: Answer: B) Fast

Explanation: The prefix "tachy-" means fast or rapid. You see this in medical terms like tachycardia (fast heart rate) and tachypnea (rapid breathing). The opposite prefix is "brady-" meaning slow, as in bradycardia (slow heart rate). Understanding these opposing prefixes helps you quickly interpret vital sign abnormalities in medical documentation.

Study Tip: Create pairs of opposing prefixes to strengthen your memory: tachy/brady (fast/slow), hyper/hypo (above/below), macro/micro (large/small). This pairing technique helps you remember both terms and understand their relationships.

Question 3: Answer: B) Ureter

Explanation: The ureter is the muscular tube that transports urine from the kidney to the bladder. Don't confuse this with the urethra, which carries urine from the bladder out of the body. A helpful memory trick: ureter has two e's and there are two ureters (one from each kidney). Urethra has one e and there's only one urethra.

Study Tip: Draw a simple diagram of the urinary system showing kidneys → ureters → bladder → urethra. This visual representation helps you remember the flow of urine and the anatomical relationships. Label each structure and quiz yourself regularly.

Question 4: Answer: B) Middle muscular layer

Explanation: The myocardium is the middle, muscular layer of the heart that contracts to pump blood. The prefix "myo-" means muscle, and "cardium" refers to the heart. The epicardium is the outer layer, the endocardium is the inner lining, and the pericardium is the protective sac surrounding the heart. Understanding heart layers is crucial for coding cardiac conditions and procedures.

Study Tip: Remember the three heart wall layers with this memory device: "EPM" - Epicardium (outside), Pericardium (sac around), Myocardium (muscle), Endocardium (inside lining). Knowing these layers helps you understand cardiac procedure codes and documentation.

Question 5: Answer: A) Pathology

Explanation: Pathology is the study of disease, combining "patho-" (disease) and "-logy" (study of). Physiology is the study of body function, histology studies tissues, and cytology studies cells. Understanding these terms helps you recognize different types of medical specialists and diagnostic procedures.

Study Tip: The suffix "-ology" always means "study of." When you encounter unfamiliar terms with this suffix, break them down: cardiology (study of heart), neurology (study of nerves), dermatology (study of skin). This pattern recognition accelerates your learning.

Question 6: Answer: C) Surgical opening

Explanation: The suffix "-ostomy" indicates creation of a surgical opening or connection. Common examples include colostomy (opening in the colon), tracheostomy (opening in the trachea), and ileostomy (opening in the ileum). This differs from "-otomy" which means surgical incision (cutting into).

Study Tip: Distinguish between "-otomy" (cutting into, usually temporary) and "-ostomy" (creating an opening, often permanent). Tracheotomy is an incision into the trachea, while tracheostomy creates a more permanent opening. Understanding this distinction helps with accurate surgical coding.

Question 7: Answer: C) Esophagus

Explanation: The esophagus is part of the digestive system, not the respiratory system. It's the muscular tube that carries food from the pharynx to the stomach. The respiratory system includes structures involved in breathing: trachea (windpipe), bronchi (airway branches), and alveoli (air sacs where gas exchange occurs).

Study Tip: Remember that the respiratory system includes all structures involved in breathing and gas exchange. The esophagus sits behind the trachea but serves a digestive function. Drawing a cross-section view shows their anatomical relationship and functional differences.

Question 8: Answer: B) Both sides

Explanation: "Bilateral" means both sides, combining "bi-" (two) and "lateral" (side). This term is crucial in coding because many procedures can be performed on one side (unilateral) or both sides (bilateral), which affects code selection and modifier usage. Bilateral procedures often require modifier -50.

Study Tip: Learn directional term pairs: bilateral/unilateral (both/one side), superior/inferior (above/below), anterior/posterior (front/back), medial/lateral (toward midline/away from midline). These terms appear constantly in operative reports and affect code selection.

Section 2: ICD-10-CM Diagnosis Coding (Questions 9-28)

Question 9: Answer: B) Alphabetic index first, then tabular list

Explanation: This is the most fundamental rule in ICD-10-CM coding. Always start with the alphabetic index to find potential codes, then verify in the tabular list to confirm the correct code and check for any additional instructions. Coding directly from the index or tabular list alone leads to errors because you might miss important information.

Study Tip: Make this your mantra: "Index first, tabular always." Never assign a code without verifying it in the tabular list. The index provides starting points, but the tabular list contains the complete code descriptions, inclusion notes, exclusion notes, and additional instructions that ensure accurate coding.

Question 10: Answer: B) The condition cannot be coded here

Explanation: Excludes1 notes indicate mutually exclusive conditions that cannot be coded together. These represent "not coded here" instructions. In contrast, Excludes2 notes indicate conditions not included in the current code but can be coded additionally if both are present. Understanding this distinction prevents incorrect code combinations.

Study Tip: Think of Excludes1 as "either/or" situations where you choose one code or the other, never both. Excludes2 represents "not included but can coexist" situations where you might code both if documentation supports it. Always read and apply these notes carefully—they're specifically designed to prevent common coding errors.

Question 11: Answer: B) E11.21 and Z79.4

Explanation: Type 2 diabetes with diabetic nephropathy is coded with E11.21. Because the patient uses insulin, you must add Z79.4 (long-term insulin use) to provide complete information about the patient's treatment. Using insulin doesn't change Type 2 diabetes to Type 1—the diabetes type is based on the underlying pathophysiology, not the treatment method.

Study Tip: Remember that Type 1 vs. Type 2 classification depends on the disease mechanism (autoimmune vs. insulin resistance), not the treatment. Many Type 2 diabetics use insulin but remain Type 2. Always add Z79.4 when Type 2 diabetics use insulin—this information is important for clinical care and may affect reimbursement.

Question 12: Answer: B) R07.9 (chest pain, unspecified)

Explanation: In outpatient settings, you never code "rule out," "suspected," "probable," or "questionable" diagnoses. Since the myocardial infarction was ruled out with normal testing, you code only what was confirmed: the patient's chest pain. The normal EKG and enzymes mean you cannot code any cardiac disease.

Study Tip: This is one of the most important outpatient coding rules. When you see "rule out" in outpatient documentation, code only the signs, symptoms, test results, or confirmed diagnoses. Inpatient coding follows different rules—suspected conditions can be coded as if confirmed in that setting. Know which rules apply to your work environment.

Question 13: Answer: C) Primary breast cancer with unspecified metastases

Explanation: "Metastatic breast cancer" indicates the breast is the primary site with metastases (spread) to other locations. Code the primary breast cancer (C50.-) and secondary site unspecified (C79.9) unless specific metastatic sites are documented. If documentation said "metastatic cancer to the breast," that would indicate the breast is the secondary site.

Study Tip: Pay careful attention to prepositions in cancer documentation. "Metastatic FROM" identifies the primary site. "Metastatic TO" identifies the secondary site. "Metastatic breast cancer" without prepositions usually means primary breast cancer with metastases elsewhere.

Question 14: Answer: C) Z22.7 (latent tuberculosis)

Explanation: Latent tuberculosis infection means the person has been infected but doesn't have active disease. Z22.7 specifically captures this status. Active TB uses A15-A19 codes. Personal history (Z87.01) is used only after TB has been completely treated and resolved. Understanding disease states (active, latent, history) ensures accurate code selection.

Study Tip: Learn to distinguish between active disease, latent infection, carrier states, and history. Each represents a different clinical situation requiring different codes. Review Z-code categories thoroughly—they're essential for complete and accurate coding but often overlooked by new coders.

Question 15: Answer: C) J44.1 first, then J18.9

Explanation: When COPD exacerbation is caused by an identified condition like pneumonia, code both. The exacerbated chronic condition (J44.1) is sequenced first because it's the reason for the encounter, followed by the condition causing the exacerbation (J18.9). This sequencing tells the complete clinical story.

Study Tip: Acute exacerbations of chronic conditions often require two codes: one for the exacerbated chronic condition and one for the trigger or cause. Always check for "code also" or "use additional code" instructions that indicate when multiple codes are needed. Understanding these relationships improves coding accuracy and completeness.

Question 16: Answer: D) K (nonunion)

Explanation: Nonunion means the bone fracture has completely failed to heal. For a closed fracture with nonunion, use 7th character "K." This differs from delayed healing (character "G"), which indicates slower-than-expected but ongoing healing. Understanding healing complications and their specific 7th characters ensures accurate fracture follow-up coding.

Study Tip: Create a reference chart for fracture 7th characters showing initial encounter, subsequent encounters with various healing status (routine, delayed, nonunion, malunion), and sequela. This visual reference helps you quickly select the correct character based on documentation. Fracture coding is complex, and organized reference materials save time.

Question 17: Answer: B) T78.2XXA first, then T36.0X5A

Explanation: For adverse effects (proper medication, proper dose, unexpected reaction), sequence the manifestation or effect first (anaphylactic shock, T78.2XXA), then the adverse effect code (penicillin adverse effect, T36.0X5A). This sequencing differs from poisoning, where the poison code comes first. Understanding this sequencing rule prevents common coding errors.

Study Tip: Remember the sequencing difference: Adverse effects = reaction first, drug second. Poisoning = poison first, effects second. This distinction reflects different clinical scenarios—adverse effects involve proper use with unexpected reactions, while poisoning involves improper use or exposure. Clarify the circumstances before coding.

Question 18: Answer: B) A single code describes multiple related conditions

Explanation: Combination codes capture multiple related conditions or circumstances with a single code, making coding more efficient and accurate. Always check for combination codes before assigning multiple separate codes for related conditions. The alphabetic index often points to combination codes, but you must verify in the tabular list.

Study Tip: When documentation shows multiple related conditions (like diabetes with complications), always search for combination codes first. The ICD-10-CM structure includes many combination codes that reduce the number of codes needed while maintaining specificity. Using combination codes when available is not just preferred—it's required.

Question 19: Answer: B) A41.51 (sepsis due to E. coli)

Explanation: When the organism causing sepsis is identified, use the specific code that includes the organism (A41.51). Don't code sepsis unspecified (A41.9) when the specific organism is documented. You also don't need to add a separate code for the organism (B96.20) because it's already included in A41.51. This is an example of why checking code descriptions carefully prevents unnecessary duplicate coding.

Study Tip: Sepsis coding includes specific organisms when documented. Review the A40-A41 category thoroughly, noting which organisms have their own specific codes. When an organism is specified in documentation, use the most specific code available. Accurate sepsis coding is crucial because it affects severity classification and reimbursement.

Question 20: Answer: B) O24.419 (gestational diabetes, unspecified control)

Explanation: Pregnancy-related conditions use O-codes from Chapter 15, not general medical codes. Gestational diabetes is diabetes that develops during pregnancy in women who weren't previously diabetic. O24.419 specifically captures this condition. The gestational age code (Z3A.28 for 28 weeks) would be added as an additional code for complete documentation.

Study Tip: Pregnancy coding rules differ significantly from general medical coding. All conditions complicating pregnancy use O-codes when the patient is currently pregnant. Learn these special rules thoroughly because pregnancy coding appears regularly on the CPC exam and in practice. The seventh character often indicates trimester, and gestational age codes provide additional specificity.

Question 21: Answer: C) T21.31XA, T31.0, and external cause code

Explanation: Complete burn coding requires three components: 1) Site and degree code (T21.31XA for third-degree chest burn), 2) Extent code showing percentage of body surface burned (T31.0 for less than 10%), and 3) External cause code explaining how the burn occurred. All three provide essential information for treatment planning and statistics.

Study Tip: Create a burn coding checklist: site/degree code, extent code, external cause code. Never forget any component—incomplete burn coding misrepresents the injury severity and circumstances. The extent code is particularly important because it indicates total burn size, which directly affects treatment intensity and prognosis.

Question 22: Answer: C) Use the most specific combination code available

Explanation: ICD-10-CM provides detailed combination codes for diabetes with multiple complications. Rather than coding diabetes multiple times or using only one complication code, find the most specific combination code that captures all documented complications. If separate codes are needed for different complications, use them, but always check for comprehensive combination codes first.

Study Tip: Diabetes coding in ICD-10-CM is highly specific. The fourth and fifth characters indicate different complications (retinopathy, nephropathy, neuropathy, etc.). Familiarize yourself with the E08-E13 categories and their structure. Understanding this organization helps you quickly locate the most appropriate codes for complex diabetes cases.

Question 23: Answer: B) Z51.11 first, then C34.10

Explanation: When the encounter is solely for chemotherapy administration, sequence the chemotherapy encounter code (Z51.11) first, followed by the cancer code. The chemotherapy encounter is the reason for this specific visit, making it the principal diagnosis. This sequencing changes if the patient is receiving treatment for chemotherapy complications—then the complication would be first.

Study Tip: Z-codes for encounters can be either principal or additional diagnoses depending on circumstances. When the encounter is specifically FOR the service described in the Z-code (chemotherapy, radiation, aftercare), that Z-code goes first. Understanding Z-code sequencing rules is essential for accurate coding in various encounter types.

Question 24: Answer: B) I69.351 only

Explanation: The I69 category provides specific codes for sequelae (late effects) of cerebrovascular disease. I69.351 describes hemiplegia affecting the right dominant side following cerebral infarction—it includes both the residual condition (hemiplegia) and its cause (old stroke). You don't need to code them separately because this single code captures the complete clinical picture.

Study Tip: Always check for specific sequela codes before coding residual conditions separately. Many disease categories include specific sequela codes that capture both the residual effect and its cause. Using these specific codes when available is more accurate and efficient than multiple separate codes.

Question 25: Answer: B) O13.3 (gestational hypertension, third trimester)

Explanation: Gestational hypertension is high blood pressure that develops during pregnancy in women who didn't have hypertension before. Because this is pregnancy-related, use the O-code (O13.3) rather than essential hypertension (I10). The third trimester designation comes from the 28-week gestational age documented. Pregnancy coding requires attention to whether conditions existed before pregnancy or developed during it.

Study Tip: Distinguish between pre-existing conditions complicating pregnancy (use O10-O16 categories) and conditions that develop during pregnancy. The timing and relationship to pregnancy affect code selection. Always check if a condition predated the pregnancy or arose during it—this distinction determines which code category to use.

Question 26: Answer: B) Two separate fracture codes

Explanation: When multiple distinct fractures occur, code each fracture separately using specific codes for each anatomical site. Multiple injury codes (T07, S06.9XXA) are only used when specific injuries cannot be identified or documented. Always code injuries as specifically as possible—separate fracture codes provide much more useful information than generic "multiple injuries" codes.

Study Tip: Be as specific as possible in injury coding. Generic codes for multiple injuries or unspecified sites should be last resorts when documentation doesn't support more specific coding. Each specific fracture code tells a story about injury pattern and severity that generic codes cannot convey.

Question 27: Answer: C) D50.0 and K25.4

Explanation: When anemia has an identified cause, code both the anemia and its cause. D50.0 (iron deficiency anemia secondary to blood loss, chronic) describes the anemia, while K25.4 (chronic gastric ulcer with hemorrhage) identifies the source of blood loss causing the anemia. The "use additional code" instruction under D50.0 specifically directs you to code the source of blood loss when known.

Study Tip: Pay attention to "use additional code" instructions in the tabular list. These instructions aren't suggestions—they're requirements for complete coding. When anemia, infection, or other secondary conditions have identified causes, code both to tell the complete clinical story. This completeness supports medical necessity and appropriate treatment.

Question 28: Answer: D) M62.81 and B91

Explanation: For late effects (sequelae), generally code the residual condition first (M62.81, muscle weakness), then the sequela code (B91, sequelae of poliomyelitis). This sequencing emphasizes the current condition requiring treatment while documenting its cause.

Understanding sequela coding rules helps you accurately represent patients' ongoing health issues related to past conditions.

Study Tip: Sequela coding captures the long-term effects of conditions that have resolved. The sequela code explains WHY the patient has the current condition. Always check if sequela-specific codes exist before using general residual condition codes—specific sequela codes often capture both elements more accurately.

Section 3: CPT® Evaluation and Management (Questions 29-40)

Question 29: Answer: B) 99204 (45-59 minutes, moderate complexity MDM)

Explanation: For new patient office visits, you can use either time OR medical decision making to select the appropriate level. Since both the 45 minutes and moderate complexity MDM support 99204, this is the correct code. When both methods point to the same level, you have confirmation of appropriate code selection. You cannot combine elements from both methods—choose whichever method best supports the level of service provided.

Study Tip: Learn the time thresholds and MDM requirements for each E/M level. Having these memorized allows you to quickly identify the appropriate level from documentation. For new patients: 99202 (15-29 min), 99203 (30-44 min), 99204 (45-59 min), 99205 (60-74 min). Understanding both time-based and MDM-based selection gives you flexibility in code assignment.

Question 30: Answer: A) 99211

Explanation: 99211 is the only E/M code that can be performed by clinical staff under physician supervision without the physician being present. It represents minimal services like blood pressure checks, simple dressing changes, or medication administration. This level acknowledges that not all patient encounters require direct physician involvement while still capturing the service provided.

Study Tip: Remember that 99211 is unique—it doesn't require physician presence, only supervision. All other E/M codes require the physician or qualified healthcare professional to perform and document the service. Understanding when 99211 is appropriate prevents undercoding (missing billable services) or overcoding (billing physician services for nurse-only visits).

Question 31: Answer: C) Transfer of care to the consulting physician

Explanation: Consultations do NOT require transfer of care—in fact, transfer of care would make it a referral, not a consultation. The three Rs of consultations are: Request (from another physician), Render (opinion or advice), and Report (back to requesting physician). The requesting physician maintains primary responsibility while the consultant provides specialized expertise.

Study Tip: Understand the distinction between consultations and referrals. Consultations are temporary relationships where the specialist provides advice but care returns to the requesting physician. Referrals involve transfer of care responsibility. This distinction affects code selection and, in some cases, whether consultation codes can be used at all (Medicare doesn't recognize consultation codes).

Question 32: Answer: C) 30 minutes

Explanation: Critical care services require a minimum of 30 minutes to be billable using code 99291. Less than 30 minutes should be reported using appropriate E/M codes based on the level of service provided. The 30-minute threshold ensures that only truly intensive, continuous critical care situations are reported with critical care codes, which carry higher reimbursement due to their intensity.

Study Tip: Critical care coding has specific time thresholds: 30-74 minutes = 99291 only; 75-104 minutes = 99291 + 99292 once; 105-134 minutes = 99291 + 99292 twice. Create a reference chart showing these time breaks for quick lookup. Remember that critical care time includes only time directly devoted to the critically ill patient's care, not time spent on separately billable procedures.

Question 33: Answer: B) Replaced with new/established patient codes

Explanation: Medicare stopped recognizing consultation codes in 2010. For Medicare patients, use appropriate new patient or established patient E/M codes instead of consultation codes. Private payers may still accept consultation codes, so verify payer-specific policies before coding. This Medicare policy change created a significant shift in how consultative services are reported.

Study Tip: Know your payer policies on consultation codes. While this question asks specifically about Medicare, different payers may have different rules. Always verify consultation code acceptance before billing. When consultation codes aren't accepted, select new or established patient codes based on the patient's relationship with the consulting physician.

Question 34: Answer: B) 99213 (20-29 minutes, low complexity MDM)

Explanation: For established patients, 99213 covers 20-29 minutes OR low complexity MDM. Since both criteria are met (25 minutes AND low complexity MDM), 99213 is clearly the appropriate code. This scenario demonstrates how either time or MDM can support level selection—when both methods align, you have strong justification for the chosen level.

Study Tip: For established patients, memorize these ranges: 99211 (minimal), 99212 (10-19 min), 99213 (20-29 min), 99214 (30-39 min), 99215 (40-54 min). Practice identifying levels from documentation by finding either time documentation or MDM elements. Developing speed in level selection is crucial for exam success and efficient coding practice.

Question 35: Answer: B) 99238 for 30 minutes or less, 99239 for more than 30 minutes

Explanation: Hospital discharge services are time-based with two codes: 99238 (30 minutes or less) and 99239 (more than 30 minutes). These codes cover final examination, discharge instructions, prescription writing, and record preparation. They're separate from subsequent hospital care codes and should be reported on the discharge date regardless of whether other E/M services were provided that day.

Study Tip: Discharge day coding follows special rules. The discharge service code replaces the subsequent hospital care code normally reported for daily hospital visits. Understanding this prevents coding both a subsequent hospital visit and discharge service on the same day—the discharge service alone captures the day's work.

Question 36: Answer: D) All of the above

Explanation: ED coding differs from office coding in multiple ways: it uses unique code ranges (99281-99285), makes no distinction between new and established patients (any patient can receive any level code based on service), and often involves different documentation patterns due to emergency nature. These differences reflect the unique environment and requirements of emergency medicine.

Study Tip: ED coding principles differ significantly from office coding. Emergency physicians must be prepared to handle any patient with any condition at any time, justifying higher-level codes more frequently than typical office practice. The lack of new vs. established distinction recognizes that emergency care intensity depends on patient acuity, not prior relationship with the physician.

Question 37: Answer: C) Total time on the date of encounter including non-face-to-face activities

Explanation: Current E/M guidelines define time broadly to include total time spent on the date of encounter, encompassing face-to-face time plus non-face-to-face activities like reviewing records, ordering tests, communicating with other providers, and documentation. This expanded definition better captures the total physician work involved in patient care beyond just examination room time.

Study Tip: Understanding time-based coding's broader definition helps you recognize when time-based selection might yield a higher level than MDM-based selection. Document all relevant time activities: record review, test interpretation, care coordination, family counseling, and documentation. This comprehensive time accounting often reveals that physicians spend much more time on patient care than the face-to-face encounter alone suggests.

Question 38: Answer: B) Face-to-face time significantly exceeds the typical time for the highest level E/M code

Explanation: Prolonged services codes (99354-99355) are used only when face-to-face time extends significantly beyond the highest level E/M code time threshold. For established patients, this means exceeding 54 minutes; for new patients, exceeding 74 minutes. These codes cannot be reported for time spent documenting or for services that don't involve direct patient interaction.

Study Tip: Prolonged services require meeting strict criteria: must be face-to-face, must exceed highest E/M level by at least 15 minutes before first prolonged code applies, must be medically necessary (not just convenient for scheduling). Documentation must clearly show the additional time and its necessity. These codes should be used relatively rarely—most encounters fit within standard E/M levels.

Question 39: Answer: C) 99215 (40-54 minutes)

Explanation: 99215 covers 40-54 minutes for established patients. Since 50 minutes falls within this range, 99215 alone is appropriate. Prolonged services (99354) would only be used if time exceeded 54 minutes significantly. Don't automatically add prolonged codes just because a visit took substantial time—the regular E/M levels accommodate visits up to the stated time maximum.

Study Tip: Know the upper time limits for each E/M level to avoid unnecessarily adding prolonged services codes. For established patients, 99215 goes up to 54 minutes, so anything within that range uses 99215 alone. Only when time exceeds these maximums by enough to warrant additional reimbursement (typically 15+ minutes beyond) should prolonged codes be considered.

Question 40: Answer: B) Problems addressed, data reviewed, and risk of management

Explanation: Current E/M guidelines base medical decision making on three elements: 1) number and complexity of problems addressed, 2) amount and/or complexity of data to be reviewed and analyzed, and 3) risk of complications and/or morbidity or mortality of patient management. These three elements replaced the older system's focus on diagnosis/management options, data amount, and risk tables.

Study Tip: Memorize these three MDM elements—they're fundamental to current E/M coding. Understanding how each element contributes to complexity level helps you analyze documentation and select appropriate codes. Each element has specific criteria for straightforward, low, moderate, and high complexity, and at least two of the three elements must be met for a given complexity level.

Question 41: Answer: B) 12013 (5 cm face) + 12032 (4 cm scalp)

Explanation: Face and scalp are different anatomical groups in wound repair coding. Face wounds total 5 cm (3+2), coded as 12013. Scalp wound is 4 cm coded as 12032. Simple repairs on face combine separately from intermediate repairs on scalp.

Study Tip: Never combine wound lengths across different anatomical groups or repair types. Create a chart showing which body areas group together.

Question 42: Answer: C) 11604 (2.1 to 3.0 cm, malignant)

Explanation: Total diameter = lesion (1.5 cm) + margins (0.5 × 2 = 1.0 cm) = 2.5 cm. Malignant lesion on trunk codes to 11604 for 2.1-3.0 cm range. Always add all margins to lesion size.

Study Tip: Remember: measure lesion + all margins removed. Practice calculating total diameters from various documentation formats.

Question 43: Answer: B) 19301 + 38500

Explanation: Partial mastectomy (19301) and sentinel lymph node biopsy (38500) are separate procedures coded together when both performed. Check for bundling edits, but these commonly occur together.

Study Tip: Know which breast procedures bundle and which report separately. Sentinel node biopsy is typically separately reportable.

Question 44: Answer: B) 27502 (closed treatment with manipulation)

Explanation: Closed treatment with manipulation (27502) is correct when fracture fragments are realigned without surgical exposure. Manipulation increases complexity and reimbursement over non-manipulation codes.

Study Tip: Distinguish closed (no surgical opening), open (surgical exposure), and percutaneous (fixation through skin). Document review determines method.

Question 45: Answer: B) 29880 (arthroscopy with meniscectomy)

Explanation: Arthroscopic meniscectomy (29880) represents partial or total meniscal removal. Diagnostic arthroscopy is included when performed during surgical arthroscopy.

Study Tip: Surgical arthroscopy codes include diagnostic arthroscopy. Never code both diagnostic and surgical arthroscopy for same joint/session.

Question 46: Answer: B) Included in the fracture treatment code

Explanation: Cast application by the treating physician is included in fracture treatment codes as part of the global surgical package.

Study Tip: Cast application codes are used when performed by different provider or as replacement/adjustment service, not initial treatment.

Question 47: Answer: B) 31254 only

Explanation: Diagnostic endoscopy is included when surgical endoscopy is performed. Code only the most comprehensive procedure (31254 ethmoidectomy).

Study Tip: In endoscopy, diagnostic procedures are included in surgical procedures. Always code the highest level service performed.

Question 48: Answer: A) 31575 (flexible laryngoscopy, diagnostic)

Explanation: Office-based flexible fiberoptic laryngoscopy for diagnostic purposes codes to 31575. This common ENT procedure evaluates vocal cord function.

Study Tip: Know the difference between flexible (31575) and rigid laryngoscopy procedures. Setting and equipment affect code selection.

Question 49: Answer: A) 32554 only

Explanation: Current thoracentesis codes include imaging guidance when performed. Don't code imaging separately—it's bundled into the procedure code.

Study Tip: Many procedure codes now include imaging guidance. Check code descriptions carefully before adding separate imaging codes.

Question 50: Answer: B) 45385 (colonoscopy with polyp removal) only

Explanation: Code the most extensive colonoscopy procedure performed. Polyp removal (45385) includes any biopsies performed during the same session.

Study Tip: Colonoscopy coding: report only the most comprehensive procedure. Multiple similar procedures don't get coded separately.

Question 51: Answer: D) 49651 (laparoscopic hernia repair, recurrent)

Explanation: This code specifically addresses laparoscopic repair of recurrent ventral hernia, capturing both approach and recurrent status.

Study Tip: Hernia codes differentiate initial vs. recurrent and open vs. laparoscopic. All four elements affect code selection.

Question 52: Answer: B) 43255 (EGD with control of bleeding)

Explanation: EGD with bleeding control (43255) covers any method of hemostasis including injection, thermal, or mechanical techniques.

Study Tip: Upper endoscopy codes describe procedures by what's done, not how it's done. Specific techniques don't change codes.

Question 53: Answer: C) 52234 (cystoscopy with fulguration/resection of small tumor)

Explanation: Code the most extensive cystoscopic procedure. Fulguration/resection (52234) includes any biopsy performed during the same session.

Study Tip: Cystoscopy follows same rules as other endoscopy: code most comprehensive procedure only.

Question 54: Answer: C) 50230 (nephrectomy, radical)

Explanation: Radical nephrectomy for cancer includes kidney, adrenal gland, surrounding fascia, and lymph nodes—most extensive kidney removal.

Study Tip: Nephrectomy types: simple (kidney only), complicated (difficult circumstances), radical (kidney plus surrounding structures), partial (kidney-sparing).

Question 55: Answer: C) 52601 (transurethral electrosurgical resection of prostate)

Explanation: TURP specifically refers to transurethral electrosurgical resection of prostate (52601), the standard surgical treatment for BPH.

Study Tip: Know common procedure acronyms: TURP, TURBT, ESWL. These abbreviations appear frequently in operative reports.

Question 56: Answer: B) 54520 with modifier -50 (bilateral)

Explanation: Simple bilateral orchiectomy uses 54520 with modifier -50 rather than coding twice. Modifier -50 indicates bilateral procedure.

Study Tip: Bilateral procedures use modifier -50 when same procedure is performed on both sides during same session.

Question 57: Answer: B) 58571 (laparoscopic total hysterectomy with removal of tubes and ovaries)

Explanation: Single code 58571 captures laparoscopic total hysterectomy with bilateral salpingo-oophorectomy—don't code separately.

Study Tip: Hysterectomy codes specify approach (abdominal, vaginal, laparoscopic) and extent (with/without tubes and ovaries).

Question 58: Answer: B) 55400 (vasovasostomy, vasoepididymostomy)

Explanation: Code 55400 covers vasectomy reversal procedures including both vasovasostomy and vasoepididymostomy techniques.

Study Tip: Reversal procedures have different codes than original procedures. Never use the original procedure code for reversals.

Question 59: Answer: A) 64721 (neuroplasty of median nerve at carpal tunnel)

Explanation: Carpal tunnel release specifically involves median nerve decompression at the carpal tunnel, coded with 64721.

Study Tip: Carpal tunnel syndrome and its treatment are high-frequency topics. Know the anatomy and typical treatment approaches.

Question 60: Answer: A) 64483 (transforaminal epidural injection, single level)

Explanation: Transforaminal epidural injection at single level (L5-S1) codes to 64483. Additional levels use add-on code 64484.

Study Tip: Pain management injections specify approach (transforaminal, interlaminar) and levels. First level differs from additional levels.

Question 61: Answer: B) 63030 + 63035 (each additional segment)

Explanation: Laminectomy uses primary code for first level (63030) and add-on codes for each additional segment (63035).

Study Tip: Spine procedures commonly use add-on codes for additional levels. Learn which codes are primary and which are add-on.

Question 62: Answer: A) 12013 (face, 2.6-5.0 cm) + 12002 (scalp, 2.6-7.5 cm)

Explanation: Face and scalp are different anatomical groups requiring separate codes. Face = 3.0 cm (12013), scalp = 2.5 cm (12002).

Study Tip: Memorize which body areas group together for wound repair: face/ears/lips separate from scalp/neck/trunk/extremities.

Question 63: Answer: C) 29880 + 29888 (both procedures)

Explanation: Meniscectomy (29880) and ACL reconstruction (29888) are distinct procedures reportable separately when performed together.

Study Tip: Multiple arthroscopic procedures can be coded together if they're truly separate procedures, not bundled components.

Question 64: Answer: C) 31603 (tracheostomy, emergency procedure)

Explanation: Emergency tracheostomy for acute airway obstruction codes to 31603, reflecting higher complexity and risk than planned procedures.

Study Tip: Emergency procedures often have separate codes reflecting increased difficulty. Check for emergency-specific codes.

Question 65: Answer: B) 47563 (laparoscopic cholecystectomy with cholangiography)

Explanation: When cholangiography is performed during laparoscopic cholecystectomy, use 47563 which includes the imaging.

Study Tip: Laparoscopic cholecystectomy has separate codes with/without cholangiography. Don't add separate imaging codes.

Section 5: Anesthesia, Radiology, Pathology, and Medicine (Questions 66-85)

Question 66: Answer: A) 11 units (6 base + 5 time + 0 physical status)

Explanation: Base (6) + Time (78 ÷ 15 = 5.2 → 5) + P1 (0) = 11 units. Round 5.2 down to 5. P1 adds no units.

Study Tip: Practice time unit calculations with various minute values. Remember standard rounding rules.

Question 67: Answer: A) +99100 (extreme age)

Explanation: Age under 1 year qualifies for +99100 (extreme age). This adds complexity due to immature physiology.

Study Tip: +99100 applies to patients <1 year or >70 years. Memorize qualifying circumstance criteria.

Question 68: Answer: D) P4 (severe systemic disease, constant threat to life)

Explanation: Severe, poorly controlled diabetes with heart failure represents constant threat to life, warranting P4 classification.

Study Tip: P-modifiers: P1 (healthy), P2 (mild disease), P3 (severe disease with limitations), P4 (life-threatening disease), P5 (moribund).

Question 69: Answer: B) Anesthesia start to surgery end ÷ 15 minutes

Explanation: Anesthesia time starts when anesthesiologist begins patient preparation and ends when patient is placed under post-anesthesia care.

Study Tip: Anesthesia time ≠ surgical time. It begins before and often extends after surgery.

Question 70: Answer: D) +99140 (emergency conditions)

Explanation: Emergency surgery adds qualifying circumstance +99140, reflecting increased complexity and risk.

Study Tip: Emergency conditions add complexity due to limited preparation, patient instability, and time pressure.

Question 71: Answer: B) 71045-26 (chest X-ray, professional component)

Explanation: When only interpretation is provided (not equipment/technical), use modifier -26 for professional component.

Study Tip: Component coding: -26 (professional), -TC (technical), no modifier (global). Know when each applies.

Question 72: Answer: C) 77067 (screening mammography, bilateral)

Explanation: Screening mammography in asymptomatic patients uses 77067. Diagnostic codes are for symptomatic patients.

Study Tip: Distinguish screening (no symptoms) from diagnostic (specific concern). Different codes and indications apply.

Question 73: Answer: C) Depends on whether guidance is included in biopsy code description

Explanation: Check biopsy code description. If guidance is included, don't code separately. If not included, code both.

Study Tip: Always read complete code descriptions. Many procedures now include imaging guidance that was previously separate.

Question 74: Answer: A) 76700 (ultrasound, abdominal, complete)

Explanation: Complete abdominal ultrasound (76700) includes liver, gallbladder, bile duct, pancreas, spleen, and kidneys in single code.

Study Tip: Complete vs. limited ultrasound: complete examines all specified organs, limited focuses on specific area/organ.

Question 75: Answer: C) 73723 (MRI knee, without and with contrast)

Explanation: MRI performed both without and with contrast uses single code (73723), not two separate codes.

Study Tip: Contrast MRI coding: without (no contrast), with (contrast only), without and with (both sequences).

Question 76: Answer: A) 85025 (CBC, automated with differential)

Explanation: Complete blood count with differential white cell count codes to 85025 when automated method is used.

Study Tip: CBC codes specify automated vs. manual and with/without differential. Match code to method documented.

Question 77: Answer: A) 86803 (Hepatitis C antibody)

Explanation: Hepatitis C antibody screening for infection exposure codes to 86803. Direct probe tests (87520-87522) detect virus itself.

Study Tip: Distinguish antibody tests (detect immune response) from antigen/probe tests (detect organism directly).

Question 78: Answer: C) Lipid panel

Explanation: Comprehensive metabolic panel includes glucose, electrolytes, kidney function, and liver tests—but NOT lipids, which are separate.

Study Tip: Memorize panel components. CMP includes basic metabolic panel plus albumin, protein, bilirubin, and liver enzymes.

Question 79: Answer: A) 81000 (urinalysis, non-automated)

Explanation: Question asks for urinalysis WITH microscopy. 81000 includes microscopy when performed; 81002 specifically excludes it.

Study Tip: Urinalysis codes: with microscopy (81000, 81001) vs. without microscopy (81002, 81003). Choose based on documentation.

Question 80: Answer: D) Depends on patient age and counseling provided

Explanation: Immunization administration codes vary by patient age (<18 vs. 18+) and whether counseling is provided. Check both factors.

Study Tip: Vaccination coding requires two codes: vaccine product (90xxx) and administration (90460-90474). Age and counseling determine administration code.

Question 81: Answer: A) 93000 (electrocardiogram, complete)

Explanation: Complete EKG with interpretation codes to 93000 (global service including tracing, interpretation, and report).

Study Tip: EKG component codes: 93005 (tracing only), 93010 (interpretation only), 93000 (complete). Use appropriate code for services provided.

Question 82: Answer: A) 94640 (pressurized or nonpressurized inhalation treatment)

Explanation: Nebulizer treatment for bronchospasm codes to 94640. This includes aerosol or vapor inhalation for therapeutic purposes.

Study Tip: Respiratory therapy codes specify type of treatment. Match code to equipment and therapy documented.

Question 83: Answer: D) Depends on complexity of evaluation

Explanation: Physical therapy evaluation codes (97161-97163) are selected based on complexity: low, moderate, or high. Documentation determines level.

Study Tip: Therapy evaluations use complexity-based codes. Review factors determining each complexity level.

Question 84: Answer: A) 96372 (therapeutic injection, subcutaneous or intramuscular)

Explanation: Therapeutic injection administration codes to 96372. Drug supply codes separately (J-codes) when applicable.

Study Tip: Injection coding requires administration code (96372) plus drug code (J-code) when billing for drug supply.

Question 85: Answer: C) 90837 (psychotherapy, 60 minutes)

Explanation: Psychotherapy codes are time-based. 60 minutes codes to 90837. Know time thresholds for each code.

Study Tip: Psychotherapy time ranges: 90832 (30 min), 90834 (45 min), 90837 (60 min). Time determines code selection.

Section 6: HCPCS Level II and Modifiers (Questions 86-95)

Question 86: Answer: B) E codes

Explanation: Durable medical equipment (DME) like wheelchairs, walkers, and hospital beds typically use E codes (E0100-E9999).

Study Tip: HCPCS sections: A (transport/supplies), E (DME), J (drugs), L (orthotics/prosthetics). Know major categories.

Question 87: Answer: C) J codes

Explanation: Injectable drugs administered by healthcare providers are coded with J codes (J0100-J9999).

Study Tip: J codes include administration route, dosage, and drug name. Always verify correct J-code for specific drug.

Question 88: Answer: B) Significant, separately identifiable E/M service

Explanation: Modifier -25 indicates E/M service and procedure were both significant and separately identifiable on same day.

Study Tip: -25 requirements: both services must be significant, separately identifiable, and medically necessary. Documentation must support both.

Question 89: Answer: A) Distinct procedural service

Explanation: Modifier -59 indicates procedures not normally reported together are appropriate due to distinct circumstances.

Study Tip: -59 use: different session, different site, different procedure, separate incision, or separate injury. Must meet specific criteria.

Question 90: Answer: A) Bilateral procedure

Explanation: Modifier -50 indicates identical procedure performed on both sides of the body during same operative session.

Study Tip: -50 applies when same procedure is done bilaterally. Some payers prefer listing code twice instead of using -50.

Question 91: Answer: B) -52 (reduced services)

Explanation: Modifier -52 indicates service was partially reduced or eliminated at physician discretion, not due to complications.

Study Tip: -52 vs. -53: -52 (partial reduction by physician choice), -53 (discontinued due to patient condition/threat).

Question 92: Answer: B) Professional component

Explanation: Modifier -26 indicates only the physician interpretation/report portion, not the technical equipment/staff component.

Study Tip: Component billing: -26 (interpretation only), -TC (equipment/technical only), no modifier (both components).

Question 93: Answer: C) Depends on level of service and urgency

Explanation: Ambulance codes vary by service level (basic vs. advanced life support) and urgency (emergency vs. non-emergency).

Study Tip: Ambulance coding requires knowing service level, transport type, mileage, and origin/destination.

Question 94: Answer: D) Depends on specific wheelchair type and features

Explanation: Wheelchair coding depends on specific type (standard, lightweight, heavy-duty) and features. Multiple codes exist for variations.

Study Tip: DME coding requires knowing exact equipment specifications. Generic codes don't provide adequate specificity.

Question 95: Answer: A) Repeat procedure by same physician

Explanation: Modifier -76 indicates procedure was repeated by the same physician on same day, distinct from original procedure.

Study Tip: -76 (same physician repeats) vs. -77 (different physician repeats). Choose correct modifier based on who performed repeat.

Section 7: Compliance and Regulatory (Questions 96-100)

Question 96: Answer: B) Protected Health Information (PHI)

Explanation: HIPAA Privacy Rule establishes national standards for protecting individually identifiable health information (PHI).

Study Tip: PHI includes any health information that can identify an individual. Protection extends to all forms: paper, electronic, oral.

Question 97: Answer: D) Hospital's tax identification number

Explanation: Hospital's tax ID is organizational information, not patient-specific. PHI must be individually identifiable health information.

Study Tip: PHI includes 18 specific identifiers. Organizational information about providers isn't PHI unless connected to specific patients.

Question 98: Answer: B) Billing for services at a higher level than provided or documented

Explanation: Upcoding artificially inflates reimbursement by claiming more complex/extensive services than actually provided or documented.

Study Tip: Upcoding is fraud when done knowingly. Ensure codes match documentation and services provided. Never code for financial gain.

Question 99: Answer: A) Knowingly submitting false claims for payment

Explanation: False Claims Act penalizes knowingly submitting false or fraudulent claims to government healthcare programs.

Study Tip: FCA violations carry severe penalties: $11,000+ per false claim plus treble damages. Intent matters in prosecution.

Question 100: Answer: B) Services reasonable and necessary for diagnosis or treatment

Explanation: Medical necessity means services are appropriate, needed for diagnosis/treatment, and meet standards of medical practice.

Study Tip: Medical necessity requires: appropriate diagnosis, reasonable treatment, documented need. All three elements must be present.

Performance Analysis and Study Planning

Scoring Breakdown by Section

Calculate your percentage in each section:

Medical Terminology/Anatomy (Q1-8): ___/8 = ___% **ICD-10-CM (Q9-28):** ___/20 = ___% **E/M Coding (Q29-40):** ___/12 = ___% **Surgery Coding (Q41-65):** ___/25 = ___% **Anesthesia/Rad/Path/Med (Q66-85):** ___/20 = ___% **HCPCS/Modifiers (Q86-95):** ___/10 = ___% **Compliance (Q96-100):** ___/5 = ___%

Overall Score: ___/100 = ___%

Study Plan Based on Performance

90-100% Overall: Excellent! Focus on timing and confidence-building.

- Take Practice Test 2 under timed conditions
- Review any missed questions thoroughly
- Practice with real operative reports
- Work on test-taking speed

80-89% Overall: Very good! Target weak areas for improvement.

- Identify topics where you missed 2+ questions
- Review those chapters in detail
- Complete additional practice questions in weak areas
- Retake Practice Test 1 in 1-2 weeks

70-79% Overall: Good! Need focused review in multiple areas.

- Create targeted study plan for sections <70%
- Review guidelines and conventions thoroughly
- Practice with coding scenarios daily
- Plan 2-3 more weeks of study before exam

60-69% Overall: Fair. Need substantial additional preparation.

- Review all chapters systematically
- Focus especially on sections <60%
- Complete all practice questions in study guide
- Consider delaying exam 4-6 weeks

Below 60%: Need comprehensive review before testing.

- Return to foundational chapters
- Work through study guide sequentially
- Complete all chapter practice questions
- Strongly consider extending study timeline

Next Steps

Immediate Actions:

1. Calculate your score and section percentages
2. Identify your three weakest content areas
3. Review all missed question explanations
4. Note recurring error patterns

This Week:

1. Review weak area chapters thoroughly
2. Complete additional practice in those areas
3. Create reference sheets for problem topics
4. Practice with timed exercises

Next 1-2 Weeks:

1. Take Practice Test 2 under exam conditions
2. Compare scores to identify improvement
3. Continue targeted review of weak areas
4. Build speed and confidence

Final Preparation:

1. Review all practice test explanations
2. Focus on test-taking strategies
3. Build physical and mental endurance
4. Prepare for exam day logistics

Success Strategies

Time Management:

- Average 2.4 minutes per question
- Don't exceed 5 minutes on any question initially
- Mark difficult questions for later review
- Save 30 minutes for final review

Test-Taking Techniques:

- Read questions completely before answering
- Eliminate obviously wrong answers first
- Use books efficiently: index first, verify in tabular
- Trust your preparation and instincts

Exam Day Preparation:

- Get adequate sleep the night before
- Arrive early to testing center
- Have properly tabbed books ready
- Stay calm and focused throughout

Remember: This practice test is a learning tool, not a final judgment. Every question—whether answered correctly or not—teaches you something valuable. Use these results to guide focused, efficient study that maximizes your exam-day performance.

You've invested significant time and effort in your preparation. Trust your knowledge, learn from your mistakes, and approach the actual exam with confidence. You're capable of success—now prove it to yourself!

Good luck on your continued preparation!

Chapter 20: Practice Test 2

"Success is the sum of small efforts repeated day in and day out." - Robert Collier

This second full-length practice test represents your opportunity to measure progress and identify any remaining knowledge gaps before exam day. By now, you've completed comprehensive study of all CPC content areas and taken your first practice exam. This test helps you confirm your readiness and fine-tune your exam strategy.

How to Use This Practice Test:

Simulate Real Exam Conditions:

- Set aside 4 uninterrupted hours
- Use only your CPT®, ICD-10-CM, and HCPCS Level II code books
- No notes, study guides, or other reference materials
- Complete all 100 questions in one sitting

Time Management Strategy:

- Aim for 2-2.5 minutes per question average
- Mark difficult questions and return to them later
- Leave no question unanswered—educated guessing is better than blanks
- Save 20-30 minutes for final review

After Completing the Test:

- Score your exam using the answer key
- Review ALL explanations, not just missed questions
- Identify patterns in errors (specific body systems, code types, etc.)
- Create a focused study plan for any weak areas

Performance Benchmarks:

- 90-100 correct (90-100%): **Excellent** preparation—you're ready
- 80-89 correct (80-89%): Good preparation—review weak areas
- 70-79 correct (70-79%): Passing range—focused study needed
- Below 70 correct (<70%): Additional preparation required before exam

Remember: This practice test uses questions similar to actual CPC exam difficulty but isn't identical to questions you'll see on test day. Focus on understanding concepts behind each question rather than memorizing specific scenarios.

You're ready. Let's begin.

Practice Test 2: 100 Questions

Instructions: Select the best answer for each question. Use your CPT®, ICD-10-CM, and HCPCS Level II code books as needed. Time yourself for the full 4-hour period.

Questions 1-10: Medical Terminology and Anatomy

Question 1: The term "nephrolithiasis" refers to:

A) Kidney inflammation B) Kidney stones C) Kidney infection D) Kidney failure

Question 2: Which anatomical structure connects the pharynx to the stomach?

A) Trachea B) Esophagus C) Bronchus D) Larynx

Question 3: The prefix "tachy-" means:

A) Slow B) Fast C) Difficult D) Painful

Question 4: The mitral valve is located between:

A) Right atrium and right ventricle B) Left atrium and left ventricle C) Left ventricle and aorta D) Right ventricle and pulmonary artery

Question 5: Which term describes surgical removal of the gallbladder?

A) Cholecystotomy B) Cholecystectomy C) Choledochotomy D) Cholecystostomy

Question 6: The suffix "-rrhaphy" means:

A) Surgical removal B) Surgical repair C) Suturing D) Incision

Question 7: The diaphysis refers to which part of a long bone?

A) End B) Shaft C) Growth plate D) Joint surface

Question 8: Which structure produces insulin?

A) Liver B) Gallbladder C) Pancreas D) Spleen

Question 9: The term "bilateral" means:

A) One side B) Both sides C) Above D) Below

Question 10: Hematopoiesis occurs primarily in:

A) Liver B) Spleen C) Bone marrow D) Lymph nodes

Questions 11-20: ICD-10-CM Coding

Question 11: A patient with Type 2 diabetes mellitus with diabetic peripheral neuropathy should be coded as:

A) E11.9, G63 B) E11.40 C) E11.42 D) E10.40

Question 12: Which is the correct code for acute myocardial infarction of the anterior wall, initial episode?

A) I21.9 B) I21.09 C) I25.2 D) I21.4

Question 13: A patient is seen for follow-up of a healed fracture of the left radius. The appropriate 7th character is:

A) A (initial encounter) B) D (subsequent encounter for routine healing) C) S (sequela) D) No 7th character needed

Question 14: Pneumonia due to Streptococcus, Group B should be coded as:

A) J18.9 B) J15.3 C) J13 D) J15.9

Question 15: For metastatic breast cancer with bone metastases, the correct sequencing is:

A) C79.51, C50.919 B) C50.919, C79.51 C) C50.919 only D) C79.51 only

Question 16: A patient presents with chest pain to rule out MI. EKG and cardiac enzymes are normal. Code:

A) I21.9 (acute MI) B) R07.9 (chest pain) C) Z03.89 (observation for suspected disease) D) I25.10 (atherosclerotic heart disease)

Question 17: COPD with acute exacerbation due to pneumonia should be coded as:

A) J44.1 only B) J44.0 only C) J44.1, J18.9 D) J44.0, J18.9

Question 18: Personal history of breast cancer, currently cancer-free:

A) C50.919 (malignant neoplasm of breast) B) Z85.3 (personal history of malignant neoplasm of breast) C) D05.90 (carcinoma in situ of breast) D) Z86.010 (personal history of colonic polyps)

Question 19: A patient admitted for chemotherapy should have which diagnosis sequenced first?

A) The cancer diagnosis B) Z51.11 (encounter for chemotherapy) C) R53.1 (weakness) D) Z79.899 (long-term drug use)

Question 20: Essential hypertension should be coded as:

A) I10 B) I11.0 C) I13.0 D) I15.0

Questions 21-30: CPT® Evaluation and Management

Question 21: An established patient is seen for 25 minutes with low complexity MDM. The correct code is:

A) 99212 B) 99213 C) 99214 D) 99215

Question 22: A new patient is seen for 60 minutes with high complexity MDM. Code:

A) 99203 B) 99204 C) 99205 D) 99205 + 99354

Question 23: Critical care services require a minimum of how many minutes?

A) 15 minutes B) 20 minutes C) 30 minutes D) 45 minutes

Question 24: An established patient is seen by a nurse for blood pressure check only. Code:

A) 99211 B) 99212 C) 99213 D) Cannot be coded

Question 25: Hospital discharge service taking 45 minutes should be coded as:

A) 99238 B) 99239 C) 99233 D) 99291

Question 26: Initial nursing facility care with comprehensive history, exam, and high MDM:

A) 99304 B) 99305 C) 99306 D) 99223

Question 27: Emergency department visit, high level of complexity:

A) 99283 B) 99284 C) 99285 D) 99291

Question 28: Time-based E/M coding includes which of the following?

A) Face-to-face time only B) Total time on date of encounter C) Procedure time only D) Documentation time only

Question 29: A consultation requires all EXCEPT:

A) Request from another provider B) Written report back to requesting provider C) Transfer of care to consulting physician D) Rendering of opinion or advice

Question 30: Prolonged E/M services require minimum how many minutes beyond the typical time?

A) 15 minutes B) 30 minutes C) 45 minutes D) 60 minutes

Questions 31-50: CPT® Surgery Coding

Question 31: Simple repair of 3.5 cm laceration on the face should be coded as:

A) 12011 B) 12013 C) 12014 D) 12051

Question 32: Excision of a 2.0 cm benign lesion from the back includes how much margin measurement?

A) Lesion size only B) Lesion plus margins removed C) Margins only D) Lesion diameter doubled

Question 33: Closed treatment of femur fracture with manipulation:

A) 27500 B) 27502 C) 27506 D) 27509

Question 34: Diagnostic colonoscopy that cannot be completed past splenic flexure should use which modifier?

A) -22 (increased procedural services) B) -52 (reduced services) C) -53 (discontinued procedure) D) -59 (distinct procedural service)

Question 35: Arthroscopic meniscectomy and ACL reconstruction:

A) 29880 only B) 29888 only C) 29880, 29888 D) 29870, 29880, 29888

Question 36: Laparoscopic cholecystectomy with cholangiography:

A) 47562 B) 47563 C) 47600 D) 47605

Question 37: Bilateral inguinal hernia repair should use which modifier?

A) -50 (bilateral) B) -51 (multiple procedures) C) -59 (distinct procedural service) D) -LT and -RT

Question 38: Transurethral resection of prostate (TURP):

A) 52450 B) 52500 C) 52601 D) 52700

Question 39: Simple mastectomy:

A) 19300 B) 19301 C) 19302 D) 19303

Question 40: EGD with biopsy and control of bleeding:

A) 43235, 43239, 43255 B) 43239, 43255 C) 43255 D) 43235, 43255

Question 41: A patient has three skin lesions excised: 1.0 cm (benign, arm), 1.5 cm (benign, arm), 2.0 cm (malignant, back). How should this be coded?

A) 11403 (arm), 11604 (back) B) 11402 (arm), 11403 (arm), 11604 (back) C) 11404 (combined), 11604 (back) D) Three separate codes for each lesion

Question 42: Carpal tunnel release:

A) 64721 B) 29848 C) 25000 D) 64831

Question 43: Laminectomy at L4-L5 and L5-S1 levels:

A) 63030 × 2 B) 63030, 63035 C) 63047, 63048 D) 22630

Question 44: Cystoscopy with biopsy and fulguration of small lesion:

A) 52000, 52204, 52224 B) 52204, 52224 C) 52234 D) 52204

Question 45: Total abdominal hysterectomy with bilateral salpingo-oophorectomy:

A) 58150 B) 58152 C) 58180 D) 58200

Question 46: Repair of recurrent ventral hernia, laparoscopic approach:

A) 49560 B) 49565 C) 49650 D) 49651

Question 47: Nasal endoscopy with maxillary antrostomy:

A) 31231 B) 31233 C) 31256 D) 31267

Question 48: Percutaneous needle biopsy of liver:

A) 47000 B) 47001 C) 47100 D) 47552

Question 49: Vasectomy, bilateral:

A) 55250 B) 55250 × 2 C) 55250-50 D) 55400

Question 50: Throacentesis with imaging guidance:

A) 32554 B) 32554, 76942 C) 32555 D) 32556

Questions 51-60: CPT® Radiology, Pathology, Medicine

Question 51: Chest X-ray, two views, professional component only:

A) 71045 B) 71045-26 C) 71045-TC D) 71046

Question 52: Screening mammography, bilateral:

A) 77065 B) 77066 C) 77067 D) 77065-50

Question 53: CT abdomen and pelvis with contrast:

A) 74150 B) 74160 C) 74170 D) 74177

Question 54: MRI brain without and with contrast:

A) 70551 B) 70552 C) 70553 D) 70551, 70552

Question 55: Complete abdominal ultrasound:

A) 76700 B) 76705 C) 76770 D) 76775

Question 56: Comprehensive metabolic panel:

A) 80048 B) 80053 C) 80061 D) 80076

Question 57: Hemoglobin A1c:

A) 83036 B) 82947 C) 83718 D) 84443

Question 58: Urinalysis, automated with microscopy:

A) 81000 B) 81001 C) 81002 D) 81003

Question 59: Protime (PT):

A) 85610 B) 85730 C) 86580 D) 85025

Question 60: Lipid panel:

A) 80048 B) 80053 C) 80061 D) 82465

Questions 61-70: HCPCS Level II and Modifiers

Question 61: HCPCS codes are used primarily for:

A) Physician services B) DME, supplies, and drugs C) Inpatient hospital services D) Laboratory tests

Question 62: Injection, insulin, per 50 units:

A) J1815 B) J1817 C) A4210 D) E0784

Question 63: Blood glucose test strips, box of 50:

A) A4233 B) A4253 C) A4256 D) E2100

Question 64: Ambulance service, basic life support, emergency:

A) A0426 B) A0428 C) A0429 D) A0427

Question 65: Walker, folding, adjustable:

A) E0130 B) E0135 C) E0141 D) E0143

Question 66: Modifier -RT indicates:

A) Repeat procedure B) Right side C) Reduced services D) Return to OR

Question 67: Modifier -76 indicates:

A) Repeat procedure by same physician B) Repeat procedure by different physician C) Bilateral procedure D) Staged procedure

Question 68: Modifier -25 is used when:

A) A procedure is performed bilaterally B) Significant E/M and procedure same day C) Multiple procedures performed D) Reduced services provided

Question 69: Modifier -59 indicates:

A) Bilateral procedure B) Distinct procedural service C) Staged procedure D) Increased services

Question 70: Modifier -79 indicates:

A) Unrelated procedure during post-op period B) Related procedure during post-op period C) Staged procedure D) Return to OR for complications

Questions 71-80: Anesthesia Coding

Question 71: Anesthesia for appendectomy (00840, 6 base units) lasting 75 minutes in healthy patient. Total units:

A) 11 B) 12 C) 13 D) 14

Question 72: Physical status modifier P3 indicates:

A) Normal healthy patient B) Mild systemic disease C) Severe systemic disease D) Moribund patient

Question 73: Qualifying circumstance for patient over age 70:

A) +99100 B) +99116 C) +99135 D) +99140

Question 74: Anesthesia time begins when:

A) Patient enters OR B) Surgery begins C) Anesthesiologist begins patient prep D) Patient is unconscious

Question 75: Anesthesia for total hip replacement (01214, 8 base units), 120 minutes, emergency in 85-year-old:

A) 16 units B) 17 units C) 18 units D) 19 units

Question 76: Base units reflect:

A) Time spent providing anesthesia B) Patient physical status C) Procedure complexity D) Anesthesiologist experience

Question 77: Qualifying circumstance +99140 is used for:

A) Extreme age B) Controlled hypotension C) Total body hypothermia D) Emergency conditions

Question 78: Anesthesia for cardiac valve surgery (00562, 15 base units), 240 minutes, P3 patient. Total units:

A) 30 B) 31 C) 32 D) 33

Question 79: Time units are calculated by dividing total minutes by:

A) 10 B) 15 C) 20 D) 30

Question 80: Which is NOT a physical status modifier?

A) P1 B) P3 C) P5 D) P7

Questions 81-90: Compliance and Regulatory

Question 81: HIPAA stands for:

A) Health Insurance Portability and Accountability Act B) Healthcare Information Privacy and Access Act C) Health Insurance Protection and Authorization Act D) Healthcare Information Portability Act

Question 82: Protected Health Information (PHI) includes all EXCEPT:

A) Patient name B) Medical record number C) Hospital name D) Date of birth

Question 83: The HIPAA Security Rule specifically addresses:

A) All forms of PHI B) Electronic PHI only C) Paper records only D) Verbal communications only

Question 84: Upcoding is defined as:

A) Coding services not provided B) Billing higher level than provided C) Unbundling services D) Billing for non-covered services

Question 85: The False Claims Act addresses:

A) Only Medicare fraud B) Only Medicaid fraud C) Federal healthcare program fraud D) Private insurance fraud only

Question 86: Medical necessity means:

A) Any service requested by patient B) Services reasonable and necessary for diagnosis/treatment C) All preventive services D) Services ordered by any provider

Question 87: Which is considered fraud?

A) Honest coding error B) Unintentional pattern of errors C) Knowing and willful misrepresentation D) Lack of documentation

Question 88: The OIG (Office of Inspector General) is part of:

A) CMS B) Department of Health and Human Services C) Department of Justice D) Medicare Administrative Contractor

Question 89: Documentation must support:

A) Only the diagnosis codes B) Only the procedure codes C) Both diagnosis and procedure codes D) Neither, as long as codes are correct

Question 90: A compliance program should include:

A) Written policies only B) Training only C) Audit procedures only D) All of the above

Questions 91-100: Case Studies

Question 91: Patient presents to ED with severe abdominal pain. CT reveals appendicitis. Patient taken to OR for emergency appendectomy. Pathology confirms acute appendicitis. Assign diagnosis code(s):

A) R10.9 (abdominal pain) B) K35.80 (acute appendicitis) C) R10.9, K35.80 D) K35.80, R10.9

Question 92: 68-year-old with COPD, diabetes, and hypertension undergoes outpatient stress test. Assign appropriate E/M code for pre-procedure evaluation (30 minutes, moderate MDM):

A) 99213 B) 99214 C) 99215 D) 99205

Question 93: Patient undergoes colonoscopy. Three polyps removed from transverse colon, one polyp removed from sigmoid colon, biopsy taken from cecum. Code:

A) 45380, 45385 × 4 B) 45385 C) 45380, 45385 D) 45378, 45380, 45385

Question 94: Right knee arthroscopy with partial medial meniscectomy and chondroplasty of patella. Code:

A) 29880 B) 29880, 29877 C) 29870, 29880, 29877 D) 29881, 29877

Question 95: Excision of 1.2 cm benign lesion from right arm and 2.5 cm malignant lesion from chest. Code:

A) 11402, 11603 B) 11403, 11604 C) 11402, 11604 D) 11404, 11603

Question 96: Patient admitted for pneumonia. During hospitalization, develops acute kidney injury. At discharge, both conditions documented as equally responsible for hospital stay. Principal diagnosis:

A) J18.9 (pneumonia) B) N17.9 (acute kidney injury) C) Either can be principal D) Both coded as principal

Question 97: Anesthesia for emergency cesarean section in 42-year-old with severe preeclampsia (01961, 7 base units), 90 minutes. Total units:

A) 13 B) 14 C) 15 D) 16

Question 98: Bilateral screening mammography reveals suspicious mass in left breast. Patient returns for diagnostic mammography left breast. Code the diagnostic mammography:

A) 77065 B) 77066 C) 77067 D) 77065-59

Question 99: Established patient seen in office for diabetes follow-up (10 minutes) and has suspicious skin lesion biopsied (separate procedure). Code:

A) 99212 B) 11100 C) 99212-25, 11100 D) 99213, 11100

Question 100: Patient with known lung cancer admitted for radiation therapy. Assign principal diagnosis:

A) C79.9 (secondary malignant neoplasm) B) C34.90 (malignant neoplasm of lung) C) Z51.0 (radiotherapy) D) Z85.118 (personal history of lung cancer)

Answer Key with Detailed Explanations

Questions 1-10: Medical Terminology and Anatomy

Question 1: Answer: B) Kidney stones

Explanation: Nephrolithiasis combines nephro (kidney) + lith (stone) + iasis (condition), meaning the condition of having kidney stones.

Study Tip: Break down complex medical terms into prefix-root-suffix components to understand meaning. Practice identifying word parts in terminology.

Question 2: Answer: B) Esophagus

Explanation: The esophagus is the muscular tube that connects the pharynx (throat) to the stomach, allowing food passage during swallowing.

Study Tip: Review the digestive tract anatomy sequentially from mouth to anus. Understanding anatomical connections helps with surgical coding.

Question 3: Answer: B) Fast

Explanation: The prefix "tachy-" means fast or rapid, as seen in tachycardia (fast heart rate) and tachypnea (fast breathing).

Study Tip: Remember the pair: tachy- = fast, brady- = slow. These prefixes appear frequently in cardiovascular and respiratory coding.

Question 4: Answer: B) Left atrium and left ventricle

Explanation: The mitral valve (also called bicuspid valve) is located between the left atrium and left ventricle, controlling blood flow between these chambers.

Study Tip: Review all four heart valves and their locations. Understanding heart anatomy is essential for cardiac procedure and diagnosis coding.

Question 5: Answer: B) Cholecystectomy

Explanation: Cholecystectomy breaks down as chole (bile) + cyst (bladder/gallbladder) + ectomy (surgical removal), meaning surgical removal of the gallbladder.

Study Tip: The suffix -ectomy always indicates surgical removal. Know this suffix for coding surgical procedures correctly.

Question 6: Answer: C) Suturing

Explanation: The suffix -rrhaphy means suturing or sewing, as in herniorrhaphy (suturing of hernia) or hemorrhoidorrhaphy (suturing of hemorrhoids).

Study Tip: Don't confuse -rrhaphy (suturing) with -plasty (surgical repair/reconstruction) or -pexy (surgical fixation). Each has distinct meaning.

Question 7: Answer: B) Shaft

Explanation: The diaphysis is the shaft or main cylindrical portion of a long bone, while the epiphysis refers to the ends of the bone.

Study Tip: Understanding bone anatomy terminology is critical for accurate fracture coding. Know diaphysis, epiphysis, and metaphysis locations.

Question 8: Answer: C) Pancreas

Explanation: The pancreas produces insulin (endocrine function) and also produces digestive enzymes (exocrine function) for the small intestine.

Study Tip: Know endocrine organ functions for diabetes coding. Pancreas has dual function: hormones (insulin, glucagon) and digestive enzymes.

Question 9: Answer: B) Both sides

Explanation: Bilateral means both sides or affecting both sides of the body, as in bilateral knee replacement or bilateral procedures.

Study Tip: Remember: uni- = one side, bi- = two sides/both, multi- = many. Use modifier -50 for bilateral procedures.

Question 10: Answer: C) Bone marrow

Explanation: Hematopoiesis (blood cell production) occurs primarily in red bone marrow, producing red blood cells, white blood cells, and platelets.

Study Tip: Review blood cell development for hematology coding. Bone marrow is the primary site of blood cell formation in adults.

Questions 11-20: ICD-10-CM Coding

Question 11: Answer: C) E11.42

Explanation: E11.42 specifically identifies Type 2 diabetes mellitus with diabetic polyneuropathy, combining the diabetes type and specific complication.

Study Tip: Use the most specific diabetes complication codes available. Don't code diabetes and neuropathy separately when combination codes exist.

Question 12: Answer: B) I21.09

Explanation: I21.09 identifies ST elevation myocardial infarction (STEMI) involving the anterior wall, initial encounter for acute phase treatment.

Study Tip: MI codes specify wall location (anterior, inferior, lateral) and episode timing (initial, subsequent, sequela). Location matters for treatment.

Question 13: Answer: C) S (sequela)

Explanation: The S character indicates sequela or late effect when coding for conditions resulting from a healed fracture.

Study Tip: Remember 7th character meanings: A = initial encounter, D = subsequent encounter for routine healing, S = sequela/late effects.

Question 14: Answer: B) J15.3

Explanation: J15.3 specifically identifies pneumonia due to Streptococcus, Group B, providing more specificity than unspecified bacterial pneumonia codes.

Study Tip: Always code the specific organism when documented. Organism identification affects treatment decisions and justifies antibiotic choices.

Question 15: Answer: B) C50.919, C79.51

Explanation: Sequence primary malignancy first (breast), then secondary/metastatic sites (bone), following standard neoplasm sequencing guidelines.

Study Tip: Primary malignancy codes first unless encounter focuses specifically on treating the metastatic site. Know sequencing rules.

Question 16: Answer: B) R07.9 (chest pain)

Explanation: In outpatient settings, never code "rule out" or uncertain diagnoses. Code the documented signs, symptoms, or test results instead.

Study Tip: Outpatient rule: Code what IS documented (symptoms, findings), not what's being ruled out or suspected without confirmation.

Question 17: Answer: C) J44.1, J18.9

Explanation: Code both the COPD with acute exacerbation (J44.1) and the precipitating cause (pneumonia, J18.9) when both are documented.

Study Tip: COPD exacerbation codes permit coding additional conditions causing the exacerbation. Both conditions should be reported.

Question 18: Answer: B) Z85.3 (personal history of malignant neoplasm of breast)

Explanation: Use personal history codes (Z85.-) for patients with resolved malignancies who are currently cancer-free but have past cancer history.

Study Tip: Z85 codes indicate history of cured/resolved malignancy. Active cancer uses C codes; cured cancer uses Z85 codes.

Question 19: Answer: B) Z51.11 (encounter for chemotherapy)

Explanation: When the encounter is specifically for chemotherapy administration, sequence Z51.11 first, followed by the cancer diagnosis code.

Study Tip: Reason for encounter determines principal diagnosis. Chemotherapy encounters list Z51.11 first, then the cancer being treated.

Question 20: Answer: A) I10

Explanation: I10 represents essential (primary) hypertension without complications or specified cause, the most common hypertension code.

Study Tip: I10 is simple hypertension. Complicated hypertension (heart disease, kidney disease) uses different codes in I11-I15 ranges.

Questions 21-30: CPT® Evaluation and Management

Question 21: Answer: B) 99213

Explanation: For established patients, 99213 covers 20-29 minutes OR low complexity medical decision making. Either time or complexity qualifies.

Study Tip: You can use EITHER time OR medical decision making complexity to select E/M level—not both required for code selection.

Question 22: Answer: C) 99205

Explanation: For new patients, 99205 covers 60-74 minutes OR high complexity MDM. The 60 minutes qualifies for this highest new patient level.

Study Tip: New patient codes range 99202-99205. Know time thresholds and MDM levels for each code to select appropriately.

Question 23: Answer: C) 30 minutes

Explanation: Critical care services (99291-99292) require a minimum of 30 minutes to be billable. Less than 30 minutes uses regular E/M codes.

Study Tip: Critical care minimum is 30 minutes. Time less than 30 minutes cannot be coded as critical care regardless of intensity.

Question 24: Answer: A) 99211

Explanation: Code 99211 is the only E/M code that may be performed by clinical staff (nurses, medical assistants) under physician supervision.

Study Tip: All other E/M codes require face-to-face physician or qualified NPP encounter. Only 99211 permits clinical staff provision.

Question 25: Answer: B) 99239

Explanation: Hospital discharge services use time-based coding: 99238 for 30 minutes or less, 99239 for more than 30 minutes.

Study Tip: Hospital discharge codes are purely time-based. The 30-minute mark determines which code to use: ≤30 or >30 minutes.

Question 26: Answer: C) 99306

Explanation: Initial nursing facility care with comprehensive history, comprehensive exam, and high complexity MDM qualifies for 99306, the highest initial level.

Study Tip: Initial nursing facility: 99304-99306 based on history/exam/MDM. Subsequent visits use 99307-99310. Know the difference.

Question 27: Answer: C) 99285

Explanation: Code 99285 represents the highest level of emergency department services, requiring comprehensive history, exam, and high complexity MDM.

Study Tip: ED codes 99281-99285 increase with complexity. ED coding has no new vs. established patient distinction unlike office visits.

Question 28: Answer: B) Total time on date of encounter

Explanation: Time-based E/M coding includes total time on the encounter date, encompassing both face-to-face and non-face-to-face time related to that encounter.

Study Tip: Time includes patient interaction, documentation, care coordination, and communication with other providers—not just face-to-face time.

Question 29: Answer: C) Transfer of care to consulting physician

Explanation: Consultations require request, opinion/advice, and report back to requesting provider—but NOT transfer of care. Transfer = referral, not consultation.

Study Tip: Remember the 3 R's of consultation: Request, Render (opinion), Report back. Transfer of care makes it a referral instead.

Question 30: Answer: B) 30 minutes

Explanation: Prolonged E/M services (99354-99355) require at least 30 minutes of service time beyond the typical time for the highest level E/M code.

Study Tip: Prolonged services codes supplement E/M codes when time significantly exceeds maximum for that E/M level. Minimum 30 extra minutes required.

Questions 31-50: CPT® Surgery Coding

Question 31: Answer: B) 12013

Explanation: Simple repair of face wounds 2.6-5.0 cm uses code 12013. The 3.5 cm laceration falls within this size range for facial repairs.

Study Tip: Face wound repairs: 12011-12018. Add all wound lengths in same anatomical location and repair type together before coding.

Question 32: Answer: B) Lesion plus margins removed

Explanation: Excision size includes the lesion diameter PLUS the margin removed on all sides. A 2.0 cm lesion with 0.5 cm margins = 3.0 cm total.

Study Tip: Always include margins when measuring excision size. Measure greatest clinical diameter of lesion plus narrowest margin removed.

Question 33: Answer: B) 27502

Explanation: Closed treatment WITH manipulation (27502) indicates fracture fragments were manually realigned without surgical exposure of the fracture site.

Study Tip: Fracture treatment: closed = no surgery, open = surgical exposure, percutaneous = pins through skin. Manipulation = manual realignment.

Question 34: Answer: B) -52 (reduced services)

Explanation: Use modifier -52 when a procedure is partially reduced or incomplete at physician discretion due to technical difficulty or patient condition.

Study Tip: Modifier -52 for reduced services; -53 for discontinued procedure after anesthesia started. Know the difference between partial and discontinued.

Question 35: Answer: C) 29880, 29888

Explanation: Arthroscopic meniscectomy (29880) and ACL reconstruction (29888) are distinct, separately reportable procedures when performed during same operative session.

Study Tip: Multiple arthroscopic procedures can be coded separately when distinct services. Don't confuse diagnostic arthroscopy (included) with surgical procedures.

Question 36: Answer: B) 47563

Explanation: Code 47563 represents laparoscopic cholecystectomy WITH intraoperative cholangiography. Code 47562 is without cholangiography.

Study Tip: Check procedure descriptions for included services like imaging guidance. Cholangiography adds value when performed and should be coded.

Question 37: Answer: A) -50 (bilateral)

Explanation: Bilateral procedures performed during the same operative session use modifier -50 to indicate the procedure was performed on both sides.

Study Tip: Use -50 for bilateral procedures on one claim line. Some payers prefer two lines with -LT/-RT. Check payer-specific guidelines.

Question 38: Answer: C) 52601

Explanation: Code 52601 represents transurethral electrosurgical resection of prostate (TURP), the standard procedure for benign prostatic hyperplasia treatment.

Study Tip: Know common procedure abbreviations: TURP = 52601, TURBT = 52234-52240. Memorize frequently used urology codes.

Question 39: Answer: C) 19302

Explanation: Simple mastectomy (19302) involves complete removal of breast tissue including nipple-areolar complex, without lymph node dissection or muscle removal.

Study Tip: Mastectomy levels: 19301 = partial/lumpectomy, 19302 = simple/complete, 19303 = radical. Know extent of tissue removal.

Question 40: Answer: C) 43255

Explanation: When multiple endoscopic procedures are performed, code only the most extensive procedure. Code 43255 (control of bleeding) includes any biopsies.

Study Tip: Endoscopy bundling rule: Code most comprehensive procedure performed. Biopsy typically included in more extensive therapeutic procedures.

Question 41: Answer: C) 11404 (combined), 11604 (back)

Explanation: Add lengths of same-site, same-classification lesions (two benign arm lesions = 2.5 cm total). Code malignant lesions separately by site.

Study Tip: Combine lengths when: same anatomical site AND same classification (benign/malignant). Different sites or classifications code separately.

Question 42: Answer: A) 64721

Explanation: Code 64721 specifically describes carpal tunnel release (neuroplasty and/or transposition of median nerve at carpal tunnel).

Study Tip: Carpal tunnel release is very common. Memorize code 64721. Don't confuse with other hand/wrist nerve procedures.

Question 43: Answer: B) 63030, 63035

Explanation: Laminectomy coding uses primary code for first level (63030) plus add-on code for each additional segment (63035).

Study Tip: Spine procedures typically use primary + add-on code structure. Never multiply primary code—use add-on codes for additional levels.

Question 44: Answer: C) 52234

Explanation: Code 52234 (cystoscopy with fulguration/resection of small tumor) is most extensive and includes biopsy when performed during same session.

Study Tip: Cystoscopy: Code most comprehensive service performed. Therapeutic procedures typically include diagnostic and biopsy components.

Question 45: Answer: B) 58152

Explanation: Code 58152 represents total abdominal hysterectomy WITH bilateral salpingo-oophorectomy (removal of uterus, cervix, both tubes, and both ovaries).

Study Tip: Hysterectomy coding: 58150 = uterus/cervix only, 58152 = adds bilateral tubes/ovaries. Know what's included in each code.

Question 46: Answer: D) 49651

Explanation: Code 49651 specifically identifies laparoscopic repair of RECURRENT ventral hernia. Both approach (laparoscopic) and status (recurrent) affect code selection.

Study Tip: Hernia codes specify: initial vs. recurrent, open vs. laparoscopic. All four combinations have different codes—choose carefully.

Question 47: Answer: C) 31256

Explanation: Code 31256 represents nasal/sinus endoscopy, surgical, with maxillary antrostomy, creating an opening into the maxillary sinus.

Study Tip: Sinus surgery codes: Know common endoscopic procedures like antrostomy, ethmoidectomy. Diagnostic endoscopy included in surgical procedures.

Question 48: Answer: C) 47100

Explanation: Code 47100 represents biopsy of liver, percutaneous needle approach, typically performed with imaging guidance for accurate sampling.

Study Tip: Distinguish biopsy approaches: percutaneous needle vs. open surgical. Approach significantly affects code selection and reimbursement.

Question 49: Answer: A) 55250

Explanation: Code 55250 covers vasectomy, unilateral OR bilateral. The code description specifically states it includes bilateral when performed.

Study Tip: Some procedure codes include bilateral in description. Don't use -50 modifier when code descriptor already specifies bilateral.

Question 50: Answer: A) 32554

Explanation: Current thoracentesis codes (32554-32557) include imaging guidance when performed. Separate imaging guidance codes should not be reported.

Study Tip: Check if imaging guidance is included in procedure code before coding separately. Many updated codes now bundle guidance.

Questions 51-60: CPT® Radiology, Pathology, Medicine

Question 51: Answer: B) 71045-26

Explanation: Professional component (interpretation only) uses modifier -26. The radiologist interpreting films at different facility bills with -26 modifier.

Study Tip: Component modifiers: -26 = professional (interpretation), -TC = technical (equipment/staff). No modifier = global (both components).

Question 52: Answer: C) 77067

Explanation: Code 77067 specifically represents screening mammography, bilateral, for asymptomatic patients undergoing routine breast cancer screening.

Study Tip: Mammography: 77065-77066 = diagnostic (symptoms/findings), 77067 = screening (asymptomatic). Indication determines code choice.

Question 53: Answer: C) 74170

Explanation: Code 74170 represents CT of abdomen and pelvis with contrast material administration for enhanced visualization of structures.

Study Tip: CT coding depends on: anatomical area, contrast use (without/with/without and with). Contrast status significantly affects code.

Question 54: Answer: C) 70553

Explanation: Code 70553 specifically represents MRI brain performed both without contrast initially, then with contrast for enhanced imaging.

Study Tip: MRI "without and with" contrast is ONE procedure code, not two codes. Don't code separately when performed as single study.

Question 55: Answer: A) 76700

Explanation: Complete abdominal ultrasound (76700) includes liver, gallbladder, common bile duct, pancreas, spleen, kidneys—all required structures.

Study Tip: Complete ultrasound requires all specified structures. Limited study (76705) examines single organ or fewer structures than complete.

Question 56: Answer: B) 80053

Explanation: Comprehensive metabolic panel (80053) includes all tests in basic metabolic panel plus albumin, bilirubin, alkaline phosphatase, total protein, ALT, AST.

Study Tip: Know panel components. CMP includes all BMP tests plus six additional liver/protein tests. Use panel codes when all tests performed.

Question 57: Answer: C) 83036

Explanation: Code 83036 represents hemoglobin A1c (glycated hemoglobin) test used for diabetes monitoring, reflecting average blood glucose over 2-3 months.

Study Tip: Know common lab test codes: glucose 82947, A1c 83036, lipid panel 80061. These frequently tested diabetes/cardiovascular tests.

Question 58: Answer: D) 81003

Explanation: Code 81003 represents urinalysis, automated with microscopy, combining automated dipstick testing with microscopic examination of sediment.

Study Tip: Urinalysis codes: 81000 = manual dipstick, 81001 = automated dipstick, 81002 = microscopy only, 81003 = automated with microscopy.

Question 59: Answer: B) 85610

Explanation: Code 85610 represents prothrombin time (PT), a coagulation test measuring blood clotting time, commonly monitored in patients on warfarin.

Study Tip: Common coagulation tests: PT 85610, PTT 85730, INR included in PT. Know tests for anticoagulation monitoring.

Question 60: Answer: C) 80061

Explanation: Lipid panel (80061) includes total cholesterol, HDL, triglycerides, and calculated LDL for cardiovascular risk assessment.

Study Tip: Panel codes save documentation and are cost-effective when all components performed. Know common panels: CMP, BMP, lipid, hepatic.

Questions 61-70: HCPCS Level II and Modifiers

Question 61: Answer: B) DME, supplies, and drugs

Explanation: HCPCS Level II codes primarily cover durable medical equipment, supplies, drugs, and services not included in CPT® code set.

Study Tip: HCPCS supplements CPT®. Use for DME, prosthetics, orthotics, medical supplies, drugs, ambulance services not in CPT®.

Question 62: Answer: A) J1815

Explanation: Code J1815 represents injection, insulin, per 5 units. Calculate units administered and divide by 5 to determine quantity billed.

Study Tip: Drug codes specify dosage units. Always check "per" amount in code descriptor to calculate correct quantity for billing.

Question 63: Answer: B) A4253

Explanation: Code A4253 represents blood glucose test or reagent strips for home blood glucose monitor, box of 50 strips.

Study Tip: Know common diabetic supply codes: test strips, lancets, syringes. A4 codes cover many medical supplies.

Question 64: Answer: C) A0429

Explanation: Code A0429 represents ambulance service, basic life support (BLS), emergency transport to nearest appropriate facility.

Study Tip: Ambulance codes specify service level (BLS, ALS) and type (emergency, non-emergency). Level and urgency determine code.

Question 65: Answer: C) E0143

Explanation: Code E0143 represents walker, folding, wheeled, adjustable or fixed height, allowing patient mobility assistance.

Study Tip: E codes cover durable medical equipment. Know common DME: walkers, wheelchairs, hospital beds, oxygen equipment.

Question 66: Answer: B) Right side

Explanation: Modifier -RT indicates right side, used to specify laterality when procedure performed on right side of paired anatomical structures.

Study Tip: Laterality modifiers: -LT = left, -RT = right. Use when procedure code doesn't already specify laterality in description.

Question 67: Answer: A) Repeat procedure by same physician

Explanation: Modifier -76 indicates procedure was repeated by same physician on same day, distinct from original procedure performed.

Study Tip: Repeat procedure modifiers: -76 = same physician repeats, -77 = different physician repeats. Choose based on who performed repeat.

Question 68: Answer: B) Significant E/M and procedure same day

Explanation: Modifier -25 indicates significant, separately identifiable E/M service performed on same day as procedure by same physician.

Study Tip: Use -25 when E/M service is above and beyond usual pre/post procedure work. Both services must be significant and documented.

Question 69: Answer: B) Distinct procedural service

Explanation: Modifier -59 identifies procedures/services not normally reported together but appropriate under circumstances due to different session, site, or procedure.

Study Tip: Use -59 cautiously for unbundling. Must meet criteria: different session, site, organ system, incision, or separate injury/lesion.

Question 70: Answer: A) Unrelated procedure during post-op period

Explanation: Modifier -79 indicates unrelated procedure/service by same physician during postoperative period of original procedure.

Study Tip: Post-op modifiers: -78 = related return to OR, -79 = unrelated procedure during post-op. Different diagnosis typically required for -79.

Questions 71-80: Anesthesia Coding

Question 71: Answer: A) 11 units

Explanation: Base units (6) + Time units (75 ÷ 15 = 5) + Physical status P1 (0) = 11 total anesthesia units.

Study Tip: Anesthesia formula: Base + Time + Physical status + Qualifying circumstances. Remember to divide minutes by 15 for time units.

Question 72: Answer: C) Severe systemic disease

Explanation: P3 indicates patient with severe systemic disease causing functional limitation but not constant threat to life.

Study Tip: Physical status: P1 = normal, P2 = mild disease, P3 = severe disease, P4 = life-threatening disease, P5 = moribund, P6 = brain dead.

Question 73: Answer: A) +99100

Explanation: Qualifying circumstance +99100 applies to patients of extreme age: under 1 year or over 70 years old.

Study Tip: Qualifying circumstances add complexity: +99100 = extreme age, +99116 = hypothermia, +99135 = hypotension, +99140 = emergency.

Question 74: Answer: C) Anesthesiologist begins patient prep

Explanation: Anesthesia time starts when anesthesiologist begins preparing patient for anesthesia induction (placing monitors, starting IV, etc.).

Study Tip: Time = anesthesiologist presence, not patient presence or surgery time. Starts with patient prep, ends when patient transferred to recovery.

Question 75: Answer: C) 18 units

Explanation: Base units (8) + Time units (120 ÷ 15 = 8) + Age >70 (+99100 = 1) + Emergency (+99140 = 1) = 18 total units.

Study Tip: Add all applicable qualifying circumstances. Emergency + extreme age both apply here, each adding 1 unit to total.

Question 76: Answer: C) Procedure complexity

Explanation: Base units reflect inherent complexity of providing anesthesia for specific surgical procedure, considering typical risk and monitoring needs.

Study Tip: Base units assigned by procedure complexity, not patient condition or time. Patient factors captured in physical status modifiers.

Question 77: Answer: D) Emergency conditions

Explanation: Qualifying circumstance +99140 is used when anesthesia complicated by emergency conditions requiring immediate surgical intervention.

Study Tip: Emergency means immediate surgery required without adequate preparation time. Not all urgent cases qualify—must be true emergency.

Question 78: Answer: B) 31 units

Explanation: Base units (15) + Time units (240 ÷ 15 = 16) + Physical status P3 (0) = 31 total anesthesia units.

Study Tip: High base units reflect cardiac surgery complexity. Physical status modifiers don't add units in most reimbursement systems.

Question 79: Answer: B) 15

Explanation: Time units calculated by dividing total anesthesia minutes by 15, then rounding to nearest whole number.

Study Tip: Always divide by 15 for time units. Round 0.5 and above up, below 0.5 down. Example: 67 min = 4.47 = 4 units.

Question 80: Answer: D) P7

Explanation: Physical status modifiers range from P1-P6 only. There is no P7 modifier in the anesthesia coding system.

Study Tip: Six physical status levels: P1-P6. Each describes patient condition from normal healthy (P1) to brain dead (P6).

Questions 81-90: Compliance and Regulatory

Question 81: Answer: A) Health Insurance Portability and Accountability Act

Explanation: HIPAA (Health Insurance Portability and Accountability Act) of 1996 establishes national standards for protecting patient health information.

Study Tip: Know HIPAA basics: Privacy Rule (PHI protection), Security Rule (ePHI), Breach Notification Rule. Foundation of healthcare compliance.

Question 82: Answer: C) Hospital name

Explanation: Hospital name alone is not PHI. PHI must be individually identifiable health information—hospital name doesn't identify specific individuals.

Study Tip: PHI = individually identifiable health information. 18 identifiers must be removed to de-identify. Hospital name not in list.

Question 83: Answer: B) Electronic PHI only

Explanation: HIPAA Security Rule specifically addresses protection of electronic protected health information (ePHI), not paper or verbal PHI.

Study Tip: Privacy Rule = all PHI (paper, electronic, verbal). Security Rule = electronic PHI only. Know which rule applies to what.

Question 84: Answer: B) Billing higher level than provided

Explanation: Upcoding means billing for higher level of service than actually provided or documented, resulting in inappropriate increased reimbursement.

Study Tip: Common fraud schemes: upcoding (higher level), unbundling (separate components), billing for services not provided. Know definitions.

Question 85: Answer: C) Federal healthcare program fraud

Explanation: False Claims Act addresses fraud against federal healthcare programs (Medicare, Medicaid, TRICARE), imposing penalties for false claims.

Study Tip: False Claims Act = federal programs. Violations carry treble damages plus penalties per false claim. Serious consequences.

Question 86: Answer: B) Services reasonable and necessary for diagnosis/treatment

Explanation: Medical necessity means services are reasonable and necessary for diagnosis or treatment of illness/injury, meeting accepted standards of medical practice.

Study Tip: Medical necessity requires: appropriate for condition, not excessive, meets standards of care. Documentation must support medical necessity.

Question 87: Answer: C) Knowing and willful misrepresentation

Explanation: Fraud requires knowing and willful execution of scheme to defraud or obtain money through false pretenses—intent is key element.

Study Tip: Fraud = intentional deception. Abuse = poor practices without intent. Mistakes = unintentional errors. Intent determines categorization.

Question 88: Answer: B) Department of Health and Human Services

Explanation: Office of Inspector General (OIG) is part of Department of Health and Human Services, overseeing Medicare/Medicaid program integrity.

Study Tip: OIG issues compliance guidance, work plans, exclusion lists. Key enforcement agency for healthcare fraud and abuse.

Question 89: Answer: C) Both diagnosis and procedure codes

Explanation: Documentation must support all codes assigned—both diagnosis codes (medical necessity) and procedure codes (services actually performed).

Study Tip: "If it's not documented, it wasn't done." Documentation must justify every code submitted for reimbursement.

Question 90: Answer: D) All of the above

Explanation: Effective compliance program includes written policies/procedures, regular training, audit procedures, and multiple other elements working together.

Study Tip: Seven elements of compliance program: policies, leadership, training, communication, monitoring, enforcement, response. All components essential.

Questions 91-100: Case Studies

Question 91: Answer: B) K35.80 (acute appendicitis)

Explanation: Code the confirmed diagnosis (acute appendicitis) after pathology confirmation. Don't code symptoms (abdominal pain) when definitive diagnosis established.

Study Tip: When definitive diagnosis confirmed, code diagnosis only—not symptoms that led to it. Symptoms integral to diagnosis not coded separately.

Question 92: Answer: B) 99214

Explanation: Established patient, 30 minutes with moderate complexity MDM qualifies for 99214 (30-39 minutes OR moderate MDM).

Study Tip: Pre-procedure evaluation can be coded when significant, separately identifiable service beyond procedure's usual pre-op work.

Question 93: Answer: B) 45385

Explanation: Colonoscopy with polyp removal (45385) is most extensive service and includes biopsy. Code once regardless of number of polyps removed.

Question 94: Answer: B) 29880, 29877

Explanation: Arthroscopic partial medial meniscectomy (29880) and chondroplasty of patella (29877) are distinct procedures performed during same operative session.

Study Tip: Multiple arthroscopic procedures on same knee can be coded separately when distinct services. Diagnostic arthroscopy is included—don't code separately.

Question 95: Answer: C) 11402, 11604

Explanation: Benign lesion on arm 1.1-2.0 cm (11402), malignant lesion on trunk 2.1-3.0 cm (11604). Different sites and classifications require separate codes.

Study Tip: Never combine benign and malignant lesion measurements. Different classifications always code separately regardless of location.

Question 96: Answer: C) Either can be principal

Explanation: When documentation indicates two conditions are equally responsible for admission, either may be selected as principal diagnosis per coding guidelines.

Study Tip: When documentation states conditions are "equal" or "both responsible," coder may choose either as principal. Query if unclear which was primary reason.

Question 97: Answer: C) 15 units

Explanation: Base units (7) + Time units (90 ÷ 15 = 6) + P3 severe preeclampsia (0) + Emergency (+99140 = 1) + Age qualifier not applicable (42 years) = 14 units. Note: If P3 adds unit in your system, answer would be 15.

Study Tip: Emergency cesarean qualifies for +99140. Patient under 70, so +99100 doesn't apply. Calculate each component carefully.

Question 98: Answer: A) 77065

Explanation: Diagnostic mammography of one breast (unilateral) following abnormal screening uses code 77065. Bilateral diagnostic would be 77066.

Study Tip: Screening (77067) for asymptomatic patients. Diagnostic (77065-77066) when symptoms or follow-up of abnormality. Know the indication difference.

Question 99: Answer: C) 99212-25, 11100

Explanation: Diabetes follow-up is significant E/M service (99212) requiring modifier -25 when performed same day as biopsy procedure (11100).

Study Tip: Use -25 when E/M service goes beyond typical pre/post procedure work. Both services must be significant and separately documented.

Question 100: Answer: C) Z51.0 (radiotherapy)

Explanation: When encounter is solely for radiation therapy, Z51.0 is principal diagnosis. The cancer diagnosis (C34.90) is listed as secondary.

Study Tip: Therapy encounter codes (Z51.-) are principal when encounter is specifically for that therapy. Cancer diagnosis becomes secondary.

Performance Analysis Guide

Scoring Your Practice Test

Total Correct: ______ / 100

Percentage Score: ______ %

Performance Categories:

90-100 Correct (90-100%): Excellent Preparation You're demonstrating strong mastery across all content areas. Your performance indicates you're ready for the CPC exam. Focus your remaining study time on:

- Reviewing any missed questions to understand why you selected incorrect answers
- Practicing time management to ensure you can complete 100 questions in 4 hours

- Taking one more practice test under timed conditions for final confidence building

80-89 Correct (80-89%): Good Preparation You're showing solid understanding of most concepts but have room for improvement. Focus on:

- Identifying specific content areas where you missed multiple questions
- Reviewing those topics thoroughly using your study materials
- Taking additional practice questions in weak areas
- Improving speed while maintaining accuracy

70-79 Correct (70-79%): Passing Range but More Study Needed You're in the passing range but should strengthen your knowledge before exam day. Focus on:

- Conducting a thorough review of all missed questions
- Identifying patterns in errors (specific body systems, code types, guidelines)
- Creating a focused study plan for weak areas
- Allowing more time before scheduling your exam
- Considering additional practice tests

Below 70 Correct (<70%): Additional Preparation Required Your score indicates more comprehensive preparation is needed. Consider:

- Postponing your exam if already scheduled
- Reviewing all study guide chapters systematically
- Working through additional practice questions with detailed explanations
- Joining a study group or finding a study partner
- Considering a CPC preparation course if available
- Focusing on fundamentals: medical terminology, anatomy, ICD-10-CM and CPT® basics

Content Area Analysis

Calculate your percentage correct in each content area:

Medical Terminology and Anatomy (Questions 1-10): Correct: ______ / 10 = ______ %

ICD-10-CM Diagnosis Coding (Questions 11-20): Correct: ______ / 10 = ______ %

CPT® E/M Coding (Questions 21-30): Correct: ______ / 10 = ______ %

CPT® Surgery Coding (Questions 31-50): Correct: ______ / 20 = ______ %

CPT® Radiology, Path/Lab, Medicine (Questions 51-60): Correct: ______ / 10 = ______ %

HCPCS and Modifiers (Questions 61-70): Correct: ______ / 10 = ______ %

Anesthesia Coding (Questions 71-80): Correct: ______ / 10 = ______ %

Compliance and Regulatory (Questions 81-90): Correct: ______ / 10 = ______ %

Case Studies (Questions 91-100): Correct: ______ / 10 = ______ %

Identifying Your Weak Areas

For each content area where you scored below 70%, create a focused study plan:

Priority 1 (Scored below 50%): These areas need immediate, intensive review

- Dedicate 2-3 hours to comprehensive chapter review
- Complete all practice questions in study guide
- Create summary notes or flashcards
- Quiz yourself daily until proficient

Priority 2 (Scored 50-69%): These areas need significant improvement

- Dedicate 1-2 hours to targeted review
- Focus on concepts behind missed questions
- Complete additional practice questions
- Review related coding guidelines

Priority 3 (Scored 70-79%): These areas need minor reinforcement

- Dedicate 30-60 minutes to quick review
- Focus specifically on question types missed
- Review relevant coding examples
- Ensure understanding of key concepts

Strength Areas (Scored 80% or higher): Maintain proficiency

- Quick 15-minute review to stay sharp
- Focus on maintaining speed and accuracy
- Use these areas to boost confidence

Common Error Patterns to Review

Check if you're making any of these common mistakes:

Pattern 1: Rushing Through Questions

- Missing key words like "NOT," "EXCEPT," or "initial encounter"
- Not reading all answer options before selecting
- **Solution:** Slow down, read carefully, eliminate wrong answers systematically

Pattern 2: Not Using Code Books Effectively

- Coding from memory instead of verifying in books
- Not reading complete code descriptions
- Missing instructional notes
- **Solution:** Always verify codes in books, read all instructions and notes

Pattern 3: Misunderstanding Guidelines

- Confusing bundling rules
- Incorrect modifier usage
- Sequencing errors

- **Solution:** Review CPT® and ICD-10-CM guidelines sections thoroughly

Pattern 4: Weak Foundational Knowledge

- Medical terminology errors
- Anatomy confusion
- Basic coding principle misunderstanding
- **Solution:** Return to foundational chapters for comprehensive review

Pattern 5: Time Management Issues

- Spending too long on difficult questions
- Not having time to review answers
- Leaving questions blank
- **Solution:** Practice timed sessions, skip and return to difficult questions

Creating Your Final Study Plan

Based on your performance, create a customized study schedule for the remaining time before your exam:

4+ Weeks Until Exam:

- Week 1: Focus on Priority 1 weak areas with comprehensive review
- Week 2: Address Priority 2 areas with targeted practice
- Week 3: Quick review of Priority 3 areas and strengthen all areas
- Week 4: Take Practice Test 3, final review, build confidence

2-3 Weeks Until Exam:

- Days 1-7: Intensive review of all weak areas (Priority 1 and 2)
- Days 8-14: Take Practice Test 3, review all errors thoroughly
- Days 15-21: Final review, practice time management, mental preparation

1 Week Until Exam:

- Days 1-4: Light review of weak areas, practice questions
- Days 5-6: Take Practice Test 3, review any remaining gaps
- Day 7: Light review only, rest, and mental preparation

Day Before Exam:

- Light review of summary notes only
- Organize materials (code books, ID, directions)
- Get good sleep
- Eat healthy meals
- Stay positive and confident

Test-Taking Strategies to Improve

Apply these strategies on your next practice test:

Strategy 1: Time Allocation

- First pass: Answer all questions you know immediately (60-70 questions)
- Second pass: Return to marked questions, use elimination method
- Final pass: Review all answers if time permits
- Always leave 15-20 minutes for final review

Strategy 2: Elimination Method

- Cross out obviously wrong answers
- Look for key words that make options incorrect
- Choose best answer from remaining options
- Never leave questions blank—educated guessing beats no answer

Strategy 3: Code Book Navigation

- Use tabs and highlighting effectively
- Start with alphabetic index, verify in tabular
- Read all instructional notes before finalizing code
- Check for additional codes, modifiers, or exclusions

Strategy 4: Managing Anxiety

- Take deep breaths if feeling overwhelmed
- Remember that 70% correct is passing
- Focus on one question at a time
- Trust your preparation and knowledge

Strategy 5: Final Review Checklist

- Verify you answered all 100 questions
- Double-check any questions you marked for review
- Ensure proper bubbling on answer sheet
- Don't second-guess yourself excessively—first instinct usually correct

Building Confidence for Exam Day

Your preparation is working. Trust the process:

You've completed comprehensive study covering all CPC exam content areas. This practice test shows you what to expect and where to focus remaining efforts.

Every practice question you complete strengthens your coding knowledge and builds the pattern recognition that makes exam questions easier.

Mistakes are learning opportunities. Each error you identify and correct now is a question you'll get right on the actual exam.

You're not alone. Thousands of coders pass the CPC exam every year with similar preparation. Your systematic approach positions you for success.

The exam is challenging but fair. Questions test practical coding knowledge you'll use in your career. Your preparation prepares you not just for the exam, but for professional success.

Next Steps

Before taking Practice Test 3:

1. **Complete your targeted review** of all weak areas identified in this test
2. **Review all missed questions** until you understand why the correct answer is right
3. **Practice time management** by taking shorter, timed quizzes
4. **Strengthen your code book navigation** skills through daily practice
5. **Build confidence** by recognizing your progress and preparation

Remember: This practice test is a learning tool, not a prediction of your exam score. Use it to identify gaps, strengthen weak areas, and build the confidence you need for success.

You're on the right path. Continue your focused preparation, trust your knowledge, and approach exam day with confidence. You've got this!

Congratulations on Completing Practice Test 2!

You've now worked through 200 practice questions across two full-length exams. This substantial practice builds the skills, speed, and confidence you need for CPC exam success.

Your next milestone: Review this test thoroughly, address any weak areas, and prepare for Practice Test 3—your final dress rehearsal before the real exam.

Every question you practice, every concept you review, every weak area you strengthen brings you closer to your goal of becoming a Certified Professional Coder.

Keep pushing forward. Success is within reach!

Chapter 21: Practice Test 3

"Success is the sum of small efforts repeated day in and day out." - Robert Collier

Welcome to your third full-length CPC practice examination. This test represents your final comprehensive assessment before taking the actual CPC exam. By now, you've completed two practice tests, identified your strengths and weaknesses, and focused your study efforts on areas needing improvement.

This practice test presents 100 questions that mirror the actual CPC exam in content, difficulty, and format. Time yourself for exactly 4 hours to simulate real testing conditions. Resist the temptation to look up answers or reference materials during the test—save that for the detailed review afterward.

Your performance on this test provides the clearest indication of your readiness for the actual CPC exam. A score of 70% or higher suggests you're prepared for certification, though higher scores obviously indicate greater confidence and preparation. Scores below 70% identify specific areas requiring additional focused study before scheduling your exam.

Remember: This practice test is a learning tool, not a final judgment. Every question you miss teaches you something valuable. Review all explanations carefully, even for questions you answered correctly, as they often contain insights that deepen your understanding.

Testing Instructions:

1. **Time Limit:** 4 hours (240 minutes)
2. **Passing Score:** 70% (70 questions correct)
3. **Materials Allowed:** CPT®, ICD-10-CM, and HCPCS Level II code books
4. **Calculator:** Basic four-function calculator permitted
5. **Environment:** Find a quiet space free from distractions

Before You Begin:

- Gather all necessary materials
- Set a timer for 4 hours
- Have blank paper for calculations
- Ensure good lighting and comfortable seating
- Silence all electronic devices
- Begin only when you can dedicate the full 4 hours

Good luck! Your preparation has brought you to this point. Trust your knowledge and approach each question systematically.

Practice Test 3: Questions

Medical Terminology and Anatomy (Questions 1-8)

Question 1: The suffix "-ectomy" means:

A) Surgical incision B) Surgical removal C) Surgical repair D) Inflammation

Question 2: The term "lateral" refers to:

A) Toward the midline B) Away from the midline C) Above D) Below

Question 3: The myocardium is:

A) The outer layer of the heart B) The middle muscular layer of the heart C) The inner lining of the heart D) The sac surrounding the heart

Question 4: Which organ is NOT part of the digestive system?

A) Pancreas B) Gallbladder C) Spleen D) Liver

Question 5: The prefix "brady-" means:

A) Fast B) Slow C) Difficult D) Excessive

Question 6: The clavicle is commonly known as the:

A) Shoulder blade B) Collarbone C) Breastbone D) Kneecap

Question 7: Which plane divides the body into right and left halves?

A) Transverse plane B) Frontal plane C) Sagittal plane D) Coronal plane

Question 8: The term "proximal" means:

A) Closer to the point of attachment B) Farther from the point of attachment C) On the same side D) On the opposite side

ICD-10-CM Diagnosis Coding (Questions 9-20)

Question 9: When should you code a "rule out" diagnosis in the outpatient setting?

A) Always code as if confirmed B) Use appropriate "rule out" code C) Code the signs and symptoms instead D) Do not code anything

Question 10: An "Excludes1" note in ICD-10-CM means:

A) The condition may be coded with others B) The condition cannot be coded here C) Additional codes are required D) The code is being deleted

Question 11: What is the correct code for Type 2 diabetes mellitus with diabetic nephropathy?

A) E11.9 B) E11.21 C) E10.21 D) E11.29

Question 12: For a patient with primary lung cancer with liver metastases, how should you sequence the codes?

A) Liver metastasis first, then lung primary B) Lung primary first, then liver metastasis C) Code only the metastatic site D) Code only the primary site

Question 13: Which character in an ICD-10-CM code indicates the chapter?

A) First character B) Second character C) Third character D) Fourth character

Question 14: A patient presents with acute exacerbation of COPD due to pneumonia. How should this be coded?

A) J44.1 only B) J18.9 only C) J44.1 and J18.9 D) J44.0 only

Question 15: What does "NOS" stand for in ICD-10-CM?

A) Not Otherwise Specified B) Not Elsewhere Classified C) New Official Standard D) No Other Symptoms

Question 16: For a fracture with nonunion, the appropriate 7th character for a closed fracture is:

A) A (initial encounter) B) D (routine healing) C) K (nonunion) D) S (sequela)

Question 17: A patient with gestational diabetes at 28 weeks should be coded with:

A) E11.9 (Type 2 diabetes) B) O24.419 (Gestational diabetes, unspecified control) C) Z87.59 (Personal history) D) R73.09 (Abnormal glucose)

Question 18: When coding burns, which should be sequenced first?

A) The burn with the largest body surface area B) The burn with the highest degree C) The burn causing the most pain D) The external cause code

Question 19: How many diagnosis codes are in the Basic Metabolic Panel (80048)?

A) This is not a diagnosis code B) 6 codes C) 8 codes D) 10 codes

Question 20: For sepsis with acute kidney injury, the acute kidney injury should be coded:

A) First, before the sepsis code B) After the sepsis code as additional diagnosis C) Only if causing symptoms D) As the principal diagnosis only

CPT® Evaluation and Management (Questions 21-32)

Question 21: A new patient office visit lasting 45 minutes with moderate complexity MDM should be coded as:

A) 99203 B) 99204 C) 99205 D) 99214

Question 22: An established patient visit for routine blood pressure check by a nurse should be coded as:

A) 99211 B) 99212 C) 99213 D) Cannot be coded separately

Question 23: Critical care services require a minimum of how many minutes?

A) 15 minutes B) 20 minutes C) 30 minutes D) 45 minutes

Question 24: For Medicare patients, consultation codes should be:

A) Used as normal B) Replaced with new/established patient codes C) Used only for office consultations D) Used only for inpatient consultations

Question 25: Time-based E/M coding includes:

A) Only face-to-face time B) Only time in examination room C) Total time on date of encounter D) Only documentation time

Question 26: An emergency department visit for a life-threatening condition should be coded as:

A) 99281 B) 99283 C) 99284 D) 99285

Question 27: Hospital discharge services taking 35 minutes should be coded as:

A) 99238 B) 99239 C) 99232 D) 99233

Question 28: Modifier -25 is used when:

A) A procedure is bilateral B) E/M and procedure both performed same day C) Service is reduced D) Procedure is discontinued

Question 29: Medical decision making complexity is based on:

A) History, examination, time B) Problems addressed, data reviewed, risk C) Patient age, diagnosis, treatment D) Documentation length, complexity, detail

Question 30: A subsequent hospital care visit with detailed interval history and moderate complexity MDM should be coded as:

A) 99231 B) 99232 C) 99233 D) 99238

Question 31: Prolonged services code 99354 requires how much time beyond the highest E/M level?

A) 15 minutes B) 30 minutes C) 45 minutes D) 60 minutes

Question 32: For established patient office visits, code 99213 covers:

A) 10-19 minutes B) 20-29 minutes C) 30-39 minutes D) 40-54 minutes

CPT® Surgery Coding (Questions 33-50)

Question 33: Simple repair of a 4 cm laceration on the face should be coded as:

A) 12011 B) 12013 C) 12014 D) 12051

Question 34: Excision of a 2.0 cm malignant lesion from the back with 0.5 cm margins should be coded as:

A) 11602 B) 11603 C) 11604 D) 11606

Question 35: Closed treatment of a displaced femur fracture with manipulation should be coded as:

A) 27500 B) 27502 C) 27506 D) 27507

Question 36: Arthroscopic meniscectomy of the knee should be coded as:

A) 29870 B) 29875 C) 29880 D) 29881

Question 37: A colonoscopy with biopsy and polyp removal should be coded as:

A) 45380 only B) 45385 only C) 45378 and 45380 D) 45380 and 45385

Question 38: Laparoscopic cholecystectomy with cholangiography should be coded as:

A) 47562 B) 47563 C) 47564 D) 47600

Question 39: Cystoscopy with fulguration of bladder tumor should be coded as:

A) 52000 B) 52204 C) 52224 D) 52234

Question 40: TURP (transurethral resection of prostate) should be coded as:

A) 52450 B) 52500 C) 52601 D) 52630

Question 41: Diagnostic nasal endoscopy followed by ethmoidectomy should be coded as:

A) 31231 and 31254 B) 31254 only C) 31231 only D) 31255 only

Question 42: Emergency tracheostomy should be coded as:

A) 31600 B) 31601 C) 31603 D) 31605

Question 43: Bilateral inguinal hernia repair in an adult should be coded as:

A) 49505 B) 49505 with modifier -50 C) 49505 × 2 D) 49507

Question 44: Carpal tunnel release should be coded as:

A) 64721 B) 25000 C) 64831 D) 20526

Question 45: A partial mastectomy should be coded as:

A) 19300 B) 19301 C) 19302 D) 19303

Question 46: Open reduction internal fixation (ORIF) of a fracture involves:

A) No surgical exposure B) Surgical exposure with internal fixation C) Fixation through skin D) External stabilization only

Question 47: Modifier -50 indicates:

A) Reduced services B) Bilateral procedure C) Multiple procedures D) Discontinued procedure

Question 48: The global surgical package includes:

A) Only the surgery itself B) Preoperative, intraoperative, and routine postoperative care C) Surgery and complications D) Surgery and all follow-up care

Question 49: An "add-on" code is identified by:

A) The ⊕ symbol B) The + symbol C) The letter T D) Ending in -99

Question 50: Laminectomy at L4-L5 and L5-S1 should be coded as:

A) 63030 × 2 B) 63030 and 63035 C) 63030 only D) 63047 and 63048

CPT® Anesthesia (Questions 51-56)

Question 51: Anesthesia base units reflect:

A) Time spent providing anesthesia B) Complexity of anesthesia management C) Patient's medical conditions D) Surgeon's skill level

Question 52: Anesthesia time starts when:

A) Surgery begins B) Patient enters OR C) Anesthesiologist begins patient preparation D) Patient is unconscious

Question 53: A patient with well-controlled diabetes and hypertension should be assigned which physical status modifier?

A) P1 B) P2 C) P3 D) P4

Question 54: Qualifying circumstance +99100 applies to:

A) Emergency surgery B) Extreme age (under 1 or over 70) C) Controlled hypotension D) Total body hypothermia

Question 55: Anesthesia for appendectomy (00840, 6 base units) lasting 90 minutes in a healthy patient results in total units of:

A) 11 B) 12 C) 13 D) 14

Question 56: Emergency surgery adds which qualifying circumstance?

A) +99100 B) +99116 C) +99135 D) +99140

CPT® Radiology (Questions 57-62)

Question 57: A radiologist interprets a chest X-ray performed at a hospital. The radiologist should bill:

A) 71045 (global) B) 71045-26 (professional component) C) 71045-TC (technical component) D) Cannot bill separately

Question 58: Screening mammography for both breasts should be coded as:

A) 77065 × 2 B) 77066 C) 77067 D) 77065-50

Question 59: CT guidance for needle biopsy should be coded:

A) 77012 always B) Depends on biopsy code description C) Never separately D) 77011

Question 60: Complete abdominal ultrasound should be coded as:

A) 76700 B) 76705 C) 76770 D) Multiple organ codes

Question 61: MRI of knee without and with contrast should be coded as:

A) 73721 B) 73722 C) 73723 D) 73721 and 73722

Question 62: Modifier -26 indicates:

A) Technical component B) Professional component C) Bilateral procedure D) Multiple procedures

CPT® Pathology and Laboratory (Questions 63-68)

Question 63: The Basic Metabolic Panel (80048) includes how many tests?

A) 6 B) 8 C) 10 D) 12

Question 64: When should you use a panel code?

A) When any tests from panel performed B) When all tests in panel performed C) When physician orders panel D) When most tests performed

Question 65: The Comprehensive Metabolic Panel adds which tests to the Basic Metabolic Panel?

A) 2 additional tests B) 4 additional tests C) 6 additional tests D) 8 additional tests

Question 66: A lipid panel includes all EXCEPT:

A) Total cholesterol B) HDL cholesterol C) Triglycerides D) Hemoglobin A1c

Question 67: Urinalysis by dipstick, automated, should be coded as:

A) 81000 B) 81001 C) 81002 D) 81003

Question 68: A complete blood count (CBC) with automated differential should be coded as:

A) 85025 B) 85027 C) 85004 D) 85007

CPT® Medicine (Questions 69-74)

Question 69: An immunization administration for a single vaccine should be coded with:

A) The vaccine code only B) The administration code only C) Both vaccine and administration codes D) Neither code

Question 70: Chemotherapy administration, intravenous infusion, first hour should be coded as:

A) 96365 B) 96409 C) 96413 D) 96374

Question 71: Routine ECG with interpretation should be coded as:

A) 93000 B) 93005 C) 93010 D) 93040

Question 72: Pulmonary function testing (spirometry) should be coded as:

A) 94010 B) 94060 C) 94375 D) 94726

Question 73: Physical therapy evaluation, low complexity, should be coded as:

A) 97161 B) 97162 C) 97163 D) 97164

Question 74: Acupuncture with electrical stimulation, 15 minutes, should be coded as:

A) 97810 B) 97813 C) 97814 D) 97820

HCPCS Level II (Questions 75-80)

Question 75: HCPCS Level II codes are identified by:

A) Five numeric digits B) One letter and four numbers C) Four numbers and one letter D) Two letters and three numbers

Question 76: Ambulance transport, basic life support should be coded with:

A) A0426 B) A0428 C) A0429 D) A0430

Question 77: Injection of insulin should be coded with a code from which HCPCS section?

A) A codes B) E codes C) J codes D) Q codes

Question 78: Durable medical equipment includes:

A) Disposable supplies B) Single-use items C) Reusable equipment D) Pharmaceuticals

Question 79: Modifier -LT indicates:

A) Left side B) Lower extremity C) Long-term use D) Limited service

Question 80: HCPCS Level II codes are used when:

A) No CPT® code exists B) Medicare requires specific code C) Supplies or equipment needed D) All of the above

Compliance and Regulatory (Questions 81-86)

Question 81: HIPAA protects:

A) Only electronic health information B) Only paper records C) All individually identifiable health information D) Only diagnostic information

Question 82: The minimum necessary standard requires:

A) Accessing all available patient information B) Limiting PHI access to what's needed for job C) Reviewing complete medical history D) Sharing all information with healthcare team

Question 83: Upcoding is defined as:

A) Billing for services not provided B) Billing at higher level than documented C) Billing same service twice D) Billing incorrect patient

Question 84: The False Claims Act addresses:

A) Only criminal fraud B) Civil and criminal fraud against government C) Only billing errors D) Only intentional fraud

Question 85: An advance beneficiary notice (ABN) is required when:

A) Medicare likely won't cover service B) Patient has no insurance C) Service is experimental D) All services provided

Question 86: The OIG Compliance Program recommends:

A) Coding only to maximize reimbursement B) Regular auditing and monitoring C) Delegating compliance to one person D) Avoiding documentation of errors

Modifiers and Guidelines (Questions 87-92)

Question 87: Modifier -22 indicates:

A) Increased procedural services B) Reduced services C) Bilateral procedure D) Multiple procedures

Question 88: Modifier -51 should NOT be used with:

A) Primary procedure B) Add-on codes C) Bilateral procedures D) Reduced services

Question 89: Modifier -59 indicates:

A) Distinct procedural service B) Bilateral procedure C) Multiple surgeons D) Staged procedure

Question 90: Modifier -62 indicates:

A) Two surgeons performing same procedure B) Co-surgeons performing different parts C) Assistant surgeon D) Multiple procedures

Question 91: Modifier -78 indicates:

A) Unplanned return to OR during global period B) Staged procedure during global period C) Related procedure during global period D) Unrelated procedure during global period

Question 92: Modifier -79 indicates:

A) Staged procedure during global period B) Related procedure during global period C) Unrelated procedure by same physician during postop period D) Repeat procedure

Integrated Coding Scenarios (Questions 93-100)

Question 93: A patient with acute appendicitis undergoes laparoscopic appendectomy. ICD-10-CM code:

A) K35.80 B) K35.89 C) K37 D) K35.2

Question 94: Same patient, laparoscopic appendectomy CPT® code:

A) 44950 B) 44960 C) 44970 D) 44979

Question 95: A 75-year-old patient with severe COPD undergoes emergency bowel resection lasting 180 minutes (00840, 6 base units). Total anesthesia units:

A) 18 B) 19 C) 20 D) 21

Question 96: A patient has simple repair of 3 cm forehead laceration and 2 cm cheek laceration. Total length for coding:

A) Code separately B) 5 cm total C) 3 cm (code highest) D) Cannot combine

Question 97: Colonoscopy reaches cecum but no biopsy or polyp removal performed. Code:

A) 45378 B) 45380 C) 45385 D) 45330

Question 98: Type 2 diabetic patient on long-term insulin. Codes needed:

A) E11.9 only B) E10.9 and Z79.4 C) E11.9 and Z79.4 D) E11.65

Question 99: Cataract surgery on right eye with IOL insertion. Code:

A) 66984 B) 66984-RT C) 66982 D) 66982-RT

Question 100: Patient has chest pain, EKG shows acute MI. Code:

A) R07.9 (chest pain) B) I21.9 (acute MI) C) I21.4 (non-STEMI) D) Both chest pain and MI

Practice Test 3 - Complete Answer Key with Explanations

Total Questions: 100
Passing Score: 70% (70 correct answers)
Time Allowed: 4 hours (240 minutes)

Score Interpretation Guide

- **90-100%:** Excellent! You're ready for the CPC exam
- **80-89%:** Very Good. Review missed questions and weak areas
- **70-79%:** Passing. Focus additional study on identified weaknesses
- **Below 70%:** Additional preparation needed. Review all sections thoroughly

Detailed Answer Explanations

Medical Terminology and Anatomy (Questions 1-8)

Question 1: Answer: B) Surgical removal
Explanation: The suffix "-ectomy" means surgical removal or excision of an organ, tissue, or body part.
Study Tip: Common surgical suffixes: -ectomy (removal), -otomy (incision), -plasty (repair), -rrhaphy (suturing).

Question 2: Answer: B) Away from the midline
Explanation: Lateral means away from the body's midline; medial means toward the midline.
Study Tip: Think "lateral" = "to the side" away from center. Opposite of medial.

Question 3: Answer: B) The middle muscular layer of the heart
Explanation: Myocardium is the heart muscle layer between epicardium (outer) and endocardium (inner lining).
Study Tip: "Myo" = muscle. Myocardium is the muscular pumping layer of the heart.

Question 4: Answer: C) Spleen
Explanation: The spleen is part of the lymphatic/immune system, not the digestive system, though located near digestive organs.
Study Tip: Digestive system = organs that process food. Spleen filters blood (lymphatic system).

Question 5: Answer: B) Slow
Explanation: The prefix "brady-" means slow, as in bradycardia (slow heart rate).
Study Tip: Brady = slow; Tachy = fast. Remember these opposites together.

Question 6: Answer: B) Collarbone
Explanation: Clavicle is the medical term for collarbone, connecting sternum to scapula (shoulder blade).
Study Tip: Clavicle sounds like "claw" - connects arm to body like a claw.

Question 7: Answer: C) Sagittal plane
Explanation: Sagittal plane divides body into right and left portions; transverse divides upper/lower.
Study Tip: Sagittal = "side to side" division. Think of an arrow (sagitta) going through sideways.

Question 8: Answer: A) Closer to the point of attachment
Explanation: Proximal means closer to center/point of attachment; distal means farther away.
Study Tip: Proximal = proximity (close to center); distal = distance (far from center).

ICD-10-CM Diagnosis Coding (Questions 9-20)

Question 9: Answer: C) Code the signs and symptoms instead
Explanation: In outpatient settings, uncertain diagnoses ("rule out," "suspected") are not coded; code documented signs/symptoms instead.
Study Tip: Outpatient rule: Never code "rule out." Use actual signs/symptoms until diagnosis confirmed.

Question 10: Answer: B) The condition cannot be coded here
Explanation: Excludes1 notes indicate mutually exclusive conditions that cannot be coded together at same encounter.
Study Tip: Excludes1 = exclusive (choose one); Excludes2 = may coexist (can code both).

Question 11: Answer: B) E11.21
Explanation: E11.21 specifically identifies Type 2 diabetes mellitus with diabetic nephropathy (kidney complication).
Study Tip: E11 = Type 2 DM; fourth/fifth characters specify complications. Learn common complications.

Question 12: Answer: B) Lung primary first, then liver metastasis
Explanation: When both primary malignancy and metastatic sites are known, sequence primary first, then secondary sites.
Study Tip: Primary before secondary when both documented. Primary determines treatment approach.

Question 13: Answer: A) First character
Explanation: The first character (always a letter A-Z) indicates the ICD-10-CM chapter.
Study Tip: First character = chapter identifier. Letters organize diseases by body system or etiology.

Question 14: Answer: C) J44.1 and J18.9
Explanation: Code both COPD with acute exacerbation (J44.1) and precipitating cause pneumonia (J18.9) when documented.
Study Tip: Acute exacerbation + documented cause = code both conditions separately.

Question 15: Answer: A) Not Otherwise Specified
Explanation: NOS means insufficient documentation exists for more specific code assignment.
Study Tip: NOS = not specified (vague documentation); NEC = not elsewhere classified (no specific code exists).

Question 16: Answer: C) K (nonunion)
Explanation: Seventh character K indicates closed fracture with nonunion (complete failure to heal).
Study Tip: Fracture 7th characters: A=initial, D=routine healing, K=nonunion, S=sequela.

Question 17: Answer: B) O24.419 (Gestational diabetes, unspecified control)
Explanation: Gestational diabetes in currently pregnant patient requires O-code from pregnancy chapter.
Study Tip: Current pregnancy conditions always use O codes, not general medical codes.

Question 18: Answer: B) The burn with the highest degree
Explanation: When multiple burns present, sequence highest-degree burn first.
Study Tip: Burn coding order: 1) highest degree, 2) extent code (T31), 3) external cause.

Question 19: Answer: A) This is not a diagnosis code
Explanation: 80048 is a CPT® laboratory panel code for testing, not an ICD-10-CM diagnosis code.
Study Tip: 80000-89000 series = CPT® Path/Lab codes. Don't confuse with ICD-10-CM diagnoses.

Question 20: Answer: B) After the sepsis code as additional diagnosis
Explanation: Sepsis codes first; complications like acute kidney injury coded as additional diagnoses.
Study Tip: Sepsis sequencing: A41.- (sepsis) first, then organ dysfunction codes.

CPT® Evaluation and Management (Questions 21-32)

Question 21: Answer: B) 99204
Explanation: New patient with 45 minutes OR moderate complexity MDM qualifies for 99204 (45-59 minutes).
Study Tip: 99204 = new patient, 45-59 min OR moderate MDM. Either criterion qualifies.

Question 22: Answer: A) 99211
Explanation: 99211 represents minimal E/M service, only code that can be performed by clinical staff under physician supervision.
Study Tip: 99211 = minimal service, nurse visit for blood pressure check, injection, etc.

Question 23: Answer: C) 30 minutes
Explanation: Critical care services (99291) require minimum 30 minutes to report.
Study Tip: Critical care minimum = 30 minutes. First 30-74 minutes = 99291.

Question 24: Answer: B) Replaced with new/established patient codes
Explanation: Medicare no longer recognizes consultation codes; use appropriate new or established patient E/M codes.
Study Tip: Medicare = no consultations. Use 99202-99205 (new) or 99211-99215 (established).

Question 25: Answer: C) Total time on date of encounter
Explanation: Time-based E/M includes both face-to-face and non-face-to-face work on encounter date.
Study Tip: Current E/M time = total time on date, including documentation, coordination, review.

Question 26: Answer: D) 99285
Explanation: Life-threatening conditions requiring immediate intervention qualify for highest ED level (99285).
Study Tip: ED levels: 99281 (lowest/minor) to 99285 (highest/life-threatening).

Question 27: Answer: B) 99239
Explanation: Hospital discharge services taking more than 30 minutes use 99239; 30 minutes or less use 99238.
Study Tip: Discharge time-based: 99238 (≤30 min), 99239 (>30 min).

Question 28: Answer: B) E/M and procedure both performed same day
Explanation: Modifier -25 indicates significant, separately identifiable E/M service same day as procedure.
Study Tip: -25 = E/M + procedure same day. Both must be significant and separately identifiable.

Question 29: Answer: B) Problems addressed, data reviewed, risk
Explanation: MDM complexity determined by: 1) problems addressed, 2) data reviewed/analyzed, 3) risk of management.
Study Tip: MDM = 3 elements: problems, data, risk. Know all three for level selection.

Question 30: Answer: B) 99232
Explanation: Subsequent hospital care with detailed interval history and moderate complexity MDM = 99232.
Study Tip: Subsequent hospital: 99231 (low), 99232 (moderate), 99233 (high complexity).

Question 31: Answer: B) 30 minutes
Explanation: Prolonged services (99354) require 30+ minutes beyond highest E/M service level.
Study Tip: Prolonged = minimum 30 min beyond typical time for highest code level.

Question 32: Answer: B) 20-29 minutes
Explanation: Established patient code 99213 covers 20-29 minutes OR low complexity

MDM.
Study Tip: Established times: 99212 (10-19), 99213 (20-29), 99214 (30-39), 99215 (40-54).

CPT® Surgery Coding (Questions 33-50)

Question 33: Answer: B) 12013
Explanation: Simple repair of face wounds 2.6-5.0 cm uses 12013. Total = 4 cm (forehead) falls in this range.
Study Tip: Face simple repairs: 12011 (≤2.5), 12013 (2.6-5.0), 12014 (7.6-12.5).

Question 34: Answer: C) 11604
Explanation: Excision of malignant lesion requires lesion size + margins. 2.0 + 0.5 + 0.5 = 3.0 cm total = 11604 (2.1-3.0).
Study Tip: Excision measurement = lesion diameter + all margins removed. Sum determines code.

Question 35: Answer: B) 27502
Explanation: Closed treatment with manipulation means realigning fracture fragments without surgical opening.
Study Tip: Fracture treatment: closed (no surgery), open (surgical exposure), percutaneous (pins through skin).

Question 36: Answer: C) 29880
Explanation: Arthroscopic meniscectomy (partial or total cartilage removal) = 29880.
Study Tip: Knee arthroscopy: 29870 (diagnostic), 29880 (meniscectomy), 29881 (meniscus repair).

Question 37: Answer: B) 45385 only
Explanation: When multiple endoscopic procedures performed, code most extensive. Polyp removal includes any biopsy.
Study Tip: Colonoscopy bundling: Most extensive procedure includes lesser procedures.

Question 38: Answer: B) 47563
Explanation: Laparoscopic cholecystectomy with intraoperative cholangiography (bile duct imaging) = 47563.
Study Tip: Lap chole: 47562 (without cholangiography), 47563 (with cholangiography).

Question 39: Answer: D) 52234
Explanation: Cystoscopy with fulguration (destruction) of bladder tumor = 52234 for small tumors.
Study Tip: Cystoscopy: 52000 (diagnostic), 52204 (biopsy), 52234 (fulguration/resection small tumor).

Question 40: Answer: C) 52601
Explanation: TURP (transurethral resection of prostate) = 52601, standard treatment for benign prostatic hyperplasia.
Study Tip: TURP = 52601. Transurethral means through urethra, not open surgery.

Question 41: Answer: B) 31254 only
Explanation: Diagnostic endoscopy included when performed with more extensive surgical endoscopy. Code surgery only.
Study Tip: Endoscopy bundling: diagnostic included in surgical procedure, don't code separately.

Question 42: Answer: C) 31603
Explanation: Emergency tracheostomy for acute airway obstruction = 31603, higher complexity than planned.
Study Tip: Tracheostomy: 31600 (planned), 31603 (emergency). Emergency = higher risk/urgency.

Question 43: Answer: B) 49505 with modifier -50
Explanation: Bilateral procedures of same code use modifier -50 rather than listing code twice.
Study Tip: Bilateral same procedure = single code + modifier -50. Not separate codes.

Question 44: Answer: A) 64721
Explanation: Carpal tunnel release = neuroplasty of median nerve at carpal tunnel = 64721.
Study Tip: Carpal tunnel syndrome = median nerve compression. Release = 64721.

Question 45: Answer: B) 19301
Explanation: Partial mastectomy (lumpectomy) removes tumor with surrounding breast tissue = 19301.
Study Tip: Mastectomy types: 19301 (partial/lumpectomy), 19302 (simple/complete), 19303 (radical).

Question 46: Answer: B) Surgical exposure with internal fixation
Explanation: ORIF = open reduction (surgical opening), internal fixation (screws, plates, rods).
Study Tip: ORIF always involves surgical opening and internal hardware placement.

Question 47: Answer: B) Bilateral procedure
Explanation: Modifier -50 indicates identical procedure performed on both sides of body.
Study Tip: -50 = bilateral. Use when same procedure done on both sides same session.

Question 48: Answer: B) Preoperative, intraoperative, and routine postoperative care
Explanation: Global surgical package includes related E/M day before/of surgery, surgery itself, and routine follow-up.
Study Tip: Global package = pre-op, surgery, routine post-op. Complications billed separately.

Question 49: Answer: B) The + symbol
Explanation: Add-on codes marked with + symbol cannot be reported alone, always with primary procedure.
Study Tip: + = add-on code. Must have primary procedure code. Exempt from modifier -51.

Question 50: Answer: B) 63030 and 63035
Explanation: Laminectomy at multiple levels: primary code (63030) + add-on for each additional segment (63035).
Study Tip: Multi-level procedures: primary code + add-on codes for additional levels.

CPT® Anesthesia (Questions 51-56)

Question 51: Answer: B) Complexity of anesthesia management
Explanation: Base units reflect inherent complexity, risk, and intensity of anesthesia for specific procedure.
Study Tip: Base units = procedure complexity. Time units = duration. Don't confuse.

Question 52: Answer: C) Anesthesiologist begins patient preparation
Explanation: Anesthesia time starts when anesthesiologist begins preparing patient for anesthesia (monitors, IV, pre-med).
Study Tip: Start time = begin patient preparation, not surgery start or OR entry.

Question 53: Answer: B) P2
Explanation: Well-controlled diabetes and mild hypertension = mild systemic disease with no functional limitation = P2.
Study Tip: P1=healthy, P2=mild disease controlled, P3=severe disease/limitation, P4=life threat.

Question 54: Answer: B) Extreme age (under 1 or over 70)
Explanation: +99100 applies to patients under 1 year old or over 70 years old.
Study Tip: Age qualifying circumstances: +99100 for under 1 year or over 70 years.

Question 55: Answer: B) 12
Explanation: Base (6) + Time (90÷15=6) + P1 physical status (0) = 12 total units.
Study Tip: Formula: Base + Time + Physical Status + Qualifying Circumstances = Total.

Question 56: Answer: D) +99140
Explanation: Emergency surgery without adequate preparation time adds qualifying circumstance +99140.
Study Tip: Emergency qualifying = +99140. Adds 1 unit for urgent surgery.

CPT® Radiology (Questions 57-62)

Question 57: Answer: B) 71045-26 (professional component)
Explanation: When radiologist only interprets (not performing technical), use modifier -26 for professional component.
Study Tip: -26 = professional (interpretation). -TC = technical (equipment/staff). No modifier = global.

Question 58: Answer: C) 77067
Explanation: Screening mammography for asymptomatic patients, bilateral = 77067.
Study Tip: Screening mammo (asymptomatic) = 77067. Diagnostic (symptoms) = 77065/77066.

Question 59: Answer: B) Depends on biopsy code description
Explanation: Check biopsy code description. If includes guidance, don't code separately. If not, code both.
Study Tip: Always verify if procedure code includes imaging guidance before coding separately.

Question 60: Answer: A) 76700
Explanation: Complete abdominal ultrasound examining all required structures = 76700.
Study Tip: 76700 = complete (all organs). 76705 = limited (single organ/area).

Question 61: Answer: C) 73723
Explanation: MRI performed both without and with contrast = single code 73723, not two separate codes.
Study Tip: MRI "without and with" = single comprehensive code, not separate codes.

Question 62: Answer: B) Professional component
Explanation: Modifier -26 indicates professional component (physician interpretation and report).
Study Tip: -26 always = professional component. Used when only interpreting, not providing equipment.

CPT® Pathology and Laboratory (Questions 63-68)

Question 63: Answer: B) 8
Explanation: Basic Metabolic Panel (80048) includes 8 tests: calcium, CO2, chloride, creatinine, glucose, potassium, sodium, BUN.
Study Tip: Remember BMP = 8 tests. CMP = 14 tests (BMP + 6 liver tests).

Question 64: Answer: B) When all tests in panel performed
Explanation: Panel codes require ALL listed tests performed. Missing one test means use individual codes.
Study Tip: Panel rule: all tests or nothing. Cannot substitute or skip any component.

Question 65: Answer: C) 6 additional tests
Explanation: CMP adds 6 liver function tests to BMP's 8 tests: albumin, bilirubin (total), alkaline phosphatase, protein, ALT, AST.
Study Tip: CMP = BMP (8) + liver tests (6) = 14 total tests.

Question 66: Answer: D) Hemoglobin A1c
Explanation: Lipid panel includes total cholesterol, HDL, triglycerides, and calculated LDL. Not A1c (diabetes test).
Study Tip: Lipid panel = cholesterol, HDL, triglycerides, calculated LDL. For cardiac risk.

Question 67: Answer: B) 81001
Explanation: Urinalysis by dipstick or tablet reagent, automated with microscopy = 81001.
Study Tip: UA codes: 81000 (manual), 81001 (automated dipstick), 81002 (non-automated), 81003 (automated with micro).

Question 68: Answer: A) 85025
Explanation: Complete blood count with automated differential (CBC with diff) = 85025.
Study Tip: CBC: 85027 (without differential), 85025 (with automated differential).

CPT® Medicine (Questions 69-74)

Question 69: Answer: C) Both vaccine and administration codes
Explanation: Immunization coding requires two codes: vaccine product code AND administration code.
Study Tip: Immunization = always two codes: product (90000s) + administration (90460-90474).

Question 70: Answer: C) 96413
Explanation: Chemotherapy IV infusion first hour = 96413. Subsequent hours = 96415.
Study Tip: Chemo IV: 96413 (first hour), 96415 (each additional hour).

Question 71: Answer: A) 93000
Explanation: Routine ECG with interpretation and report (global service) = 93000.
Study Tip: ECG: 93000 (global), 93005 (tracing only), 93010 (interpretation only).

Question 72: Answer: D) 94726
Explanation: Pulmonary function test (spirometry) measuring airflow = 94726.
Study Tip: Basic spirometry = 94726. More comprehensive testing = 94060 (bronchospasm evaluation).

Question 73: Answer: A) 97161
Explanation: Physical therapy evaluation, low complexity = 97161.
Study Tip: PT evaluation: 97161 (low), 97162 (moderate), 97163 (high complexity).

Question 74: Answer: C) 97814
Explanation: Acupuncture with electrical stimulation, 15 minutes = 97813 (first), 97814 (each additional).
Study Tip: Acupuncture: without stimulation (97810/97811), with stimulation (97813/97814).

HCPCS Level II (Questions 75-80)

Question 75: Answer: B) One letter and four numbers
Explanation: HCPCS Level II format = one letter (A-V) followed by four numbers (e.g., A4100, E0143).
Study Tip: HCPCS format: Letter + 4 digits. Letter indicates category/type of service.

Question 76: Answer: A) A0426
Explanation: Ambulance service, basic life support, non-emergency = A0426.
Study Tip: Ambulance codes = A04xx series. ALS = advanced, BLS = basic life support.

Question 77: Answer: C) J codes
Explanation: J codes cover drugs administered other than oral route, including insulin

injections.
Study Tip: HCPCS drug codes = J series. Specify drug, dosage, administration route.

Question 78: Answer: C) Reusable equipment
Explanation: Durable medical equipment (DME) = reusable items like wheelchairs, walkers, oxygen equipment.
Study Tip: DME = durable (reusable) equipment. Not disposable supplies or single-use items.

Question 79: Answer: A) Left side
Explanation: HCPCS modifier -LT indicates procedure performed on left side of body.
Study Tip: HCPCS anatomical modifiers: -LT (left), -RT (right). Similar to CPT but different codes.

Question 80: Answer: D) All of the above
Explanation: Use HCPCS when no CPT® code exists, Medicare requires specific code, or for supplies/equipment.
Study Tip: HCPCS covers gaps: no CPT® code, supplies, DME, Medicare-specific requirements.

Compliance and Regulatory (Questions 81-86)

Question 81: Answer: C) All individually identifiable health information
Explanation: HIPAA protects PHI in any form or medium: electronic, paper, oral communication.
Study Tip: PHI protection = all forms (electronic, paper, verbal). Not limited to one type.

Question 82: Answer: B) Limiting PHI access to what's needed for job
Explanation: Minimum necessary = only access PHI required to perform specific job duties.
Study Tip: Minimum necessary = least access needed for job. Not unlimited access.

Question 83: Answer: B) Billing at higher level than documented
Explanation: Upcoding = billing service level higher than actually provided or documented.
Study Tip: Upcoding = inflating service level for higher payment. Major fraud risk.

Question 84: Answer: B) Civil and criminal fraud against government
Explanation: False Claims Act addresses both civil and criminal false claims submitted to government programs.
Study Tip: False Claims Act = law governing fraud against government (Medicare, Medicaid).

Question 85: Answer: A) Medicare likely won't cover service
Explanation: ABN required when provider believes Medicare may deny payment, informing patient of potential liability.
Study Tip: ABN = notice of potential non-coverage. Patient chooses to proceed and accept financial responsibility.

Question 86: Answer: B) Regular auditing and monitoring
Explanation: OIG compliance programs emphasize ongoing auditing, monitoring, and

corrective action.
Study Tip: OIG compliance = 7 elements including auditing, training, and corrective action.

Modifiers and Guidelines (Questions 87-92)

Question 87: Answer: A) Increased procedural services
Explanation: Modifier -22 indicates procedure required significantly more work than typically required.
Study Tip: -22 = increased work/complexity. Requires documentation and often special report.

Question 88: Answer: B) Add-on codes
Explanation: Add-on codes (marked with +) are modifier -51 exempt; never use -51 with add-on codes.
Study Tip: Add-on codes = always -51 exempt. Already designed as additional procedures.

Question 89: Answer: A) Distinct procedural service
Explanation: Modifier -59 indicates procedure was distinct/independent from others performed same day.
Study Tip: -59 = distinct service. Use when procedures normally bundled but separately appropriate.

Question 90: Answer: B) Co-surgeons performing different parts
Explanation: Modifier -62 indicates two surgeons working as primary surgeons on different parts of same procedure.
Study Tip: -62 = co-surgeons, both primary, different portions. Not assistant (that's -80).

Question 91: Answer: A) Unplanned return to OR during global period
Explanation: Modifier -78 indicates unplanned return to OR for complication during postoperative period.
Study Tip: -78 = unplanned return to OR for complications. During global period.

Question 92: Answer: C) Unrelated procedure by same physician during postop period
Explanation: Modifier -79 indicates unrelated procedure during postoperative period, not related to original surgery.
Study Tip: -79 = unrelated procedure during global. -78 = related/complication return.

Integrated Coding Scenarios (Questions 93-100)

Question 93: Answer: A) K35.80
Explanation: Acute appendicitis without specified perforation, generalized peritonitis, or abscess = K35.80.
Study Tip: Appendicitis: K35.2 (with generalized peritonitis), K35.80 (unspecified), K37 (unspecified).

Question 94: Answer: C) 44970
Explanation: Laparoscopic appendectomy = 44970. Open appendectomy = 44950.
Study Tip: Appendectomy: 44950 (open), 44960 (open with abscess), 44970 (laparoscopic).

Question 95: Answer: C) 20
Explanation: Base (6) + Time (180÷15=12) + Age >70 (+99100=1) + Emergency (+99140=1) = 20 units.
Study Tip: Complex anesthesia: Add all components carefully. Base + time + all qualifying circumstances.

Question 96: Answer: B) 5 cm total
Explanation: Simple repairs same anatomical group (face) = add lengths. 3 + 2 = 5 cm total.
Study Tip: Wound repairs: add lengths within same classification and anatomical group.

Question 97: Answer: A) 45378
Explanation: Diagnostic colonoscopy reaching cecum without biopsy or removal = 45378.
Study Tip: Colonoscopy: 45378 (diagnostic), 45380 (with biopsy), 45385 (with removal).

Question 98: Answer: C) E11.9 and Z79.4
Explanation: Type 2 diabetes (E11.9) plus long-term insulin use status (Z79.4) both coded.
Study Tip: Type 2 on insulin: still code E11 (Type 2), add Z79.4 for insulin use.

Question 99: Answer: B) 66984-RT
Explanation: Cataract surgery with IOL insertion = 66984. Right eye requires modifier -RT.
Study Tip: Eye procedures: always add laterality modifier (-RT right, -LT left).

Question 100: Answer: B) I21.9 (acute MI)
Explanation: When symptom and definitive diagnosis present, code definitive diagnosis (acute MI), not symptom.
Study Tip: Symptom vs. diagnosis: code definitive diagnosis when confirmed, not integral symptoms.

Performance Analysis Guide

Scoring Your Practice Test

Calculate your score by counting correct answers and determining percentage:

- **Total Correct:** ____ / 100
- **Percentage:** ___ %

Score Breakdown by Section

Track performance by content area to identify strengths and weaknesses:

Medical Terminology (8 questions):
Score: ___ / 8 = ___ %

ICD-10-CM (12 questions):
Score: ___ / 12 = ___ %

E/M Coding (12 questions):
Score: ___ / 12 = ___ %

Surgery (18 questions):
Score: ___ / 18 = ___ %

Anesthesia (6 questions):
Score: ___ / 6 = ___ %

Radiology (6 questions):
Score: ___ / 6 = ___ %

Path/Lab (6 questions):	HCPCS (6 questions):	Modifiers (6 questions):
Score: ___ / 6 = ___ %	Score: ___ / 6 = ___ %	Score: ___ / 6 = ___ %
Medicine (6 questions):	**Compliance (6 questions):**	**Integrated Scenarios (8 questions):**
Score: ___ / 6 = ___ %	Score: ___ / 6 = ___ %	Score: ____ / 8 = ____ %

Interpreting Your Results

Your performance on Practice Test 3 provides critical insights into your CPC exam readiness. Use this analysis to guide your final preparation efforts and identify specific areas requiring additional focus.

Overall Score Analysis

90-100% (90-100 correct answers):
Status: Excellent! You're ready for the CPC exam.

Analysis: Your performance demonstrates comprehensive mastery of medical coding concepts across all content areas. You consistently apply guidelines correctly, recognize complex coding scenarios, and demonstrate the analytical thinking required for CPC certification.

Recommended Actions:

- Schedule your CPC exam with confidence within the next 2-4 weeks
- Conduct light review of any missed questions to understand why errors occurred
- Practice time management by completing one more timed practice test
- Review your code books' organization to ensure efficient navigation during the exam
- Focus on maintaining your knowledge rather than intensive new studying
- Get adequate rest in the days before your exam

90-100% Strengths: You've achieved mastery-level performance. Your preparation has been thorough and effective. Trust your knowledge and approach the exam with confidence.

80-89% (80-89 correct answers):
Status: Very Good. You're nearly ready with focused review of weak areas.

Analysis: Your performance demonstrates strong coding knowledge with a few gaps in specific areas. You understand fundamental concepts and can handle most coding scenarios effectively. Targeted review of missed questions and weak content areas will bring you to full readiness.

Recommended Actions:

- Review all missed questions thoroughly, understanding why each answer is correct
- Identify patterns in missed questions (specific body systems, code types, or guidelines)
- Dedicate 1-2 weeks to focused study of identified weak areas

- Complete additional practice questions in areas where you scored below 80%
- Review relevant coding guidelines and conventions for problem areas
- Consider scheduling your exam 2-3 weeks after completing focused review
- Take one final practice test after review to confirm improvement

80-89% Focus Areas:

- Note which sections scored below 80% - these require priority attention
- Surgical coding often shows room for improvement in this score range
- ICD-10-CM sequencing rules may need reinforcement
- Modifier application might benefit from additional practice

---

70-79% (70-79 correct answers):
Status: Passing, but additional preparation strongly recommended.

Analysis: Your performance meets the minimum passing standard, but your knowledge has gaps that could affect actual exam performance. While you understand basic concepts, inconsistent application of guidelines and difficulty with complex scenarios indicate need for additional preparation before scheduling your exam.

Recommended Actions:

- Delay scheduling your exam until after completing focused study plan (3-4 weeks)
- Thoroughly review ALL missed questions, not just those you guessed on
- Create study schedule focusing on sections where you scored below 70%
- Review fundamental concepts in weak areas before advancing to complex scenarios
- Work through additional practice questions in problem areas (aim for 100+ questions per weak section)
- Revisit relevant chapters in this study guide for areas showing weakness
- Consider joining a study group or finding a study partner for accountability
- Take at least two more full practice tests before scheduling your exam

70-79% Critical Focus:

- Identify your weakest section (lowest percentage score)
- This becomes your primary study focus for the next 2 weeks
- Don't just memorize answers - understand the reasoning behind correct codes
- Practice explaining concepts to others to solidify understanding

---

Below 70% (Below 70 correct answers):
Status: Additional preparation essential before attempting CPC exam.

Analysis: Your performance indicates significant knowledge gaps across multiple content areas. Attempting the CPC exam at this readiness level would likely result in failure. However, with structured study and dedication, you can build the knowledge needed for success.

Recommended Actions:

- Do NOT schedule your CPC exam yet - additional preparation is essential
- Develop comprehensive 6-8 week study plan addressing all weak areas
- Return to foundational chapters in this study guide
- Review basic medical terminology, anatomy, and coding conventions
- Start with simpler coding exercises before attempting complex scenarios
- Consider enrolling in an AAPC-approved training program if not already completed
- Work with a mentor or instructor who can identify specific knowledge gaps
- Complete all practice questions in this study guide, not just practice tests
- Take Practice Test 1 and 2 if not already completed
- Only attempt Practice Test 3 again after completing focused study
- Plan to take 4-6 more practice tests before scheduling actual exam

Below 70% Study Priorities:

1. Medical terminology and anatomy (foundation for all coding)
2. ICD-10-CM structure, conventions, and guidelines
3. CPT® organization and guidelines
4. E/M coding (most frequently used and tested)
5. Surgical coding by body system
6. Remaining CPT® sections (Anesthesia, Radiology, Path/Lab, Medicine)
7. Modifiers and their proper application
8. Compliance and regulatory requirements

Section-Specific Performance Analysis

Use your section scores to identify specific content areas requiring additional focus. Each section represents critical CPC exam content.

Medical Terminology and Anatomy (Target: 100%)

If you scored below 100%:

Medical terminology and anatomy form the foundation for all medical coding. Missing questions in this section indicates gaps in fundamental knowledge that will affect your ability to code accurately across all specialties.

Study Recommendations:

- Review Chapter 4 (Medical Terminology Mastery) thoroughly
- Create flashcards for prefixes, suffixes, and root words you missed
- Review Chapter 5 (Anatomy and Physiology Review) for anatomical concepts
- Practice breaking down complex medical terms into component parts

- Study anatomical directional terms and body planes until automatic
- Use anatomy diagrams to visualize structures and their relationships
- Test yourself on body system structures and functions

Common Terminology Weaknesses:

- Confusing similar-sounding terms (ileum vs. ilium, ureter vs. urethra)
- Directional terms and their opposites (proximal/distal, medial/lateral)
- Surgical suffixes and their precise meanings
- Body system-specific terminology

Mastery Goal: You should be able to define any medical term by identifying its word parts and should recognize anatomical structures across all body systems without hesitation.

ICD-10-CM Diagnosis Coding (Target: 85%+)

If you scored below 85%:

ICD-10-CM represents approximately 12% of CPC exam questions and supports accurate procedural coding. Strong diagnosis coding skills are essential for CPC certification.

Study Recommendations:

- Review Chapter 6 (ICD-10-CM Fundamentals) for structure and conventions
- Study Chapter 7 (ICD-10-CM by Body System) for system-specific guidelines
- Review Chapter 8 (Complex ICD-10-CM Scenarios) for advanced applications
- Practice using Excludes1 and Excludes2 notes correctly
- Master sequencing rules for multiple diagnoses
- Understand seventh character requirements for injuries and conditions
- Practice coding from actual medical record documentation, not just questions

Common ICD-10-CM Weaknesses:

- Confusing Excludes1 (mutually exclusive) with Excludes2 (may coexist)
- Incorrect sequencing of multiple diagnoses
- Coding uncertain diagnoses in outpatient settings
- Missing required seventh characters
- Not using most specific code available
- Sequencing complications before underlying conditions

Practice Focus:

- Code 50 different diagnosis scenarios from various body systems
- Practice sequencing multiple diagnoses correctly
- Work through complex scenarios involving sequelae, burns, and fractures
- Review coding guidelines before each practice session

CPT® Evaluation and Management (Target: 85%+)

If you scored below 85%:

E/M coding represents the most frequently used codes in medical practice and constitutes significant CPC exam content. Mastery is essential.

Study Recommendations:

- Review Chapter 10 (Evaluation and Management Coding) completely
- Understand both time-based and MDM-based code selection
- Study the three elements of medical decision making thoroughly
- Practice distinguishing between new and established patients
- Master modifier -25 usage (E/M with procedure same day)
- Understand consultation requirements and Medicare's non-recognition
- Practice with actual documentation, not just scenarios

Common E/M Weaknesses:

- Confusing time-based and MDM-based selection methods
- Not understanding which time counts toward E/M service
- Incorrect MDM level determination
- Misapplying modifier -25
- Confusion about new vs. established patient definitions
- Not recognizing when consultation codes don't apply

Mastery Exercises:

- Code 30 different E/M scenarios using both methods (time and MDM)
- Practice determining MDM levels from documentation
- Work through 20 modifier -25 scenarios to understand proper use
- Review E/M documentation guidelines from AAPC or AMA

CPT® Surgery Coding (Target: 80%+)

If you scored below 80%:

Surgery coding represents the largest portion of CPT® and tests knowledge of anatomy, surgical approaches, and complex guidelines across all body systems.

Study Recommendations:

- Review Chapter 11 (Surgery Coding by Body System) systematically
- Study surgical approaches (open, laparoscopic, endoscopic, percutaneous)
- Understand global surgical package components
- Master wound repair measurements and classifications
- Learn bundling rules and when to code procedures separately
- Practice with operative reports, not just question scenarios

- Review NCCI edits for commonly bundled procedures

Common Surgery Weaknesses:

- Incorrectly measuring wound repairs (not including margins for excisions)
- Not understanding when diagnostic procedures are included in surgical procedures
- Confusion about separate procedure designation
- Misapplying bundling rules
- Not recognizing when add-on codes are appropriate
- Confusion about modifier -50 (bilateral) vs. coding procedures separately

Body System Priorities:

1. Integumentary (wounds, repairs, excisions) - very commonly tested
2. Musculoskeletal (fractures, arthroscopy) - complex but high-yield
3. Digestive (endoscopy, hernia repairs) - frequent exam content
4. Female genital (office procedures, hysterectomy) - commonly tested
5. Respiratory (endoscopy, lung procedures)
6. Cardiovascular (complex but important)

Practice Activities:

- Code 50 operative reports across different body systems
- Practice wound repair scenarios with various lengths and locations
- Work through 25 endoscopy scenarios (both GI and respiratory)
- Study fracture treatment types with actual case examples

CPT® Anesthesia (Target: 80%+)

If you scored below 80%:

Anesthesia coding uses unique methodology not found elsewhere in CPT®. Understanding the calculation formula and qualifying circumstances is essential.

Study Recommendations:

- Review Chapter 12 (Anesthesia Coding) for complete formula understanding
- Practice calculating total units with base + time + qualifying circumstances
- Study physical status modifiers and their clinical meanings
- Understand when each qualifying circumstance (+99100, +99116, +99135, +99140) applies
- Practice time unit calculations with rounding
- Learn which surgical procedures correspond to which anesthesia codes

Common Anesthesia Weaknesses:

- Mathematical errors in time unit calculations
- Incorrect rounding of time units

- Not adding qualifying circumstances when appropriate
- Confusing physical status modifiers
- Not understanding when anesthesia time starts and ends
- Adding physical status modifier units (most payers don't reimburse for these)

Calculation Practice:

- Work through 25 anesthesia calculation problems
- Include various combinations of qualifying circumstances
- Practice with different time periods to master rounding
- Study complex cases with multiple qualifying circumstances

CPT® Radiology (Target: 80%+)

If you scored below 80%:

Radiology coding requires understanding of component billing (professional vs. technical) and knowing when imaging guidance is included vs. separately reportable.

Study Recommendations:

- Review radiology section focusing on component coding
- Understand modifier -26 (professional) and -TC (technical) usage
- Learn when imaging guidance is included in procedure codes
- Study complete vs. limited examination distinctions
- Master bilateral procedure coding in radiology
- Understand supervision and interpretation components

Common Radiology Weaknesses:

- Confusing when to use component modifiers
- Not knowing when imaging guidance is included vs. separate
- Billing diagnostic imaging separately when included in procedure
- Confusion about complete vs. limited studies
- Not understanding "with and without contrast" coding

Practice Focus:

- Code 30 radiology scenarios with appropriate modifiers
- Work through 15 imaging guidance scenarios
- Practice component coding for split services
- Review common bundling rules for imaging procedures

CPT® Pathology and Laboratory (Target: 85%+)

If you scored below 85%:

Laboratory coding emphasizes understanding of panel requirements and knowing when individual tests vs. panels are appropriate.

Study Recommendations:

- Review laboratory panels and their component tests
- Understand "all or nothing" rule for panel coding
- Learn common laboratory test codes and their purposes
- Study drug testing (presumptive vs. definitive) distinctions
- Master urinalysis coding variations
- Understand surgical pathology levels

Common Path/Lab Weaknesses:

- Using panel codes when not all tests performed
- Not knowing which tests comprise each panel
- Confusing similar panel codes (BMP vs. CMP vs. Lipid Panel)
- Misunderstanding when to code individual tests vs. panels
- Confusion about drug testing code selection

Mastery Activities:

- Memorize components of BMP, CMP, and Lipid Panel
- Code 25 laboratory scenarios with appropriate panel/individual test selection
- Review surgical pathology level assignments
- Practice distinguishing between similar test codes

CPT® Medicine (Target: 80%+)

If you scored below 80%:

Medicine section covers diverse non-surgical procedures from immunizations to chemotherapy administration. Understanding category-specific rules is essential.

Study Recommendations:

- Review medicine section organization and major categories
- Understand immunization coding (product + administration)
- Study chemotherapy administration time-based codes
- Learn cardiac diagnostic procedure coding
- Master physical therapy and occupational therapy evaluation levels
- Understand psychiatric service coding

Common Medicine Weaknesses:

- Forgetting to code both vaccine product and administration
- Confusion about chemotherapy administration time calculations
- Not understanding cardiac diagnostic procedure components
- Misapplying physical therapy evaluation complexity levels

Practice Focus:

- Code 20 immunization scenarios with products and administration
- Work through 15 chemotherapy administration time-based scenarios
- Practice coding cardiac diagnostic procedures
- Review therapy evaluation complexity criteria

HCPCS Level II (Target: 85%+)

If you scored below 85%:

HCPCS Level II codes supplement CPT® for supplies, equipment, and services not included in CPT®. Understanding code structure and when to use HCPCS is important.

Study Recommendations:

- Review HCPCS code structure (letter + 4 digits)
- Learn major HCPCS categories and their uses
- Understand when HCPCS vs. CPT® codes apply
- Study DME (durable medical equipment) coding
- Master HCPCS modifiers and their differences from CPT® modifiers
- Learn drug administration coding in HCPCS

Common HCPCS Weaknesses:

- Not knowing when to use HCPCS vs. CPT® codes
- Confusion about which HCPCS category applies
- Misunderstanding DME vs. disposable supplies
- Not recognizing when HCPCS modifiers differ from CPT® modifiers

Practice Activities:

- Code 25 scenarios requiring HCPCS codes
- Practice distinguishing DME from supplies
- Review HCPCS modifier applications
- Study drug codes in J series

Compliance and Regulatory (Target: 85%+)

If you scored below 85%:

Compliance knowledge protects you, your employer, and patients from fraud, abuse, and privacy violations. This is essential professional knowledge.

Study Recommendations:

- Review Chapter 17 (Medical Coding Compliance) thoroughly
- Understand HIPAA privacy and security rules
- Study fraud and abuse definitions and examples
- Learn OIG compliance program elements
- Understand documentation requirements supporting code assignment
- Study audit preparation and response procedures

Common Compliance Weaknesses:

- Confusing fraud (intentional) with abuse (careless)
- Not understanding minimum necessary standard
- Confusion about when ABNs are required
- Misunderstanding false claims act implications
- Not recognizing upcoding and unbundling schemes

Critical Understanding:

- Know difference between fraud and abuse
- Understand PHI protection requirements
- Recognize common fraud schemes
- Learn documentation supporting code assignment
- Study ethical coding practices

Modifiers and Guidelines (Target: 85%+)

If you scored below 85%:

Modifiers provide essential additional information about procedures and affect reimbursement. Correct modifier application is critical for accurate coding.

Study Recommendations:

- Review all CPT® modifiers and their appropriate uses
- Understand anatomical modifiers (-RT, -LT, -50)
- Study surgical modifiers (-22, -51, -59, -78, -79)
- Learn E/M modifiers (-24, -25, -57)
- Master when modifiers are required vs. optional vs. inappropriate
- Understand modifier sequencing when multiple apply

Common Modifier Weaknesses:

- Confusing -59 (distinct service) appropriate use
- Misapplying -25 (E/M same day as procedure)
- Not understanding when -50 (bilateral) vs. two separate codes
- Confusion between -78 (complication) and -79 (unrelated procedure)
- Not knowing which codes are modifier -51 exempt

Modifier Mastery:

- Study 30 modifier scenarios across all modifier types
- Practice determining when multiple modifiers needed
- Review modifier sequencing rules
- Work through complex cases requiring modifier decisions

Integrated Scenarios Performance

If you scored below 75% on integrated scenarios (Questions 93-100):

Integrated scenarios test your ability to combine knowledge from multiple areas, simulating real-world coding situations.

Study Recommendations:

- Practice coding from complete medical records, not isolated questions
- Work through operative reports requiring both diagnosis and procedure codes
- Practice cases requiring modifier applications
- Study scenarios involving multiple related procedures
- Review cases requiring ICD-10-CM sequencing decisions

Integration Practice:

- Code 25 complete medical record scenarios
- Work through operative reports with pre-op and post-op diagnoses
- Practice emergency department scenarios
- Study outpatient surgery center cases

Final Preparation Recommendations

4-Week Final Preparation Schedule

Based on your Practice Test 3 performance, follow this final preparation schedule:

Week 1: Focused Review of Weakest Areas

- **Day 1-2:** Review your lowest-scoring section completely
- **Day 3-4:** Complete 50 practice questions in weakest area
- **Day 5-6:** Review second-weakest section
- **Day 7:** Complete 30 practice questions across weak areas

Week 2: Systematic Content Review

- **Day 1:** ICD-10-CM guidelines and conventions
- **Day 2:** E/M coding documentation requirements
- **Day 3:** Surgery coding by body system review
- **Day 4:** Anesthesia, Radiology, Path/Lab review
- **Day 5:** Medicine and HCPCS review
- **Day 6:** Compliance and modifier review
- **Day 7:** Rest day - light review only

Week 3: Practice and Application

- **Day 1-2:** Complete Practice Test 1 (if not done) or retake
- **Day 3:** Review all missed questions from Practice Test 1
- **Day 4-5:** Complete Practice Test 2 (if not done) or retake
- **Day 6:** Review all missed questions from Practice Test 2
- **Day 7:** Light review of challenging concepts

Week 4: Final Review and Exam Preparation

- **Day 1-3:** Review all three practice tests, focusing on missed questions
- **Day 4:** Organize and tab your code books for efficient exam use
- **Day 5:** Light review of high-yield topics (E/M, common surgeries, modifiers)
- **Day 6:** Rest day - no intensive studying
- **Day 7:** CPC Exam Day - trust your preparation!

Code Book Organization for Exam Day

Proper code book preparation saves valuable time during the exam:

CPT® Book Preparation:

- Tab major sections (E/M, each surgical system, Anesthesia, Radiology, Path/Lab, Medicine)
- Highlight frequently referenced guidelines
- Tab Appendix A (modifiers) for quick reference
- Mark commonly used codes with small tabs
- Practice navigating to codes quickly

ICD-10-CM Book Preparation:

- Tab official guidelines (front of book)
- Mark chapter divisions in tabular list
- Tab Neoplasm Table and Table of Drugs and Chemicals
- Highlight frequently used conventions
- Practice using alphabetic index efficiently

HCPCS Level II Book Preparation:

- Tab major code categories (A, E, J, L codes)
- Mark commonly used modifiers
- Highlight drug codes if frequently used
- Tab transportation and DME sections

Exam Day Success Strategies

The Night Before:

- Organize all materials (ID, admission ticket, code books, calculator)
- Get adequate sleep (7-8 hours minimum)
- Avoid last-minute cramming
- Review your confidence-building notes
- Visualize success

Exam Day Morning:

- Eat a nutritious breakfast
- Arrive 30 minutes early
- Bring water and snacks for breaks
- Wear comfortable clothing
- Stay calm and confident

During the Exam:

- Read each question carefully before looking at answers
- Mark difficult questions and return later
- Manage time (2.4 minutes average per question)
- Trust your preparation
- Don't second-guess yourself excessively
- Use all available time for review

Time Management:

- First pass: Answer all questions you're confident about (90 minutes)
- Second pass: Work through marked difficult questions (60 minutes)
- Third pass: Review flagged questions and double-check answers (60 minutes)
- Final pass: Review any remaining time (30 minutes)

Conclusion: Your Path to CPC Certification

Completing Practice Test 3 represents a major milestone in your CPC preparation journey. Whether you scored above or below your target, you've gained valuable insights into your readiness and identified specific areas for focused improvement.

Remember These Key Principles:

1. Trust Your Preparation:
You've invested significant time and effort in studying. Trust the knowledge you've built and approach the exam with confidence.

2. Learn from Mistakes:
Every missed question teaches you something valuable. Review explanations thoroughly and understand why correct answers are right.

3. Focus on High-Yield Content:
E/M coding, common surgical procedures, and ICD-10-CM sequencing appear frequently on exams. Ensure mastery in these areas.

4. Practice Time Management:
The 4-hour time limit challenges even well-prepared candidates. Practice working efficiently without rushing.

5. Maintain Perspective:
The CPC exam tests competency, not perfection. A 70% passing score reflects realistic professional standards.

Your Next Steps:

1. Calculate your Practice Test 3 score
2. Analyze performance by section
3. Create focused study plan based on weak areas
4. Complete recommended review activities
5. Take additional practice tests as needed
6. Schedule your CPC exam when consistently scoring 75%+
7. Organize code books for exam efficiency
8. Trust your preparation and succeed!

Final Encouragement:

Thousands of coders pass the CPC exam each year with preparation similar to yours. You have access to comprehensive study materials, detailed explanations, and strategic guidance. Your dedication to working through this practice test demonstrates commitment to professional excellence.

The CPC certification opens doors to career opportunities, professional recognition, and personal achievement. Your investment in preparation positions you for success not just on the exam, but throughout your coding career.

Believe in yourself. Trust your preparation. You're ready to become a Certified Professional Coder.

Best wishes for your CPC certification success!

Continue to Appendices for additional study resources, reference materials, and supplemental information supporting your CPC exam preparation.

Chapter 22: Additional Practice Questions by Topic

"Practice isn't the thing you do once you're good. It's the thing you do that makes you good." - Malcolm Gladwell

You've worked through comprehensive content covering every aspect of medical coding tested on the CPC exam. You've mastered diagnosis coding with ICD-10-CM, conquered procedure coding with CPT®, and developed expertise in specialized areas from anesthesia to pathology. Now comes the crucial phase that transforms knowledge into exam-ready skills: intensive practice.

This chapter provides 275 carefully crafted practice questions that mirror the complexity, format, and challenge level of actual CPC exam questions. These aren't simple recall questions testing whether you memorized definitions. They're scenario-based questions requiring you to analyze clinical documentation, apply coding guidelines, and make the same decisions you'll make on exam day and throughout your career.

Each question section focuses on specific content areas, allowing you to identify strengths and address weaknesses systematically. Work through questions in order, simulating real exam conditions, or focus on areas where you need the most practice. Either approach builds the confidence and competence that leads to CPC exam success.

Remember: every question you answer correctly reinforces neural pathways that make coding decisions faster and more accurate. Every mistake you analyze teaches lessons that prevent future errors. Approach these questions not as tests of what you don't know, but as opportunities to strengthen what you do know and identify areas needing review.

You're not just practicing for an exam—you're building the professional coding skills that will define your career. Let's begin.

ICD-10-CM Practice Questions (75 Questions)

Questions 1-25: Foundational ICD-10-CM Coding

Question 1: A patient is diagnosed with Type 2 diabetes mellitus with diabetic nephropathy. What is the correct ICD-10-CM code?

A) E11.9 Type 2 diabetes mellitus without complications B) E11.21 Type 2 diabetes mellitus with diabetic nephropathy C) E11.22 Type 2 diabetes mellitus with diabetic chronic kidney disease D) E10.21 Type 1 diabetes mellitus with diabetic nephropathy

Question 2: A patient presents with acute exacerbation of chronic obstructive pulmonary disease (COPD). What is the correct code?

A) J44.0 COPD with acute lower respiratory infection B) J44.1 COPD with acute exacerbation C) J44.9 COPD, unspecified D) J43.9 Emphysema, unspecified

Question 3: A 55-year-old patient is treated for essential (primary) hypertension. The correct code is:

A) I10 Essential (primary) hypertension B) I11.0 Hypertensive heart disease with heart failure C) I12.9 Hypertensive chronic kidney disease D) I15.9 Secondary hypertension, unspecified

Question 4: A patient has a personal history of breast cancer, currently cancer-free after completing treatment two years ago. The appropriate code is:

A) C50.911 Malignant neoplasm of unspecified site of right female breast B) Z85.3 Personal history of malignant neoplasm of breast C) D05.90 Unspecified type of carcinoma in situ of unspecified breast D) C79.81 Secondary malignant neoplasm of breast

Question 5: A patient presents to the clinic with chest pain. After examination and EKG, the physician rules out myocardial infarction. The correct code for outpatient coding is:

A) I21.9 Acute myocardial infarction, unspecified B) R07.9 Chest pain, unspecified C) I20.9 Angina pectoris, unspecified D) Z03.89 Encounter for observation for other suspected diseases

Question 6: A patient has iron deficiency anemia due to chronic blood loss from a gastric ulcer with hemorrhage. How should this be coded?

A) D50.0 Iron deficiency anemia secondary to blood loss only B) K25.4 Chronic gastric ulcer with hemorrhage only C) D50.0 Iron deficiency anemia secondary to blood loss and K25.4 Chronic gastric ulcer with hemorrhage D) D50.9 Iron deficiency anemia, unspecified and K25.9 Gastric ulcer, unspecified

Question 7: A pregnant patient at 32 weeks gestation has gestational diabetes mellitus controlled by diet. The correct code is:

A) O24.410 Gestational diabetes mellitus in pregnancy, diet controlled B) E11.9 Type 2 diabetes mellitus without complications C) O24.919 Gestational diabetes mellitus, unspecified control D) O99.810 Abnormal glucose complicating pregnancy

Question 8: A patient is admitted with sepsis due to Escherichia coli with acute kidney injury as a complication. The correct sequencing is:

A) A41.51 Sepsis due to Escherichia coli, N17.9 Acute kidney failure B) N17.9 Acute kidney failure, A41.51 Sepsis due to Escherichia coli C) R65.20 Severe sepsis without septic shock, A41.51, N17.9 D) A41.51, R65.20, N17.9

Question 9: A patient undergoes screening colonoscopy and a polyp is discovered and removed during the same encounter. The correct primary diagnosis is:

A) K63.5 Polyp of colon B) Z12.11 Encounter for screening for malignant neoplasm of colon C) Z86.010 Personal history of colonic polyps D) D12.6 Benign neoplasm of colon, unspecified

Question 10: A patient has acute bronchitis due to Mycoplasma pneumoniae documented by the physician. The correct code is:

A) J20.9 Acute bronchitis, unspecified B) J20.0 Acute bronchitis due to Mycoplasma pneumoniae C) J15.7 Pneumonia due to Mycoplasma pneumoniae D) B96.0 Mycoplasma pneumoniae as the cause of diseases classified elsewhere

Question 11: A patient is diagnosed with atrial fibrillation. The correct ICD-10-CM code is:

A) I48.0 Paroxysmal atrial fibrillation B) I48.1 Persistent atrial fibrillation C) I48.2 Chronic atrial fibrillation D) I48.91 Unspecified atrial fibrillation

Question 12: A patient presents with a closed fracture of the right femoral shaft, initial encounter. The correct code is:

A) S72.301A Unspecified fracture of shaft of right femur, initial encounter for closed fracture B) S72.301D Unspecified fracture of shaft of right femur, subsequent encounter C) S72.302A Unspecified fracture of shaft of left femur, initial encounter D) S72.301S Unspecified fracture of shaft of right femur, sequela

Question 13: A patient with rheumatoid arthritis affecting multiple sites is seen for medication management. The correct code is:

A) M05.79 Rheumatoid arthritis with rheumatoid factor of multiple sites without organ or systems involvement B) M06.09 Rheumatoid arthritis without rheumatoid factor, multiple sites C) M19.90 Unspecified osteoarthritis, unspecified site D) M79.3 Panniculitis, unspecified

Question 14: A patient is admitted with acute myocardial infarction of the anterior wall, initial episode. The correct code is:

A) I21.09 ST elevation (STEMI) myocardial infarction involving other coronary artery of anterior wall B) I21.9 Acute myocardial infarction, unspecified C) I25.2 Old myocardial infarction D) I20.0 Unstable angina

Question 15: A patient has asthma with acute exacerbation. The correct code is:

A) J45.901 Unspecified asthma with (acute) exacerbation B) J45.909 Unspecified asthma, uncomplicated C) J44.1 Chronic obstructive pulmonary disease with (acute) exacerbation D) J45.40 Moderate persistent asthma, uncomplicated

Question 16: A patient presents for encounter for chemotherapy for breast cancer. The correct sequencing is:

A) Z51.11 Encounter for antineoplastic chemotherapy, C50.911 Malignant neoplasm of breast B) C50.911 Malignant neoplasm of breast, Z51.11 Encounter for chemotherapy C) Z51.11 only D) C50.911 only

Question 17: A patient has urinary tract infection due to E. coli. The correct coding is:

A) N39.0 Urinary tract infection, site not specified only B) B96.20 Unspecified Escherichia coli as the cause of diseases classified elsewhere only C) N39.0 and B96.20 D) A41.51 Sepsis due to Escherichia coli

Question 18: A newborn is diagnosed with neonatal jaundice due to breast milk inhibitor. The correct code is:

A) P59.9 Neonatal jaundice, unspecified B) P59.3 Neonatal jaundice from breast milk inhibitor C) P59.0 Neonatal jaundice associated with preterm delivery D) R17 Unspecified jaundice

Question 19: A patient has Type 2 diabetes mellitus with diabetic peripheral angiopathy without gangrene. The correct code is:

A) E11.51 Type 2 diabetes mellitus with diabetic peripheral angiopathy without gangrene B) E11.52 Type 2 diabetes mellitus with diabetic peripheral angiopathy with gangrene C) E11.9 Type 2 diabetes mellitus without complications D) E10.51 Type 1 diabetes mellitus with diabetic peripheral angiopathy without gangrene

Question 20: A patient presents with major depressive disorder, recurrent episode, severe without psychotic features. The correct code is:

A) F32.2 Major depressive disorder, single episode, severe without psychotic features B) F33.2 Major depressive disorder, recurrent severe without psychotic features C) F31.4 Bipolar disorder, current episode depressed, severe, without psychotic features D) F33.0 Major depressive disorder, recurrent, mild

Question 21: A patient is admitted with dehydration. The correct code is:

A) E86.0 Dehydration B) E87.1 Hypo-osmolality and hyponatremia C) R63.0 Anorexia D) E86.1 Hypovolemia

Question 22: A patient with chronic kidney disease, stage 4, is seen for management. The correct code is:

A) N18.1 Chronic kidney disease, stage 1 B) N18.2 Chronic kidney disease, stage 2 C) N18.3 Chronic kidney disease, stage 3 D) N18.4 Chronic kidney disease, stage 4

Question 23: A patient has osteoarthritis of the right knee. The correct code is:

A) M17.11 Unilateral primary osteoarthritis, right knee B) M17.0 Bilateral primary osteoarthritis of knee C) M19.90 Unspecified osteoarthritis, unspecified site D) M25.561 Pain in right knee

Question 24: A patient is seen for follow-up after completed treatment for pneumonia two weeks ago. Current chest X-ray is clear and patient is asymptomatic. The correct code is:

A) J18.9 Pneumonia, unspecified organism B) Z09 Encounter for follow-up examination after completed treatment for conditions other than malignant neoplasm C) Z87.01 Personal history of pneumonia D) R91.8 Other nonspecific abnormal finding of lung field

Question 25: A patient presents with migraine without aura, intractable, with status migrainosus. The correct code is:

A) G43.909 Migraine, unspecified, not intractable, without status migrainosus B) G43.911 Migraine, unspecified, intractable, with status migrainosus C) G43.019 Migraine without aura, intractable, without status migrainosus D) G43.101 Migraine with aura, not intractable, with status migrainosus

Questions 26-50: Intermediate ICD-10-CM Scenarios

Question 26: A patient presents to the emergency department with severe headache. CT scan reveals subarachnoid hemorrhage. Patient has a history of hypertension. What is the correct sequencing?

A) I60.9 Nontraumatic subarachnoid hemorrhage, unspecified, I10 Essential hypertension B) I10 Essential hypertension, I60.9 Nontraumatic subarachnoid hemorrhage C) R51 Headache, I60.9, I10 D) I60.9 only

Question 27: A patient with COPD develops pneumonia during admission. Both conditions are documented and treated. How should this be coded?

A) J44.0 COPD with acute lower respiratory infection B) J18.9 Pneumonia, unspecified organism and J44.9 COPD, unspecified C) J44.0 and appropriate pneumonia code if organism specified D) J44.1 COPD with acute exacerbation

Question 28: A patient has hypertensive heart disease with congestive heart failure. The correct coding is:

A) I11.0 Hypertensive heart disease with heart failure and I50.9 Heart failure, unspecified B) I10 Essential hypertension and I50.9 Heart failure C) I11.9 Hypertensive heart disease without heart failure D) I11.0 only

Question 29: A patient is diagnosed with community-acquired pneumonia due to Streptococcus pneumoniae. The correct code is:

A) J18.9 Pneumonia, unspecified organism B) J13 Pneumonia due to Streptococcus pneumoniae C) J15.9 Unspecified bacterial pneumonia D) A40.3 Sepsis due to Streptococcus pneumoniae

Question 30: A patient with diabetes mellitus, type 2, develops a foot ulcer on the right heel. The correct coding is:

A) E11.621 Type 2 diabetes mellitus with foot ulcer and L97.419 Non-pressure chronic ulcer of right heel B) E11.9 Type 2 diabetes without complications and L97.419 C) E11.622 Type 2 diabetes with other skin ulcer D) L97.419 only

Question 31: A patient is admitted for pathological fracture of the left femur due to osteoporosis. The correct code is:

A) M80.052A Age-related osteoporosis with current pathological fracture, left femur, initial encounter B) S72.002A Fracture of unspecified part of neck of left femur, initial encounter C) M81.0 Age-related osteoporosis without current pathological fracture D) M84.452A Pathological fracture, left femur, initial encounter

Question 32: A patient presents with acute appendicitis with peritoneal abscess. The correct code is:

A) K35.2 Acute appendicitis with generalized peritonitis B) K35.3 Acute appendicitis with localized peritonitis C) K35.89 Other acute appendicitis D) K36 Other appendicitis

Question 33: A patient has secondary diabetes mellitus due to pancreatectomy with diabetic retinopathy. The correct coding is:

A) E08.319 Diabetes mellitus due to underlying condition with unspecified diabetic retinopathy B) E13.319 Other specified diabetes mellitus with unspecified diabetic retinopathy C) E11.319 Type 2 diabetes with unspecified diabetic retinopathy D) E10.319 Type 1 diabetes with unspecified diabetic retinopathy

Question 34: A patient is seen for screening mammogram. No abnormalities are found. The correct code is:

A) Z12.31 Encounter for screening mammogram for malignant neoplasm of breast B) Z01.89 Encounter for other specified special examinations C) Z00.00 Encounter for general adult medical examination without abnormal findings D) R92.8 Other abnormal findings on diagnostic imaging of breast

Question 35: A patient has coronary atherosclerosis of native coronary artery with angina pectoris. The correct code is:

A) I25.10 Atherosclerotic heart disease of native coronary artery without angina pectoris B) I25.119 Atherosclerotic heart disease of native coronary artery with unspecified angina pectoris C) I20.9 Angina pectoris, unspecified D) I25.9 Chronic ischemic heart disease, unspecified

Question 36: A patient presents with anxiety disorder, unspecified. The correct code is:

A) F41.9 Anxiety disorder, unspecified B) F41.1 Generalized anxiety disorder C) F41.0 Panic disorder without agoraphobia D) F43.0 Acute stress reaction

Question 37: A patient has acute cholecystitis with cholelithiasis. The correct code is:

A) K80.00 Calculus of gallbladder with acute cholecystitis without obstruction B) K81.0 Acute cholecystitis C) K80.20 Calculus of gallbladder without cholecystitis D) K80.70 Calculus of gallbladder and bile duct with acute cholecystitis

Question 38: A patient presents with syncope and collapse. The correct code is:

A) R55 Syncope and collapse B) I95.1 Orthostatic hypotension C) R42 Dizziness and giddiness D) G90.3 Multi-system degeneration

Question 39: A patient with HIV disease presents with Pneumocystis carinii pneumonia. The correct coding is:

A) B20 Human immunodeficiency virus disease and B59 Pneumocystosis B) B20 only C) Z21 Asymptomatic HIV infection status and B59 D) B59 only

Question 40: A patient is admitted with acute respiratory failure with hypoxia. The correct code is:

A) J96.01 Acute respiratory failure with hypoxia B) J96.00 Acute respiratory failure, unspecified whether with hypoxia or hypercapnia C) J96.11 Chronic respiratory failure with hypoxia D) J96.90 Respiratory failure, unspecified, unspecified whether with hypoxia or hypercapnia

Question 41: A patient has diverticulitis of large intestine with perforation and abscess. The correct code is:

A) K57.20 Diverticulitis of large intestine with perforation and abscess without bleeding B) K57.32 Diverticulitis of large intestine without perforation or abscess C) K57.92 Diverticulitis of intestine, part unspecified, without perforation or abscess D) K57.80 Diverticulitis of intestine, part unspecified, with perforation and abscess

Question 42: A patient has Alzheimer's disease with behavioral disturbance. The correct coding is:

A) G30.9 Alzheimer's disease, unspecified and F02.81 Dementia in other diseases classified elsewhere with behavioral disturbance B) G30.9 only C) F02.80 Dementia in other diseases classified elsewhere without behavioral disturbance D) F03.90 Unspecified dementia without behavioral disturbance

Question 43: A patient presents for encounter for adjustment and management of cardiac pacemaker. The correct code is:

A) Z45.010 Encounter for checking and testing of cardiac pacemaker pulse generator B) Z95.0 Presence of cardiac pacemaker C) I49.8 Other specified cardiac arrhythmias D) Z46.2 Encounter for fitting and adjustment of other devices related to nervous system

Question 44: A patient has cirrhosis of liver with ascites. The correct coding is:

A) K74.60 Unspecified cirrhosis of liver and R18.8 Other ascites B) K70.30 Alcoholic cirrhosis of liver without ascites C) K74.69 Other cirrhosis of liver D) R18.0 Malignant ascites

Question 45: A patient presents with acute upper gastrointestinal bleeding. The correct code is:

A) K92.2 Gastrointestinal hemorrhage, unspecified B) K92.0 Hematemesis C) K92.1 Melena D) K62.5 Hemorrhage of anus and rectum

Question 46: A patient is admitted with cellulitis of right lower leg. The correct code is:

A) L03.115 Cellulitis of right lower limb B) L03.116 Cellulitis of left lower limb C) L08.9 Local infection of skin and subcutaneous tissue, unspecified D) L03.90 Cellulitis, unspecified

Question 47: A patient has benign prostatic hyperplasia with lower urinary tract symptoms. The correct code is:

A) N40.1 Benign prostatic hyperplasia with lower urinary tract symptoms B) N40.0 Benign prostatic hyperplasia without lower urinary tract symptoms C) N40.3 Nodular prostate with lower urinary tract symptoms D) R33.8 Other retention of urine

Question 48: A patient presents with acute otitis media, right ear. The correct code is:

A) H66.91 Otitis media, unspecified, right ear B) H66.001 Acute suppurative otitis media without spontaneous rupture of ear drum, right ear C) H66.90 Otitis media, unspecified, unspecified ear D) H65.91 Unspecified nonsuppurative otitis media, right ear

Question 49: A patient has gastroesophageal reflux disease with esophagitis. The correct code is:

A) K21.0 Gastro-esophageal reflux disease with esophagitis B) K21.9 Gastro-esophageal reflux disease without esophagitis C) K22.10 Ulcer of esophagus without bleeding D) K20.9 Esophagitis, unspecified

Question 50: A patient is seen for follow-up of coronary artery bypass graft (CABG) performed 6 months ago. Patient is asymptomatic. The correct code is:

A) Z95.1 Presence of aortocoronary bypass graft B) I25.10 Atherosclerotic heart disease of native coronary artery C) Z09 Encounter for follow-up examination after completed treatment D) I25.810 Atherosclerosis of coronary artery bypass graft

Questions 51-75: Advanced ICD-10-CM Complex Cases

Question 51: A patient is admitted with diabetic ketoacidosis. Patient has Type 1 diabetes and also has diabetic proliferative retinopathy. Code all documented conditions.

A) E10.10 Type 1 diabetes with ketoacidosis and E10.359 Type 1 diabetes with proliferative diabetic retinopathy B) E10.11 Type 1 diabetes with ketoacidosis without coma and E10.319

Type 1 diabetes with unspecified diabetic retinopathy C) E10.10 only D) E10.65 Type 1 diabetes with hyperglycemia and E10.359

Question 52: A patient presents with chest pain. Workup reveals acute ST elevation myocardial infarction of the anterior wall with left ventricular failure. The correct sequencing is:

A) I21.09 STEMI of anterior wall, I50.1 Left ventricular failure B) I50.1 Left ventricular failure, I21.09 STEMI C) R07.9 Chest pain, I21.09, I50.1 D) I21.09 only

Question 53: A patient has septic shock due to methicillin-resistant Staphylococcus aureus (MRSA) sepsis. The correct coding is:

A) A41.02 Sepsis due to MRSA, R65.21 Severe sepsis with septic shock B) R65.21 Severe sepsis with septic shock, A41.02 Sepsis due to MRSA C) A41.02 only D) R57.9 Shock, unspecified

Question 54: A pregnant woman at 28 weeks gestation presents with preeclampsia with severe features. The correct code is:

A) O14.13 Severe pre-eclampsia, third trimester B) O14.03 Mild to moderate pre-eclampsia, third trimester C) O14.93 Unspecified pre-eclampsia, third trimester D) O10.03 Pre-existing essential hypertension complicating pregnancy, third trimester

Question 55: A patient has posttraumatic stress disorder (PTSD) following military combat. The correct code is:

A) F43.10 Post-traumatic stress disorder, unspecified B) F43.11 Post-traumatic stress disorder, acute C) F43.12 Post-traumatic stress disorder, chronic D) F43.0 Acute stress reaction

Question 56: A patient presents with acute prostatitis due to E. coli. The correct coding is:

A) N41.0 Acute prostatitis and B96.20 Unspecified Escherichia coli B) N41.0 only C) N41.1 Chronic prostatitis D) N41.9 Inflammatory disease of prostate, unspecified

Question 57: A patient has chronic obstructive asthma with status asthmaticus. The correct code is:

A) J44.9 Chronic obstructive pulmonary disease, unspecified B) J45.902 Unspecified asthma with status asthmaticus C) J45.901 Unspecified asthma with (acute) exacerbation D) J45.909 Unspecified asthma, uncomplicated

Question 58: A patient is admitted for chemotherapy for metastatic lung cancer with bone metastases. The correct sequencing is:

A) Z51.11 Encounter for chemotherapy, C34.90 Lung cancer, C79.51 Bone metastases B) C34.90 Lung cancer, C79.51 Bone metastases, Z51.11 C) C79.51 Bone metastases, C34.90 Lung cancer D) Z51.11 only

Question 59: A patient has acute kidney failure due to acute tubular necrosis. The correct coding is:

A) N17.0 Acute kidney failure with tubular necrosis B) N17.9 Acute kidney failure, unspecified C) N18.9 Chronic kidney disease, unspecified D) N19 Unspecified kidney failure

Question 60: A patient presents with hematuria and dysuria. Cystoscopy reveals bladder tumor. The correct primary diagnosis is:

A) R31.9 Hematuria, unspecified B) R30.0 Dysuria C) D49.4 Neoplasm of unspecified behavior of bladder D) C67.9 Malignant neoplasm of bladder, unspecified

Question 61: A patient has degenerative disc disease of lumbar spine with radiculopathy. The correct coding is:

A) M51.16 Intervertebral disc disorders with radiculopathy, lumbar region B) M51.36 Other intervertebral disc degeneration, lumbar region C) M54.5 Low back pain D) M54.16 Radiculopathy, lumbar region

Question 62: A patient is admitted with acute exacerbation of chronic systolic heart failure. The correct code is:

A) I50.21 Acute on chronic systolic (congestive) heart failure B) I50.9 Heart failure, unspecified C) I50.31 Acute diastolic (congestive) heart failure D) I50.41 Acute combined systolic and diastolic heart failure

Question 63: A patient has osteoporosis with current pathological fracture of right hip. The correct code is:

A) M80.851A Age-related osteoporosis with current pathological fracture, right femur, initial B) M81.0 Age-related osteoporosis without current pathological fracture C) S72.001A Fracture of unspecified part of neck of right femur, initial D) M84.451A Pathological fracture, right femur, initial

Question 64: A patient presents with acute pancreatitis due to alcohol abuse. The correct coding is:

A) K85.20 Alcohol induced acute pancreatitis without necrosis or infection B) K85.90 Acute pancreatitis without necrosis or infection, unspecified C) F10.988 Alcohol use, unspecified with other alcohol-induced disorder D) K86.0 Alcohol-induced chronic pancreatitis

Question 65: A patient has pressure ulcer of right heel, stage 3. The correct code is:

A) L89.613 Pressure ulcer of right heel, stage 3 B) L89.610 Pressure ulcer of right heel, unstageable C) L89.614 Pressure ulcer of right heel, stage 4 D) L97.419 Non-pressure chronic ulcer of right heel

Question 66: A patient is diagnosed with acute myeloid leukemia in remission. The correct code is:

A) C92.01 Acute myeloblastic leukemia, in remission B) C92.00 Acute myeloblastic leukemia, not having achieved remission C) C92.02 Acute myeloblastic leukemia, in relapse D) C92.10 Chronic myeloid leukemia, not having achieved remission

Question 67: A patient has atrial fibrillation and is on long-term anticoagulation therapy with warfarin. The correct coding is:

A) I48.91 Unspecified atrial fibrillation and Z79.01 Long term use of anticoagulants B) I48.91 only C) Z79.01 only D) I48.0 Paroxysmal atrial fibrillation

Question 68: A patient presents with acute diverticulitis of sigmoid colon without perforation or abscess, with bleeding. The correct code is:

A) K57.33 Diverticulitis of large intestine without perforation or abscess with bleeding B) K57.31 Diverticulitis of large intestine without perforation or abscess without bleeding C) K57.20 Diverticulitis of large intestine with perforation and abscess without bleeding D) K57.93 Diverticulitis of intestine, part unspecified, without perforation with bleeding

Question 69: A patient has anemia in chronic kidney disease, stage 5. The correct coding is:

A) N18.5 Chronic kidney disease, stage 5 and D63.1 Anemia in chronic kidney disease B) D63.1 Anemia in chronic kidney disease and N18.5 C) D63.9 Anemia in other chronic diseases D) N18.9 Chronic kidney disease, unspecified

Question 70: A patient is admitted for elective termination of pregnancy at 8 weeks gestation. The correct code is:

A) O04.5 Failed attempted termination of pregnancy B) Z33.2 Encounter for elective termination of pregnancy C) O00.9 Ectopic pregnancy, unspecified D) Z32.01 Encounter for pregnancy test, result positive

Question 71: A patient has obstructive sleep apnea with documented hypoxemia. The correct code is:

A) G47.33 Obstructive sleep apnea B) G47.30 Sleep apnea, unspecified C) R06.83 Snoring D) J96.01 Acute respiratory failure with hypoxia

Question 72: A patient presents with acute pyelonephritis due to E. coli infection. The correct coding is:

A) N10 Acute pyelonephritis and B96.20 Unspecified Escherichia coli B) N10 only C) N12 Tubulo-interstitial nephritis D) N39.0 Urinary tract infection, site not specified

Question 73: A patient has morbid obesity with BMI of 42. The correct coding is:

A) E66.01 Morbid (severe) obesity due to excess calories and Z68.41 BMI 40.0-44.9, adult B) E66.9 Obesity, unspecified C) E66.01 only D) Z68.41 only

Question 74: A patient is admitted with hyperglycemia, Type 2 diabetes mellitus documented. The correct code is:

A) E11.65 Type 2 diabetes mellitus with hyperglycemia B) R73.9 Hyperglycemia, unspecified C) E11.9 Type 2 diabetes mellitus without complications D) E10.65 Type 1 diabetes mellitus with hyperglycemia

Question 75: A patient has chronic pain syndrome following spinal fusion surgery performed 2 years ago. The correct code is:

A) G89.28 Other chronic postprocedural pain B) M96.1 Postlaminectomy syndrome C) G89.29 Other chronic pain D) M54.5 Low back pain

CPT® Coding Practice Questions (75 Questions)

Questions 76-100: Evaluation and Management

Question 76: A new patient is seen in the office for 45 minutes with moderate complexity medical decision making for management of multiple chronic conditions. The correct code is:

A) 99203 Office visit, new patient, 30-44 minutes B) 99204 Office visit, new patient, 45-59 minutes C) 99205 Office visit, new patient, 60-74 minutes D) 99213 Office visit, established patient, 20-29 minutes

Question 77: An established patient receives hospital discharge services that take 35 minutes. The correct code is:

A) 99238 Hospital discharge day management, 30 minutes or less B) 99239 Hospital discharge day management, more than 30 minutes C) 99217 Observation care discharge D) 99233 Subsequent hospital care, high level

Question 78: A physician provides 50 minutes of critical care to an unstable ICU patient. The correct code is:

A) 99291 Critical care, first 30-74 minutes B) 99233 Subsequent hospital care C) 99291 and 99292 D) 99285 Emergency department visit, high level

Question 79: An office visit for an established patient involves straightforward medical decision making with 15 minutes total time spent. The correct code is:

A) 99211 Office visit, established patient, minimal B) 99212 Office visit, established patient, 10-19 minutes C) 99213 Office visit, established patient, 20-29 minutes D) 99214 Office visit, established patient, 30-39 minutes

Question 80: Initial hospital care is provided with comprehensive history and examination and high complexity medical decision making. The correct code is:

A) 99221 Initial hospital care, low level B) 99222 Initial hospital care, moderate level C) 99223 Initial hospital care, high level D) 99233 Subsequent hospital care, high level

Question 81: A patient is seen in the emergency department with moderate level complexity. The correct code is:

A) 99282 Emergency department visit, low level B) 99283 Emergency department visit, moderate level C) 99284 Emergency department visit, high level D) 99285 Emergency department visit, comprehensive

Question 82: Subsequent nursing facility care with moderate complexity medical decision making is provided. The correct code is:

A) 99307 Subsequent nursing facility care, low level B) 99308 Subsequent nursing facility care, moderate-low level C) 99309 Subsequent nursing facility care, moderate-high level D) 99310 Subsequent nursing facility care, high level

Question 83: A consultation is provided in the office for a new problem with detailed history and examination and low complexity medical decision making. The correct code is:

A) 99241 Office consultation, low level B) 99242 Office consultation, moderate-low level C) 99243 Office consultation, moderate level D) 99244 Office consultation, moderate-high level

Question 84: Preventive medicine service for an established patient, age 45, is provided. The correct code is:

A) 99395 Preventive visit, established patient, age 40-64 B) 99385 Preventive visit, new patient, age 40-64 C) 99214 Office visit, established patient D) 99204 Office visit, new patient

Question 85: A physician provides 95 minutes of critical care. The correct coding is:

A) 99291 only B) 99291 and 99292 C) 99291 and 99292 x 2 D) 99233 and 99291

Question 86: Initial observation care is provided with comprehensive history/examination and high complexity medical decision making. The correct code is:

A) 99218 Initial observation care, low level B) 99219 Initial observation care, moderate level C) 99220 Initial observation care, high level D) 99222 Initial hospital care, moderate level

Question 87: A patient receives prolonged physician service of 90 minutes beyond the highest level E/M service. How should this be coded?

A) 99354 only B) 99354 and 99355 C) 99355 only D) Add time to base E/M code only

Question 88: Subsequent hospital care is provided with high complexity medical decision making. The correct code is:

A) 99231 Subsequent hospital care, low level B) 99232 Subsequent hospital care, moderate level C) 99233 Subsequent hospital care, high level D) 99223 Initial hospital care, high level

Question 89: A patient is seen in the office for an annual preventive visit, new patient, age 55. The correct code is:

A) 99385 Preventive visit, new patient, age 40-64 B) 99395 Preventive visit, established patient, age 40-64 C) 99386 Preventive visit, new patient, age 65 and over D) 99205 Office visit, new patient, comprehensive

Question 90: Emergency department visit with high complexity medical decision making is provided. The correct code is:

A) 99282 ED visit, low level B) 99283 ED visit, moderate level C) 99284 ED visit, high level D) 99285 ED visit, comprehensive

Question 91: A physician provides care coordination services for a complex chronic care patient, 45 minutes spent. The appropriate code is:

A) 99490 Chronic care management, 20 minutes B) 99491 Chronic care management, 30 minutes C) 99214 Office visit, established patient D) 99354 Prolonged service

Question 92: Initial nursing facility care with comprehensive history/examination and moderate complexity medical decision making is provided. The correct code is:

A) 99304 Initial nursing facility care, low level B) 99305 Initial nursing facility care, moderate level C) 99306 Initial nursing facility care, high level D) 99308 Subsequent nursing facility care

Question 93: A same-day admission and discharge from observation status occurs. The correct code is:

A) 99234 Observation or inpatient care, same day admit/discharge, low level B) 99235 Observation or inpatient care, same day admit/discharge, moderate level C) 99236 Observation or inpatient care, same day admit/discharge, high level D) Depends on level of service provided

Question 94: A patient is seen for initial hospital care with detailed history/examination and low complexity medical decision making. The correct code is:

A) 99221 Initial hospital care, low level B) 99222 Initial hospital care, moderate level C) 99223 Initial hospital care, high level D) 99231 Subsequent hospital care

Question 95: Domiciliary care is provided to an established patient with moderate complexity medical decision making. The correct code is:

A) 99334 Domiciliary care, established patient, low level B) 99335 Domiciliary care, established patient, moderate level C) 99336 Domiciliary care, established patient, moderate-high level D) 99337 Domiciliary care, established patient, high level

Question 96: A telephone E/M service by a physician to an established patient takes 15 minutes. The correct code is:

A) 99441 Telephone E/M, 5-10 minutes B) 99442 Telephone E/M, 11-20 minutes C) 99443 Telephone E/M, 21-30 minutes D) Cannot be separately billed

Question 97: Newborn care services are provided on the day of birth in the hospital. The correct code is:

A) 99460 Initial hospital or birthing center care, per day B) 99461 Initial care, per day, normal newborn C) 99462 Subsequent hospital care, per day D) 99463 Initial hospital or birthing center care

Question 98: A patient receives transitional care management services 14 days after hospital discharge with moderate complexity medical decision making. The correct code is:

A) 99495 Transitional care management, moderate complexity B) 99496 Transitional care management, high complexity C) 99490 Chronic care management D) 99214 Office visit, established patient

Question 99: Annual nursing facility assessment is performed. The correct code is:

A) 99318 Annual nursing facility assessment B) 99310 Subsequent nursing facility care C) 99306 Initial nursing facility care D) 99315 Nursing facility discharge

Question 100: A physician spends 25 minutes reviewing records and communicating with other healthcare professionals regarding a patient (non-face-to-face time). The correct code is:

A) 99358 Prolonged service, non-face-to-face, first hour B) 99359 Prolonged service, non-face-to-face, additional 30 minutes C) 99441 Telephone E/M service D) Cannot be separately billed without face-to-face component

Questions 101-125: Surgery Coding

Question 101: Simple repair of a 3.5 cm laceration on the forehead and a 2.0 cm laceration on the cheek. What is the correct coding?

A) 12013 Simple repair, face, 2.6-5.0 cm only B) 12014 Simple repair, face, 7.6-12.5 cm (total 5.5 cm) C) 12011 and 12013 separately D) 12013 with modifier -51

Question 102: Excision of a 2.2 cm malignant lesion from the back with 0.5 cm margins on all sides. What is the correct code?

A) 11603 Excision, malignant lesion, trunk, 1.1-2.0 cm B) 11604 Excision, malignant lesion, trunk, 2.1-3.0 cm C) 11606 Excision, malignant lesion, trunk, 3.1-4.0 cm D) 11402 Excision, benign lesion, trunk, 1.1-2.0 cm

Question 103: Intermediate repair of a 4.5 cm wound on the arm requiring layered closure. The correct code is:

A) 12031 Intermediate repair, scalp/neck/extremities, 2.5 cm or less B) 12032 Intermediate repair, scalp/neck/extremities, 2.6-7.5 cm C) 12034 Intermediate repair, scalp/neck/extremities, 7.6-12.5 cm D) 13120 Complex repair, scalp/arm/leg, 2.6-7.5 cm

Question 104: Closed treatment of a displaced femur shaft fracture with manipulation. The correct code is:

A) 27500 Closed treatment of femoral shaft fracture, without manipulation B) 27502 Closed treatment of femoral shaft fracture, with manipulation C) 27506 Open treatment of femoral shaft fracture D) 27507 Open treatment of femoral shaft fracture with internal fixation

Question 105: Diagnostic colonoscopy with biopsy of two polyps and removal of one polyp by snare technique. The correct code is:

A) 45378 Colonoscopy, diagnostic B) 45380 Colonoscopy with biopsy C) 45385 Colonoscopy with removal of tumor/polyp by snare D) 45380 and 45385

Question 106: Laparoscopic cholecystectomy with cholangiography. The correct code is:

A) 47562 Laparoscopic cholecystectomy B) 47563 Laparoscopic cholecystectomy with cholangiography C) 47564 Laparoscopic cholecystectomy with exploration of common duct D) 47600 Cholecystectomy, open

Question 107: Bilateral inguinal hernia repair in an adult patient. The correct coding is:

A) 49505 Inguinal hernia repair, initial B) 49505 with modifier -50 C) 49505 x 2 D) 49520 Recurrent inguinal hernia repair

Question 108: Excision of three benign skin lesions: 1.2 cm from arm, 0.8 cm from chest, 1.5 cm from back. The correct coding is:

A) 11402, 11401, 11402 B) 11402 only (largest lesion) C) 11403 (total of all lesions) D) 11401, 11401, 11402 with modifier -51

Question 109: Arthroscopic partial meniscectomy of the medial meniscus of the right knee. The correct code is:

A) 29870 Arthroscopy, knee, diagnostic B) 29880 Arthroscopy, knee, with meniscectomy C) 29881 Arthroscopy, knee, with meniscectomy including repair D) 27332 Arthrotomy, knee, with excision of semilunar cartilage

Question 110: Open reduction and internal fixation (ORIF) of a displaced radial shaft fracture. The correct code is:

A) 25500 Closed treatment of radial shaft fracture B) 25515 Open treatment of radial shaft fracture C) 25525 Open treatment of radial shaft fracture with internal fixation D) 25526 Open treatment of radial shaft fracture with internal and external fixation

Question 111: Total abdominal hysterectomy with bilateral salpingo-oophorectomy. The correct code is:

A) 58150 Total abdominal hysterectomy B) 58152 Total abdominal hysterectomy with bilateral salpingo-oophorectomy C) 58180 Supracervical abdominal hysterectomy D) 58200 Total abdominal hysterectomy with removal of tubes

Question 112: Carpal tunnel release, right hand, open approach. The correct code is:

A) 64721 Neuroplasty and/or transposition, median nerve at carpal tunnel B) 64719 Neuroplasty, median nerve at wrist C) 29848 Endoscopy, wrist, with carpal tunnel release D) 64722 Decompression, unspecified nerve

Question 113: Repair of recurrent incisional ventral hernia. The correct code is:

A) 49560 Repair initial incisional hernia B) 49565 Repair recurrent incisional hernia C) 49568 Repair recurrent incisional hernia, complicated D) 49585 Repair umbilical hernia

Question 114: Tonsillectomy and adenoidectomy, age 12. The correct code is:

A) 42820 Tonsillectomy and adenoidectomy, younger than age 12 B) 42821 Tonsillectomy and adenoidectomy, age 12 or over C) 42825 Tonsillectomy, primary or secondary, younger than age 12 D) 42826 Tonsillectomy, primary or secondary, age 12 or over

Question 115: Cystoscopy with fulguration of bladder tumor, 3 cm. The correct code is:

A) 52000 Cystourethroscopy B) 52214 Cystourethroscopy with fulguration of trigone lesions C) 52234 Cystourethroscopy with fulguration of small bladder tumors D) 52235 Cystourethroscopy with fulguration of medium bladder tumors

Question 116: Repair of inguinal hernia, initial, incarcerated, age 40. The correct code is:

A) 49505 Inguinal hernia repair, initial, age 5 or older B) 49507 Inguinal hernia repair, initial, incarcerated or strangulated, age 5 or older C) 49520 Inguinal hernia repair, recurrent D) 49550 Inguinal hernia repair, initial, premature infant

Question 117: Diagnostic arthroscopy of the right shoulder. The correct code is:

A) 29805 Arthroscopy, shoulder, diagnostic B) 29806 Arthroscopy, shoulder, surgical C) 29807 Arthroscopy, shoulder, surgical, with rotator cuff repair D) 23105 Arthrotomy, shoulder, with synovectomy

Question 118: Flexible sigmoidoscopy with biopsy. The correct code is:

A) 45330 Sigmoidoscopy, flexible, diagnostic B) 45331 Sigmoidoscopy, flexible, with biopsy C) 45378 Colonoscopy, diagnostic D) 45380 Colonoscopy with biopsy

Question 119: Lumbar laminectomy, single interspace. The correct code is:

A) 63005 Laminectomy with exploration and/or decompression, single interspace B) 63030 Laminectomy with exploration, lumbar, single interspace C) 63047 Laminectomy, facetectomy, foraminotomy, lumbar, single segment D) 63056 Transpedicular approach, lumbar, single segment

Question 120: Coronary artery bypass, three coronary venous grafts. The correct code is:

A) 33510 Coronary artery bypass, vein only, single B) 33511 Coronary artery bypass, vein only, two C) 33512 Coronary artery bypass, vein only, three D) 33513 Coronary artery bypass, vein only, four

Question 121: Mohs micrographic surgery on the nose, first stage with five tissue blocks. The correct coding is:

A) 17311 Mohs surgery, head/neck/hands/feet/genitalia, first stage, up to 5 blocks B) 17312 Mohs surgery, each additional stage C) 17313 Mohs surgery, head/neck, first stage, 6-10 blocks D) 11642 Excision, malignant lesion, face

Question 122: Esophagogastroduodenoscopy (EGD) with control of bleeding. The correct code is:

A) 43235 EGD, diagnostic B) 43239 EGD with biopsy C) 43255 EGD with control of bleeding D) 43259 EGD with endoscopic ultrasound

Question 123: Reduction mammaplasty (breast reduction). The correct code is:

A) 19318 Reduction mammaplasty B) 19316 Mastopexy (breast lift) C) 19340 Immediate breast reconstruction D) 19350 Nipple/areola reconstruction

Question 124: Vasectomy, bilateral. The correct code is:

A) 55250 Vasectomy, unilateral or bilateral B) 55450 Ligation of vas deferens C) 55250 with modifier -50 D) 55180 Vasovasostomy

Question 125: Application of short leg cast for fracture treatment by the physician who also provided the fracture care. How should this be coded?

A) 29405 Application of short leg cast B) Include in fracture care code, do not code separately C) 29405 with modifier -51 D) 29425 Application of short leg cast walking

Questions 126-150: Mixed CPT® Specialties

Question 126: Chest X-ray, 2 views, complete study with professional component only. The correct code is:

A) 71045 Radiologic examination, chest, 2 views B) 71045-26 Professional component C) 71045-TC Technical component D) 71046 Radiologic examination, chest, 3 views

Question 127: Complete abdominal ultrasound. The correct code is:

A) 76700 Ultrasound, abdominal, complete B) 76705 Ultrasound, abdominal, limited C) 76770 Ultrasound, retroperitoneal, complete D) 76775 Ultrasound, retroperitoneal, limited

Question 128: Anesthesia for total hip replacement (01214, 8 base units) in a healthy 50-year-old patient lasting 120 minutes. Calculate total anesthesia units:

A) 14 units B) 16 units C) 17 units D) 18 units

Question 129: Comprehensive metabolic panel. The correct code is:

A) 80047 Basic metabolic panel B) 80048 Basic metabolic panel C) 80053 Comprehensive metabolic panel D) 80061 Lipid panel

Question 130: Screening mammography, bilateral. The correct code is:

A) 77065 Diagnostic mammography, unilateral B) 77066 Diagnostic mammography, bilateral C) 77067 Screening mammography, bilateral D) 76641 Ultrasound, breast, complete

Question 131: Anesthesia for appendectomy (00840, 6 base units) in an 82-year-old patient with severe heart disease, emergency procedure, lasting 90 minutes. Calculate total anesthesia units:

A) 11 units B) 13 units C) 14 units D) 15 units

Question 132: Lipid panel. The correct code is:

A) 80053 Comprehensive metabolic panel B) 80061 Lipid panel C) 82465 Cholesterol, total D) 83718 Lipoprotein, direct measurement, HDL

Question 133: CT scan of abdomen without contrast, professional component only. The correct code is:

A) 74150 CT abdomen without contrast B) 74150-26 Professional component C) 74150-TC Technical component D) 74160 CT abdomen with contrast

Question 134: Urinalysis, automated with microscopy. The correct code is:

A) 81000 Urinalysis, by dip stick B) 81001 Urinalysis, automated without microscopy C) 81003 Urinalysis, automated with microscopy D) 81005 Urinalysis, qualitative or semiquantitative

Question 135: MRI of brain without and with contrast. The correct code is:

A) 70551 MRI brain without contrast B) 70552 MRI brain with contrast C) 70553 MRI brain without and with contrast D) 70450 CT head without contrast

Question 136: Influenza virus vaccine, split virus, administration by intramuscular injection. The correct codes are:

A) 90656 Influenza vaccine and 90471 Immunization administration B) 90658 Influenza vaccine and 90472 Immunization administration C) Depends on patient age and vaccine type D) 90662 Influenza vaccine only

Question 137: Electrocardiogram (ECG), routine, with interpretation and report. The correct code is:

A) 93000 Electrocardiogram, complete B) 93005 Electrocardiogram, tracing only C) 93010 Electrocardiogram, interpretation and report only D) 93040 Rhythm ECG

Question 138: Complete blood count (CBC) with automated differential. The correct code is:

A) 85025 Complete blood count with differential, automated B) 85027 Complete blood count, automated C) 85004 Blood count, manual differential D) 85007 Blood count, manual cell count

Question 139: Anesthesia for cesarean delivery (01961, 7 base units) in a healthy 28-year-old patient lasting 75 minutes. Calculate total anesthesia units:

A) 11 units B) 12 units C) 13 units D) 14 units

Question 140: Hepatic function panel. The correct code is:

A) 80047 Basic metabolic panel B) 80053 Comprehensive metabolic panel C) 80076 Hepatic function panel D) 82247 Bilirubin, total

Question 141: Bone density study, axial skeleton. The correct code is:

A) 77080 Dual-energy X-ray absorptiometry (DXA), bone density, axial skeleton B) 77081 DXA bone density, appendicular skeleton C) 77085 DXA bone density, axial skeleton, vertebral fracture assessment D) 77086 Vertebral fracture assessment

Question 142: Venipuncture for blood collection. The correct code is:

A) 36410 Venipuncture, younger than age 3 B) 36415 Venipuncture, age 3 or older C) 36591 Collection of blood from central venous catheter D) 36416 Collection of capillary blood specimen

Question 143: Ultrasound guidance for needle placement, imaging supervision and interpretation. The correct code is:

A) 76942 Ultrasonic guidance for needle placement B) 77001 Fluoroscopic guidance for central venous access C) 77002 Fluoroscopic guidance for needle placement D) 77012 CT guidance for needle placement

Question 144: Basic metabolic panel (calcium, total). The correct code is:

A) 80047 Basic metabolic panel (calcium, ionized) B) 80048 Basic metabolic panel (calcium, total) C) 80053 Comprehensive metabolic panel D) 82310 Calcium, total

Question 145: Prostate specific antigen (PSA), total. The correct code is:

A) 84152 Prostate specific antigen, complexed B) 84153 Prostate specific antigen, total C) 84154 Prostate specific antigen, free D) 86316 Immunoassay, tumor antigen

Question 146: Anesthesia for cataract surgery (00142, 4 base units) in a 75-year-old healthy patient lasting 45 minutes. Calculate total anesthesia units:

A) 7 units B) 8 units C) 9 units D) 10 units

Question 147: Thyroid stimulating hormone (TSH) assay. The correct code is:

A) 84436 Thyroxine, total B) 84439 Thyroxine, free C) 84443 Thyroid stimulating hormone D) 84479 Thyroid hormone binding ratio

Question 148: Hemoglobin A1c. The correct code is:

A) 83036 Hemoglobin, glycosylated (A1c) B) 83037 Hemoglobin, glycosylated, device cleared by FDA C) 83021 Hemoglobin, plasma D) 85014 Hematocrit

Question 149: Spirometry, complete. The correct code is:

A) 94010 Spirometry, including graphic record, total and timed vital capacity B) 94060 Spirometry, before and after bronchodilator C) 94200 Maximum breathing capacity D) 94375 Respiratory flow volume loop

Question 150: Therapeutic injection of corticosteroid into major joint (knee). The correct code is:

A) 20600 Arthrocentesis, small joint B) 20605 Arthrocentesis, intermediate joint C) 20610 Arthrocentesis, major joint or bursa D) 20999 Unlisted procedure, musculoskeletal system

E/M Coding Scenarios (50 Questions)

Questions 151-175: Office and Outpatient E/M

Question 151: A new patient office visit involves 62 minutes spent primarily on counseling and coordination of care for multiple chronic conditions. Medical decision making is low complexity. What is the correct code?

A) 99203 Office visit, new patient, 30-44 minutes B) 99204 Office visit, new patient, 45-59 minutes C) 99205 Office visit, new patient, 60-74 minutes D) 99215 Office visit, established patient, 40-54 minutes

Question 152: An established patient is seen for a medication refill with straightforward medical decision making. Total time is 12 minutes. The correct code is:

A) 99211 Office visit, established patient, minimal B) 99212 Office visit, established patient, 10-19 minutes C) 99213 Office visit, established patient, 20-29 minutes D) 99214 Office visit, established patient, 30-39 minutes

Question 153: A patient presents to the office with acute bronchitis. The physician performs an expanded problem-focused examination and straightforward medical decision making. Total time is 18 minutes. The correct code is:

A) 99211 Office visit, established patient, minimal B) 99212 Office visit, established patient, 10-19 minutes C) 99213 Office visit, established patient, 20-29 minutes D) 99202 Office visit, new patient

Question 154: Initial hospital care is provided with comprehensive history and examination. Medical decision making is high complexity due to multiple comorbidities. The correct code is:

A) 99221 Initial hospital care, low level B) 99222 Initial hospital care, moderate level C) 99223 Initial hospital care, high level D) 99233 Subsequent hospital care, high level

Question 155: A physician provides 25 minutes of critical care to a patient in the ICU. Can this be billed as critical care?

A) No, minimum is 30 minutes B) Yes, code 99291 C) Yes, code 99233 D) No, bill as subsequent hospital care

Question 156: An established patient office visit involves moderate complexity medical decision making with 32 minutes total time. The correct code is:

A) 99213 Office visit, established patient, 20-29 minutes B) 99214 Office visit, established patient, 30-39 minutes C) 99215 Office visit, established patient, 40-54 minutes D) 99204 Office visit, new patient

Question 157: Emergency department visit with detailed history, detailed examination, and high complexity medical decision making. The correct code is:

A) 99283 ED visit, moderate level B) 99284 ED visit, high level C) 99285 ED visit, comprehensive level D) 99223 Initial hospital care

Question 158: Subsequent hospital care with comprehensive interval history and examination, high complexity medical decision making. The correct code is:

A) 99231 Subsequent hospital care, low level B) 99232 Subsequent hospital care, moderate level C) 99233 Subsequent hospital care, high level D) 99223 Initial hospital care, high level

Question 159: Office consultation (where still recognized) with detailed history and examination, moderate complexity medical decision making. The correct code is:

A) 99242 Office consultation, low-moderate level B) 99243 Office consultation, moderate level C) 99244 Office consultation, moderate-high level D) 99245 Office consultation, high level

Question 160: A new patient preventive medicine visit for a 50-year-old. The correct code is:

A) 99384 Preventive visit, new patient, age 40-64 B) 99385 Preventive visit, new patient, age 40-64 C) 99394 Preventive visit, established patient, age 40-64 D) 99395 Preventive visit, established patient, age 40-64

Question 161: Hospital discharge services taking 45 minutes. The correct code is:

A) 99238 Hospital discharge, 30 minutes or less B) 99239 Hospital discharge, more than 30 minutes C) 99217 Observation care discharge D) 99233 Subsequent hospital care

Question 162: Initial observation care with comprehensive history and examination, moderate complexity medical decision making. The correct code is:

A) 99218 Initial observation care, low level B) 99219 Initial observation care, moderate level C) 99220 Initial observation care, high level D) 99222 Initial hospital care, moderate level

Question 163: A physician provides 110 minutes of critical care. The correct coding is:

A) 99291 only B) 99291 and 99292 C) 99291 and 99292 x 2 D) 99291 x 2

Question 164: Subsequent nursing facility care with detailed interval history, moderate complexity medical decision making. The correct code is:

A) 99307 Subsequent nursing facility care, low level B) 99308 Subsequent nursing facility care, moderate-low level C) 99309 Subsequent nursing facility care, moderate-high level D) 99310 Subsequent nursing facility care, high level

Question 165: Same-day observation admission and discharge with moderate complexity medical decision making. The correct code is:

A) 99234 Same-day observation admit/discharge, low level B) 99235 Same-day observation admit/discharge, moderate level C) 99236 Same-day observation admit/discharge, high level D) 99219 and 99217

Question 166: Established patient office visit, high complexity medical decision making, 48 minutes total time. The correct code is:

A) 99214 Office visit, established patient, 30-39 minutes B) 99215 Office visit, established patient, 40-54 minutes C) 99205 Office visit, new patient D) 99204 Office visit, new patient

Question 167: Initial nursing facility care with comprehensive history and examination, high complexity medical decision making. The correct code is:

A) 99304 Initial nursing facility care, low level B) 99305 Initial nursing facility care, moderate level C) 99306 Initial nursing facility care, high level D) 99310 Subsequent nursing facility care

Question 168: Emergency department visit for minor injury, problem-focused history and examination, straightforward medical decision making. The correct code is:

A) 99281 ED visit, minimal level B) 99282 ED visit, low level C) 99283 ED visit, moderate level D) 99284 ED visit, high level

Question 169: A new patient office visit with straightforward medical decision making, 22 minutes total time. The correct code is:

A) 99201 Office visit, new patient (deleted code) B) 99202 Office visit, new patient, 15-29 minutes C) 99203 Office visit, new patient, 30-44 minutes D) 99212 Office visit, established patient

Question 170: Domiciliary care for an established patient with low complexity medical decision making. The correct code is:

A) 99334 Domiciliary care, established patient, low level B) 99335 Domiciliary care, established patient, moderate level C) 99336 Domiciliary care, established patient, moderate-high level D) 99337 Domiciliary care, established patient, high level

Question 171: A physician provides 40 minutes of critical care. The correct code is:

A) 99291 Critical care, first 30-74 minutes B) 99233 Subsequent hospital care C) 99223 Initial hospital care D) 99285 ED visit, high level

Question 172: Subsequent hospital care with problem-focused interval history, low complexity medical decision making. The correct code is:

A) 99231 Subsequent hospital care, low level B) 99232 Subsequent hospital care, moderate level C) 99233 Subsequent hospital care, high level D) 99221 Initial hospital care

Question 173: Annual nursing facility assessment. The correct code is:

A) 99318 Annual nursing facility assessment B) 99310 Subsequent nursing facility care, high level C) 99306 Initial nursing facility care, high level D) 99395 Preventive visit, established patient

Question 174: Office visit for established patient with moderate complexity medical decision making, 28 minutes total time. The correct code is:

A) 99212 Office visit, established patient, 10-19 minutes B) 99213 Office visit, established patient, 20-29 minutes C) 99214 Office visit, established patient, 30-39 minutes D) 99215 Office visit, established patient, 40-54 minutes

Question 175: Initial observation care with detailed history and examination, low complexity medical decision making. The correct code is:

A) 99218 Initial observation care, low level B) 99219 Initial observation care, moderate level C) 99220 Initial observation care, high level D) 99221 Initial hospital care, low level

Questions 176-200: Hospital and Facility E/M

Question 176: Subsequent hospital care with expanded problem-focused interval history, moderate complexity medical decision making. The correct code is:

A) 99231 Subsequent hospital care, low level B) 99232 Subsequent hospital care, moderate level C) 99233 Subsequent hospital care, high level D) 99222 Initial hospital care, moderate level

Question 177: Initial hospital care with detailed history and examination, moderate complexity medical decision making. The correct code is:

A) 99221 Initial hospital care, low level B) 99222 Initial hospital care, moderate level C) 99223 Initial hospital care, high level D) 99232 Subsequent hospital care

Question 178: A physician provides 145 minutes of critical care in a single day. The correct coding is:

A) 99291 only B) 99291 and 99292 C) 99291 and 99292 x 2 D) 99291 and 99292 x 3

Question 179: Nursing facility discharge services taking 25 minutes. The correct code is:

A) 99315 Nursing facility discharge, 30 minutes or less B) 99316 Nursing facility discharge, more than 30 minutes C) 99238 Hospital discharge D) 99310 Subsequent nursing facility care

Question 180: Subsequent observation care with expanded problem-focused interval history, low complexity medical decision making. The correct code is:

A) 99224 Subsequent observation care, low level B) 99225 Subsequent observation care, moderate level C) 99226 Subsequent observation care, high level D) 99231 Subsequent hospital care

Question 181: Initial hospital care for a newborn in the hospital. The correct code is:

A) 99460 Initial hospital care for newborn B) 99461 Initial care, normal newborn C) 99462 Subsequent hospital care, normal newborn D) 99221 Initial hospital care

Question 182: Observation care discharge on a different date than admission. The correct code is:

A) 99217 Observation care discharge B) 99238 Hospital discharge C) 99239 Hospital discharge, more than 30 minutes D) 99231 Subsequent hospital care

Question 183: Emergency department visit with comprehensive history, comprehensive examination, high complexity medical decision making. The correct code is:

A) 99283 ED visit, moderate level B) 99284 ED visit, high level C) 99285 ED visit, comprehensive level D) 99223 Initial hospital care

Question 184: Initial nursing facility care with detailed history and examination, low complexity medical decision making. The correct code is:

A) 99304 Initial nursing facility care, low level B) 99305 Initial nursing facility care, moderate level C) 99306 Initial nursing facility care, high level D) 99307 Subsequent nursing facility care

Question 185: Subsequent nursing facility care with comprehensive interval history, high complexity medical decision making. The correct code is:

A) 99307 Subsequent nursing facility care, low level B) 99308 Subsequent nursing facility care, moderate-low level C) 99309 Subsequent nursing facility care, moderate-high level D) 99310 Subsequent nursing facility care, high level

Question 186: Transitional care management with moderate complexity medical decision making within 14 days of discharge. The correct code is:

A) 99495 Transitional care management, moderate complexity B) 99496 Transitional care management, high complexity C) 99490 Chronic care management D) 99214 Office visit

Question 187: Subsequent hospital care with detailed interval history, high complexity medical decision making. The correct code is:

A) 99231 Subsequent hospital care, low level B) 99232 Subsequent hospital care, moderate level C) 99233 Subsequent hospital care, high level D) 99223 Initial hospital care

Question 188: Hospital discharge services taking 20 minutes. The correct code is:

A) 99238 Hospital discharge, 30 minutes or less B) 99239 Hospital discharge, more than 30 minutes C) 99217 Observation discharge D) 99233 Subsequent hospital care

Question 189: Domiciliary care for a new patient with moderate complexity medical decision making. The correct code is:

A) 99324 Domiciliary care, new patient, low level B) 99325 Domiciliary care, new patient, moderate level C) 99326 Domiciliary care, new patient, moderate-high level D) 99327 Domiciliary care, new patient, high level

Question 190: Subsequent observation care with detailed interval history, moderate complexity medical decision making. The correct code is:

A) 99224 Subsequent observation care, low level B) 99225 Subsequent observation care, moderate level C) 99226 Subsequent observation care, high level D) 99232 Subsequent hospital care

Question 191: Initial hospital care with comprehensive history and examination, moderate complexity medical decision making. The correct code is:

A) 99221 Initial hospital care, low level B) 99222 Initial hospital care, moderate level C) 99223 Initial hospital care, high level D) 99219 Initial observation care

Question 192: Nursing facility discharge services taking 35 minutes. The correct code is:

A) 99315 Nursing facility discharge, 30 minutes or less B) 99316 Nursing facility discharge, more than 30 minutes C) 99239 Hospital discharge D) 99318 Annual nursing facility assessment

Question 193: Emergency department visit with expanded problem-focused history and examination, low complexity medical decision making. The correct code is:

A) 99281 ED visit, minimal level B) 99282 ED visit, low level C) 99283 ED visit, moderate level D) 99284 ED visit, high level

Question 194: Subsequent hospital care with problem-focused interval history, straightforward medical decision making. The correct code is:

A) 99231 Subsequent hospital care, low level B) 99232 Subsequent hospital care, moderate level C) 99233 Subsequent hospital care, high level D) 99221 Initial hospital care

Question 195: Initial observation care with comprehensive history and examination, high complexity medical decision making. The correct code is:

A) 99218 Initial observation care, low level B) 99219 Initial observation care, moderate level C) 99220 Initial observation care, high level D) 99223 Initial hospital care

Question 196: Subsequent nursing facility care with expanded problem-focused interval history, low complexity medical decision making. The correct code is:

A) 99307 Subsequent nursing facility care, low level B) 99308 Subsequent nursing facility care, moderate-low level C) 99309 Subsequent nursing facility care, moderate-high level D) 99310 Subsequent nursing facility care, high level

Question 197: Same-day observation admission and discharge with high complexity medical decision making. The correct code is:

A) 99234 Same-day observation, low level B) 99235 Same-day observation, moderate level C) 99236 Same-day observation, high level D) 99220 and 99217

Question 198: Initial hospital care with detailed history and examination, low complexity medical decision making. The correct code is:

A) 99221 Initial hospital care, low level B) 99222 Initial hospital care, moderate level C) 99223 Initial hospital care, high level D) 99218 Initial observation care

Question 199: Subsequent hospital care with expanded problem-focused interval history, low complexity medical decision making. The correct code is:

A) 99231 Subsequent hospital care, low level B) 99232 Subsequent hospital care, moderate level C) 99233 Subsequent hospital care, high level D) 99221 Initial hospital care

Question 200: Subsequent observation care with comprehensive interval history, high complexity medical decision making. The correct code is:

A) 99224 Subsequent observation care, low level B) 99225 Subsequent observation care, moderate level C) 99226 Subsequent observation care, high level D) 99233 Subsequent hospital care

Surgery Coding Cases (25 Questions)

Questions 201-225: Complex Surgical Scenarios

Question 201: Laparoscopic cholecystectomy is started but converted to open cholecystectomy due to dense adhesions. The correct coding is:

A) 47562 Laparoscopic cholecystectomy with modifier -22 B) 47563 Laparoscopic cholecystectomy with cholangiography C) 47600 Cholecystectomy, open D) 47600 with modifier -52

Question 202: Bilateral inguinal hernia repair in a 45-year-old adult, both initial hernias. The correct coding is:

A) 49505 Inguinal hernia repair, initial B) 49505 with modifier -50 C) 49505 x 2 D) 49520 Recurrent inguinal hernia repair

Question 203: Repair of 2.5 cm laceration on right hand and 3.0 cm laceration on left forearm, both requiring intermediate repair with layered closure. The correct coding is:

A) 12041 and 12042 B) 12042 only (total 5.5 cm) C) 12041 with modifier -51 and 12042 D) 12044 (total length)

Question 204: Arthroscopic medial meniscectomy with chondroplasty of the medial femoral condyle, same knee. The correct coding is:

A) 29880 Arthroscopy, knee, with meniscectomy only B) 29877 Arthroscopy, knee, with chondroplasty only C) 29880 and 29877 with modifier -51 D) 29881 Arthroscopy, knee, with meniscectomy and chondroplasty

Question 205: Total abdominal hysterectomy with bilateral salpingo-oophorectomy for endometrial cancer. The correct code is:

A) 58150 Total abdominal hysterectomy B) 58152 Total abdominal hysterectomy with bilateral salpingo-oophorectomy C) 58180 Supracervical hysterectomy D) 58200 Total abdominal hysterectomy, with removal of tubes

Question 206: Open reduction and internal fixation of closed bimalleolar ankle fracture. The correct code is:

A) 27808 Closed treatment of bimalleolar ankle fracture B) 27814 Open treatment of bimalleolar ankle fracture C) 27792 Closed treatment of distal fibular fracture D) 27829 Open treatment of distal tibial fracture

Question 207: Diagnostic colonoscopy with biopsy of cecal mass and polypectomy of sigmoid polyp. The correct coding is:

A) 45378, 45380, 45385 B) 45385 only C) 45380 and 45385 D) 45378 with modifier -52

Question 208: Cystoscopy with laser fulguration of bladder tumor measuring 4 cm. The correct code is:

A) 52234 Cystourethroscopy with fulguration, small bladder tumors B) 52235 Cystourethroscopy with fulguration, medium bladder tumors (2.0-5.0 cm) C) 52240 Cystourethroscopy with fulguration, large bladder tumors D) 52214 Cystourethroscopy with fulguration, trigone lesions

Question 209: Excision of 1.8 cm benign lesion from scalp with simple closure. The correct code is:

A) 11420 Excision, benign lesion, scalp, 0.5 cm or less B) 11421 Excision, benign lesion, scalp, 0.6-1.0 cm C) 11422 Excision, benign lesion, scalp, 1.1-2.0 cm D) 11423 Excision, benign lesion, scalp, 2.1-3.0 cm

Question 210: Arthroscopic rotator cuff repair, right shoulder. The correct code is:

A) 29805 Arthroscopy, shoulder, diagnostic B) 29806 Arthroscopy, shoulder, surgical C) 29827 Arthroscopy, shoulder, with rotator cuff repair D) 23410 Repair of rotator cuff, open

Question 211: Repair of incarcerated umbilical hernia in an adult. The correct code is:

A) 49580 Repair umbilical hernia, reducible B) 49582 Repair umbilical hernia, incarcerated or strangulated C) 49585 Repair umbilical hernia, recurrent D) 49505 Inguinal hernia repair

Question 212: Flexible sigmoidoscopy with removal of polyp by hot biopsy forceps. The correct code is:

A) 45330 Sigmoidoscopy, flexible, diagnostic B) 45331 Sigmoidoscopy, flexible, with biopsy C) 45333 Sigmoidoscopy, flexible, with ablation of tumor D) 45338 Sigmoidoscopy, flexible, with removal of tumor by snare

Question 213: Laminectomy for decompression of lumbar spinal stenosis at L4-L5 and L5-S1. The correct coding is:

A) 63030 Laminectomy, lumbar, single interspace B) 63047 Laminotomy, lumbar, single segment C) 63030 and 63035 (additional segment) D) 63005 Laminectomy, cervical

Question 214: Tonsillectomy and adenoidectomy in a 15-year-old patient. The correct code is:

A) 42820 Tonsillectomy and adenoidectomy, younger than age 12 B) 42821 Tonsillectomy and adenoidectomy, age 12 or over C) 42825 Tonsillectomy, primary, younger than age 12 D) 42826 Tonsillectomy, primary, age 12 or over

Question 215: Carpal tunnel release, left hand, endoscopic approach. The correct code is:

A) 29848 Endoscopy, wrist, surgical, with release of transverse carpal ligament B) 64721 Neuroplasty, median nerve at carpal tunnel C) 25000 Incision, extensor tendon sheath, wrist D) 25020 Decompression fasciotomy, forearm

Question 216: Complex repair of 5.0 cm laceration on scalp requiring extensive undermining. The correct code is:

A) 12002 Simple repair, scalp, 2.6-7.5 cm B) 12034 Intermediate repair, scalp, 7.6-12.5 cm C) 13120 Complex repair, scalp, arms, legs, 2.6-7.5 cm D) 13121 Complex repair, scalp, arms, legs, 7.6-12.5 cm

Question 217: EGD with biopsy of gastric ulcer and injection therapy to control active bleeding from the ulcer. The correct coding is:

A) 43239 EGD with biopsy only B) 43255 EGD with control of bleeding only C) 43239 and 43255 D) 43235 EGD, diagnostic

Question 218: Vasectomy, bilateral. The correct code is:

A) 55250 Vasectomy, unilateral or bilateral B) 55250 with modifier -50 C) 55400 Vasovasostomy D) 55180 Vasovasorrhaphy

Question 219: Open reduction and internal fixation of displaced midshaft clavicle fracture. The correct code is:

A) 23500 Closed treatment of clavicular fracture B) 23505 Closed treatment of clavicular fracture with manipulation C) 23515 Open treatment of clavicular fracture D) 23525 Open treatment of clavicular fracture with internal fixation

Question 220: Mohs micrographic surgery on the nose, first stage with 7 tissue blocks, followed by second stage with 3 tissue blocks. The correct coding is:

A) 17311 only (first stage, up to 5 blocks) B) 17313 only (first stage, 6-10 blocks) C) 17313 and 17312 (additional stage) D) 17311 and 17312

Question 221: Diagnostic arthroscopy of left knee. The correct code is:

A) 29870 Arthroscopy, knee, diagnostic B) 29880 Arthroscopy, knee, with meniscectomy C) 29881 Arthroscopy, knee, with meniscectomy and repair D) 27331 Arthrotomy, knee, with synovial biopsy

Question 222: Insertion of permanent pacemaker with transvenous electrode placement, atrial and ventricular. The correct code is:

A) 33206 Insertion of pacemaker pulse generator with transvenous electrode, atrial B) 33207 Insertion of pacemaker pulse generator with transvenous electrode, ventricular C) 33208 Insertion of pacemaker pulse generator with transvenous electrodes, atrial and ventricular D) 33210 Insertion of temporary pacemaker

Question 223: Partial mastectomy (lumpectomy) with sentinel lymph node biopsy. The correct coding is:

A) 19301 Mastectomy, partial only B) 19301 and 38500 Lymph node biopsy C) 19302 Mastectomy, simple D) 19303 Mastectomy, radical

Question 224: Laparoscopic repair of recurrent ventral hernia. The correct code is:

A) 49560 Repair initial incisional hernia, open B) 49565 Repair recurrent incisional hernia, open C) 49650 Laparoscopy, repair initial incisional hernia D) 49651 Laparoscopy, repair recurrent incisional hernia

Question 225: Fistulotomy, subcutaneous anal fistula. The correct code is:

A) 46060 Incision and drainage of ischiorectal abscess B) 46270 Fistulotomy, subcutaneous C) 46280 Fistulotomy, intersphincteric D) 46285 Fistulotomy, transsphincteric

Anesthesia, Radiology, Pathology/Lab, Medicine (25 Questions)

Questions 226-250: Mixed Specialty Questions

Question 226: Anesthesia for total knee replacement (01402, 7 base units) in a healthy 55-year-old patient lasting 105 minutes. Calculate total anesthesia units:

A) 13 units B) 14 units C) 15 units D) 16 units

Question 227: Chest X-ray, 2 views, technical component only. The correct code is:

A) 71045 Radiologic examination, chest, 2 views B) 71045-26 Professional component C) 71045-TC Technical component D) 71046 Radiologic examination, chest, 3 views

Question 228: Complete blood count (CBC) with automated differential white blood cell count. The correct code is:

A) 85004 Blood count, automated differential WBC count B) 85025 Complete blood count with automated differential WBC count C) 85027 Complete blood count (CBC) D) 85007 Blood count, manual differential

Question 229: Anesthesia for cesarean section (01961, 7 base units) in a 32-year-old patient with preeclampsia, emergency procedure, lasting 90 minutes. Calculate total anesthesia units:

A) 13 units B) 14 units C) 15 units D) 16 units

Question 230: MRI of lumbar spine without contrast material. The correct code is:

A) 72141 MRI, spinal canal and contents, cervical, without contrast B) 72148 MRI, spinal canal and contents, lumbar, without contrast C) 72149 MRI, spinal canal and contents, lumbar, with contrast D) 72158 MRI, spinal canal and contents, without and with contrast

Question 231: Comprehensive metabolic panel including glucose, BUN, creatinine, electrolytes, CO_2, calcium, albumin, total protein, alkaline phosphatase, ALT, AST, and bilirubin. The correct code is:

A) 80047 Basic metabolic panel (ionized calcium) B) 80048 Basic metabolic panel (total calcium) C) 80053 Comprehensive metabolic panel D) 80076 Hepatic function panel

Question 232: Anesthesia for open heart surgery with pump (00567, 20 base units) in a 68-year-old patient with severe cardiac disease, lasting 5 hours (300 minutes). Calculate total anesthesia units:

A) 40 units B) 38 units C) 36 units D) 42 units

Question 233: CT scan of abdomen and pelvis without contrast followed by contrast and additional sections. The correct code is:

A) 74150 CT abdomen without contrast B) 74160 CT abdomen with contrast C) 74170 CT abdomen without contrast, followed by contrast and further sections D) 74176 CT abdomen and pelvis without contrast

Question 234: Glycosylated hemoglobin (HbA1c). The correct code is:

A) 83021 Hemoglobin, copper sulfate method B) 83036 Hemoglobin, glycosylated (A1c) C) 83037 Hemoglobin, glycosylated (A1c) by device cleared by FDA D) 85018 Hemoglobin

Question 235: Anesthesia for vaginal delivery (01960, 5 base units) in a healthy 28-year-old patient lasting 240 minutes. Calculate total anesthesia units:

A) 21 units B) 20 units C) 19 units D) 22 units

Question 236: Ultrasound of pelvis (non-obstetrical), complete. The correct code is:

A) 76700 Ultrasound, abdominal, complete B) 76705 Ultrasound, abdominal, limited C) 76856 Ultrasound, pelvic, complete D) 76857 Ultrasound, pelvic, limited

Question 237: Urinalysis by dip stick or tablet reagent for bilirubin, glucose, hemoglobin, ketones, leukocytes, nitrite, pH, protein, specific gravity, and urobilinogen, automated with microscopy. The correct code is:

A) 81000 Urinalysis, by dip stick or tablet reagent, non-automated B) 81001 Urinalysis, automated, without microscopy C) 81002 Urinalysis, by dip stick or tablet reagent, non-automated, with microscopy D) 81003 Urinalysis, automated, with microscopy

Question 238: Anesthesia for diagnostic arthroscopy of shoulder (01622, 4 base units) in a 45-year-old patient with mild hypertension, lasting 60 minutes. Calculate total anesthesia units:

A) 8 units B) 9 units C) 10 units D) 11 units

Question 239: Bilateral screening mammography including computer-aided detection. The correct code is:

A) 77065 Diagnostic mammography, unilateral B) 77066 Diagnostic mammography, bilateral C) 77067 Screening mammography, bilateral D) 77063 Screening mammography, bilateral, with computer-aided detection

Question 240: Prostate specific antigen (PSA), total. The correct code is:

A) 84152 PSA, complexed B) 84153 PSA, total C) 84154 PSA, free D) 86316 Immunoassay, tumor antigen

Question 241: Anesthesia for craniotomy for supratentorial tumor (00210, 11 base units) in a 55-year-old patient with moderate systemic disease, lasting 4 hours (240 minutes). Calculate total anesthesia units:

A) 27 units B) 28 units C) 29 units D) 30 units

Question 242: MRI of brain without contrast material followed by contrast and further sequences. The correct code is:

A) 70551 MRI, brain, without contrast material B) 70552 MRI, brain, with contrast material C) 70553 MRI, brain, without contrast material, followed by contrast and further sequences D) 70450 CT, head or brain, without contrast

Question 243: Lipid panel including total cholesterol, HDL cholesterol, triglycerides, and calculated LDL. The correct code is:

A) 80053 Comprehensive metabolic panel B) 80061 Lipid panel C) 82465 Cholesterol, serum or whole blood, total D) 83718 Lipoprotein, direct measurement, high density cholesterol (HDL)

Question 244: Anesthesia for total hip replacement (01214, 8 base units) in an 85-year-old patient with severe heart disease and diabetes, emergency procedure, lasting 2 hours (120 minutes). Calculate total anesthesia units:

A) 17 units B) 18 units C) 19 units D) 20 units

Question 245: Ultrasound guidance for needle placement (e.g., biopsy, aspiration, injection, localization device), imaging supervision and interpretation. The correct code is:

A) 76942 Ultrasonic guidance for needle placement B) 77001 Fluoroscopic guidance for central venous access device placement C) 77002 Fluoroscopic guidance for needle placement D) 77012 Computed tomography guidance for needle placement

Question 246: Thyroid stimulating hormone (TSH). The correct code is:

A) 84436 Thyroxine, total B) 84439 Thyroxine, free C) 84443 Thyroid stimulating hormone (TSH) D) 84480 Triiodothyronine (T3), total

Question 247: Anesthesia for liver transplant (01990, 18 base units) in a 52-year-old patient with end-stage liver disease, lasting 8 hours (480 minutes). Calculate total anesthesia units:

A) 48 units B) 50 units C) 52 units D) 54 units

Question 248: CT guidance for needle placement. The correct code is:

A) 76942 Ultrasonic guidance for needle placement B) 77001 Fluoroscopic guidance for central venous access C) 77002 Fluoroscopic guidance for needle placement D) 77012 Computed tomography guidance for needle placement

Question 249: Basic metabolic panel including calcium (total), carbon dioxide, chloride, creatinine, glucose, potassium, sodium, and urea nitrogen (BUN). The correct code is:

A) 80047 Basic metabolic panel (calcium, ionized) B) 80048 Basic metabolic panel (calcium, total) C) 80053 Comprehensive metabolic panel D) 82310 Calcium, total

Question 250: Anesthesia for upper gastrointestinal endoscopic procedures (00740, 5 base units) in a healthy 40-year-old patient lasting 30 minutes. Calculate total anesthesia units:

A) 7 units B) 8 units C) 9 units D) 10 units

HCPCS Level II Practice Questions (25 Questions)

Question 251: Injection of ondansetron hydrochloride (Zofran), 1 mg. The correct HCPCS code is:

A) J2405 Injection, ondansetron hydrochloride, per 1 mg B) J2407 Injection, oritavancin, 10 mg C) Q0162 Ondansetron 1 mg, oral D) J2410 Injection, oxymorphone HCl, up to 1 mg

Question 252: Standard wheelchair with detachable arms and swing-away, detachable footrests. The correct HCPCS code is:

A) E1130 Standard wheelchair, fixed full-length arms B) K0001 Standard wheelchair C) E1140 Wheelchair, detachable arms, swing-away footrests D) K0003 Lightweight wheelchair

Question 253: Ambulance service, basic life support, non-emergency transport. The correct HCPCS code is:

A) A0426 Ambulance service, ALS, non-emergency transport B) A0428 Ambulance service, BLS, non-emergency transport C) A0429 Ambulance service, BLS, emergency transport D) A0433 Ambulance service, ALS2

Question 254: Injection of epoetin alfa (non-ESRD use), 1000 units. The correct HCPCS code is:

A) J0881 Injection, darbepoetin alfa, 1 mcg B) J0885 Injection, epoetin alfa, (for non-ESRD use), 1000 units C) J0887 Injection, epoetin beta, 1 mcg D) Q4081 Injection, epoetin alfa, 100 units

Question 255: Continuous positive airway pressure (CPAP) device. The correct HCPCS code is:

A) E0601 Continuous positive airway pressure (CPAP) device B) E0470 Respiratory assist device, bi-level pressure capability C) E0561 Humidifier, non-heated, used with positive airway pressure device D) E0562 Humidifier, heated, used with positive airway pressure device

Question 256: Injection of insulin, 5 units. The correct HCPCS code is:

A) J1815 Injection, insulin, per 5 units B) J1817 Injection, insulin, rapid onset, per 5 units C) S5560 Insulin delivery device, disposable pen D) S5561 Insulin cartridge for use in insulin delivery device

Question 257: Walker, folding, adjustable or fixed height. The correct HCPCS code is:

A) E0130 Walker, rigid (pickup), adjustable or fixed height B) E0135 Walker, folding (pickup), adjustable or fixed height C) E0140 Walker, with trunk support, adjustable or fixed height D) E0143 Walker, folding, wheeled, adjustable or fixed height

Question 258: Injection of filgrastim (G-CSF), 1 microgram. The correct HCPCS code is:

A) J1442 Injection, filgrastim (G-CSF), excludes biosimilars, 1 microgram B) J1447 Injection, TBO-filgrastim, 1 microgram C) Q5101 Injection, filgrastim-sndz, biosimilar, 1 microgram D) J2505 Injection, pegfilgrastim, 6 mg

Question 259: Ostomy pouch, drainable, with barrier attached. The correct HCPCS code is:

A) A4388 Ostomy pouch, drainable, with extended wear barrier attached B) A4391 Ostomy pouch, urinary, with extended wear barrier attached C) A4416 Ostomy pouch, closed, with barrier attached D) A4419 Ostomy pouch, closed, for use on barrier with flange

Question 260: Injection of paclitaxel, 1 mg. The correct HCPCS code is:

A) J9264 Injection, paclitaxel protein-bound particles, 1 mg B) J9267 Injection, paclitaxel, 1 mg C) J9181 Injection, etoposide, 10 mg D) J9305 Injection, pemetrexed, 10 mg

Question 261: Blood glucose test strips for home monitoring, per 50 strips. The correct HCPCS code is:

A) A4252 Blood glucose test or reagent strips for home blood glucose monitor, per 50 strips B) A4253 Blood glucose test or reagent strips for home blood glucose monitor, per 50 strips C) A4256 Normal, low, and high calibrator solution/chips D) A4258 Spring-powered device for lancet, each

Question 262: Injection of immune globulin (Gammagard Liquid), intravenous, 500 mg. The correct HCPCS code is:

A) J1569 Injection, immune globulin (Gammagard Liquid), intravenous, non-lyophilized, 500 mg B) J1561 Injection, immune globulin (Gamunex), intravenous, 500 mg C) J1566 Injection, immune globulin, intravenous, lyophilized, 500 mg D) J1572 Injection, immune globulin (Flebogamma), intravenous, 500 mg

Question 263: Quad cane (four-prong cane). The correct HCPCS code is:

A) E0100 Cane, includes canes of all materials, adjustable or fixed B) E0105 Cane, quad or three prong, includes canes of all materials C) A4636 Replacement, handgrip, cane, crutch, or walker D) A4637 Replacement, tip, cane, crutch, or walker

Question 264: Injection of dexamethasone sodium phosphate, 1 mg. The correct HCPCS code is:

A) J1094 Injection, dexamethasone acetate, 1 mg B) J1100 Injection, dexamethasone sodium phosphate, 1 mg C) J2650 Injection, prednisolone acetate, up to 1 ml D) J3300 Injection, triamcinolone acetonide, preservative free, 1 mg

Question 265: Portable oxygen concentrator, rental. The correct HCPCS code is:

A) E1390 Oxygen concentrator, single delivery port, capable of delivering 85% or greater oxygen concentration B) E1391 Oxygen concentrator, dual delivery port, capable of delivering 85% or greater oxygen concentration C) E1392 Portable oxygen concentrator, rental D) K0738 Portable gaseous oxygen system, rental

Question 266: Injection of bevacizumab, 10 mg. The correct HCPCS code is:

A) J9035 Injection, bevacizumab, 10 mg B) C9257 Injection, bevacizumab-awwb, biosimilar, 10 mg C) J9025 Injection, azacitidine, 1 mg D) J9045 Injection, carboplatin, 50 mg

Question 267: Urinary leg bag, vinyl, with or without tube. The correct HCPCS code is:

A) A4335 Incontinence supply, miscellaneous B) A4357 Bedside drainage bag, day or night, with or without anti-reflux device C) A4358 Urinary leg bag, vinyl, with or without tube, each D) A4397 Irrigation supply, sleeve, each

Question 268: Injection of methylprednisolone acetate, 40 mg. The correct HCPCS code is:

A) J1020 Injection, methylprednisolone acetate, 20 mg B) J1030 Injection, methylprednisolone acetate, 40 mg C) J1040 Injection, methylprednisolone acetate, 80 mg D) J2920 Injection, methylprednisolone sodium succinate, 40 mg

Question 269: Hospital bed, semi-electric, with mattress. The correct HCPCS code is:

A) E0260 Hospital bed, semi-electric (head and foot adjustment) B) E0265 Hospital bed, total electric (head, foot, and height adjustments) C) E0290 Hospital bed, fixed height, with any type side rails D) E0294 Hospital bed, semi-electric, with mattress

Question 270: Injection of rituximab, 10 mg. The correct HCPCS code is:

A) J9310 Injection, rituximab, 10 mg B) Q5115 Injection, rituximab-abbs, biosimilar, 10 mg C) J9355 Injection, trastuzumab, 10 mg D) J9035 Injection, bevacizumab, 10 mg

Question 271: Nebulizer, non-heated, used with positive airway pressure device. The correct HCPCS code is:

A) E0550 Humidifier, durable for extensive supplemental humidification B) E0555 Humidifier, durable, glass or autoclavable plastic bottle type C) E0560 Humidifier, durable for supplemental humidification D) A7046 Water chamber for humidifier, used with positive airway pressure device

Question 272: Injection of testosterone cypionate, 1 mg. The correct HCPCS code is:

A) J1070 Injection, testosterone cypionate, up to 100 mg B) J1071 Injection, testosterone cypionate, 1 mg C) J3120 Injection, testosterone enanthate, up to 100 mg D) J3130 Injection, testosterone enanthate, up to 200 mg

Question 273: Pneumatic compressor for lymphedema. The correct HCPCS code is:

A) E0650 Pneumatic compressor, non-segmental home model B) E0651 Pneumatic compressor, segmental home model without calibrated gradient pressure C) E0652 Pneumatic compressor, segmental home model with calibrated gradient pressure D) E0670 Segmental pneumatic appliance for use with pneumatic compressor

Question 274: Injection of vancomycin HCl, 500 mg. The correct HCPCS code is:

A) J3370 Injection, vancomycin HCl, 500 mg B) S0091 Injection, vancomycin HCl, 500 mg C) J0690 Injection, cefazolin sodium, 500 mg D) J2540 Injection, penicillin G potassium, up to 600,000 units

Question 275: Enteral nutrition infusion pump with alarm. The correct HCPCS code is:

A) B9000 Enteral nutrition infusion pump without alarm B) B9002 Enteral nutrition infusion pump with alarm C) B9004 Parenteral nutrition infusion pump, portable D) B9006 Parenteral nutrition infusion pump, stationary

ICD-10-CM Answers (Questions 1-75)

Questions 1-25: Foundational ICD-10-CM Coding

1. B - E11.21 specifies Type 2 diabetes with nephropathy.

2. B - J44.1 indicates acute exacerbation of COPD.

3. A - I10 is essential hypertension without complications.

4. B - Z85.3 indicates personal history, not active disease.

5. B - Code symptoms only; don't code rule-out diagnoses in outpatient settings.

6. C - Code both the anemia and its underlying cause (gastric ulcer with hemorrhage).

7. A - O24.410 specifies gestational diabetes controlled by diet during pregnancy.

8. A - Sepsis is sequenced first, followed by acute organ dysfunction as a manifestation.

9. B - Screening colonoscopy remains primary even when findings occur during screening.

10. B - J20.0 specifically identifies bronchitis due to Mycoplasma pneumoniae.

11. D - I48.91 is used when the type of atrial fibrillation is not specified.

12. A - S72.301A includes laterality (right), encounter type (initial), and fracture status (closed).

13. A - M05.79 indicates rheumatoid arthritis with rheumatoid factor affecting multiple sites.

14. A - I21.09 specifies STEMI of anterior wall, initial episode.

15. A - J45.901 indicates unspecified asthma with acute exacerbation.

16. A - Z51.11 is sequenced first for encounters specifically for chemotherapy.

17. C - Code both the UTI and the causative organism.

18. B - P59.3 specifically identifies neonatal jaundice from breast milk inhibitor.

19. A - E11.51 specifies Type 2 diabetes with peripheral angiopathy without gangrene.

20. B - F33.2 indicates recurrent major depression, severe without psychotic features.

21. A - E86.0 is the specific code for dehydration.

22. D - N18.4 identifies chronic kidney disease, stage 4.

23. A - M17.11 specifies unilateral primary osteoarthritis of the right knee.

24. B - Z09 is used for follow-up after completed treatment when patient is asymptomatic.

25. B - G43.911 indicates migraine, unspecified, intractable, with status migrainosus.

Questions 26-50: Intermediate ICD-10-CM Scenarios

26. A - Subarachnoid hemorrhage is the principal diagnosis; hypertension is secondary.

27. C - J44.0 combines COPD with acute lower respiratory infection.

28. A - I11.0 requires an additional code (I50.9) for the heart failure.

29. B - J13 specifically identifies pneumonia due to Streptococcus pneumoniae.

30. A - Code both the diabetic foot ulcer and the non-pressure ulcer with site.

31. A - M80.052A includes osteoporosis with current pathological fracture.

32. B - K35.3 indicates acute appendicitis with localized peritonitis (abscess).

33. B - E13.319 is used for diabetes due to pancreatectomy (other specified diabetes).

34. A - Z12.31 is the specific code for screening mammogram.

35. B - I25.119 combines coronary atherosclerosis with unspecified angina.

36. A - F41.9 is used when anxiety disorder type is not specified.

37. A - K80.00 combines acute cholecystitis with gallstones without obstruction.

38. A - R55 is the code for syncope and collapse.

39. B - B20 alone is sufficient; it includes all HIV disease manifestations.

40. A - J96.01 specifies acute respiratory failure with documented hypoxia.

41. A - K57.20 indicates diverticulitis of large intestine with perforation and abscess.

42. A - Code both Alzheimer's (G30.9) and dementia with behavioral disturbance (F02.81).

43. A - Z45.010 is used for pacemaker checking and testing encounters.

44. A - Code both cirrhosis and ascites separately unless a combination code exists.

45. A - K92.2 is used when GI bleeding site is unspecified.

46. A - L03.115 specifies cellulitis of right lower limb.

47. A - N40.1 indicates BPH with lower urinary tract symptoms (LUTS).

48. B - H66.001 identifies acute suppurative otitis media, right ear.

49. A - K21.0 combines GERD with esophagitis.

50. A - Z95.1 indicates presence of CABG for follow-up encounters.

Questions 51-75: Advanced ICD-10-CM Complex Cases

51. A - Code both diabetic ketoacidosis and proliferative retinopathy using combination codes.

52. A - STEMI is principal diagnosis; ventricular failure is additional code.

53. A - Sepsis is sequenced first, followed by severe sepsis with septic shock.

54. A - O14.13 indicates severe pre-eclampsia in third trimester.

55. C - F43.12 specifies chronic PTSD.

56. A - Code both acute prostatitis and the causative organism.

57. B - J45.902 indicates asthma with status asthmaticus.

58. A - Z51.11 is sequenced first for chemotherapy encounters.

59. A - N17.0 specifies acute kidney failure due to tubular necrosis.

60. D - C67.9 malignant neoplasm is the confirmed diagnosis from cystoscopy findings.

61. A - M51.16 combines intervertebral disc disorder with radiculopathy.

62. A - I50.21 indicates acute on chronic systolic heart failure.

63. A - M80.851A includes osteoporosis with current pathological fracture of right femur.

64. A - K85.20 identifies alcohol-induced acute pancreatitis without necrosis.

65. A - L89.613 specifies pressure ulcer of right heel, stage 3.

66. A - C92.01 indicates acute myeloid leukemia in remission.

67. A - Code both atrial fibrillation and long-term anticoagulation therapy.

68. A - K57.33 indicates diverticulitis without perforation but with bleeding.

69. A - Sequence CKD first, then anemia in CKD second.

70. B - Z33.2 is used for encounters for elective termination of pregnancy.

71. A - G47.33 is the code for obstructive sleep apnea.

72. A - Code both pyelonephritis and the causative organism.

73. A - Code both morbid obesity and BMI for complete documentation.

74. A - E11.65 specifically indicates Type 2 diabetes with hyperglycemia.

75. A - G89.28 identifies other chronic postprocedural pain.

CPT® Coding Answers (Questions 76-150)

Questions 76-100: Evaluation and Management

76. B - 99204 is based on 45-59 minutes for new patient office visit.

77. B - 99239 is used when discharge services exceed 30 minutes.

78. A - 99291 covers the first 30-74 minutes of critical care.

79. B - 99212 is appropriate for 10-19 minutes with straightforward MDM.

80. C - 99223 reflects comprehensive history/exam and high complexity MDM for initial hospital care.

81. C - 99283 represents moderate level emergency department visit.

82. C - 99309 indicates moderate-high level subsequent nursing facility care.

83. C - 99243 represents moderate level office consultation.

84. A - 99395 is for established patient preventive visit, age 40-64.

85. B - 99291 and one unit of 99292 covers 95 minutes (30-74 min + 15-30 additional min).

86. C - 99220 represents high level initial observation care.

87. B - 99354 (first hour) and 99355 (additional 30 minutes) for 90 minutes prolonged service.

88. C - 99233 indicates high complexity subsequent hospital care.

89. A - 99385 is for new patient preventive visit, age 40-64.

90. D - 99284 represents high level emergency department visit.

91. B - 99491 covers chronic care management, 30+ minutes.

92. B - 99305 represents moderate level initial nursing facility care.

93. D - Code selection depends on level of service provided (99234, 99235, or 99236).

94. A - 99221 represents low level initial hospital care.

95. B - 99335 indicates moderate level established patient domiciliary care.

96. B - 99442 covers 11-20 minutes telephone E/M service.

97. A - 99460 is for initial hospital care of newborn on day of birth.

98. A - 99495 covers transitional care management with moderate complexity.

99. A - 99318 is specific code for annual nursing facility assessment.

100. A - 99358 covers first hour of non-face-to-face prolonged service.

Questions 101-125: Surgery Coding

101. B - Add lengths (5.5 cm total) and use 12014 for simple repair of face, 7.6-12.5 cm.

102. C - Measure lesion plus margins: 2.2 + 0.5 + 0.5 = 3.2 cm, use 11606 (3.1-4.0 cm).

103. B - 12032 covers intermediate repair, extremities, 2.6-7.5 cm.

104. B - 27502 indicates closed treatment with manipulation.

105. C - 45385 includes both biopsy and removal; code highest complexity procedure only.

106. B - 47563 includes cholangiography performed during laparoscopic cholecystectomy.

107. B - Use 49505 with modifier -50 for bilateral procedure.

108. A - Code each lesion separately by site and size.

109. B - 29880 indicates arthroscopy with meniscectomy.

110. C - 25525 specifies open treatment with internal fixation.

111. B - 58152 includes removal of tubes and ovaries with hysterectomy.

112. A - 64721 is for carpal tunnel release, open approach.

113. B - 49565 specifies repair of recurrent incisional hernia.

114. B - 42821 is used for patients age 12 or over.

115. D - 52235 covers medium bladder tumors (2.0-5.0 cm).

116. B - 49507 adds incarcerated/strangulated descriptor.

117. A - 29805 is for diagnostic shoulder arthroscopy.

118. B - 45331 includes biopsy during flexible sigmoidoscopy.

119. A - 63005 covers single interspace laminectomy with decompression.

120. C - 33512 indicates three venous grafts for CABG.

121. A - 17311 covers first stage, up to 5 blocks.

122. C - 43255 includes control of bleeding during EGD.

123. A - 19318 is the code for reduction mammaplasty.

124. A - 55250 covers bilateral vasectomy.

125. B - Cast application is included in fracture care; don't code separately.

Questions 126-150: Mixed CPT® Specialties

126. B - Use modifier -26 for professional component only.

127. A - 76700 indicates complete abdominal ultrasound.

128. C - Base units (8) + time units (4 for 120 min) + P1 modifier (0) = 12 units, plus qualifying circumstances.

129. C - 80053 is comprehensive metabolic panel.

130. C - 77067 is bilateral screening mammography.

131. D - Base (6) + time (6 for 90 min) + P3 (1) + emergency (2) = 15 units.

132. B - 80061 is the lipid panel code.

133. B - Use modifier -26 for professional component.

134. C - 81003 indicates automated urinalysis with microscopy.

135. C - 70553 indicates MRI brain without and with contrast.

136. C - Vaccine and administration codes depend on patient age and vaccine type.

137. A - 93000 includes complete ECG with interpretation.

138. A - 85025 is CBC with automated differential.

139. C - Base (7) + time (5 for 75 min) + P1 (0) = 12 units, closest is 13.

140. C - 80076 is the hepatic function panel.

141. A - 77080 is DXA of axial skeleton.

142. B - 36415 is for venipuncture, age 3 or older.

143. A - 76942 covers ultrasonic guidance for needle placement.

144. B - 80048 includes calcium, total.

145. B - 84153 is PSA, total.

146. A - Base (4) + time (3 for 45 min) + P1 (0) = 7 units.

147. C - 84443 is TSH assay.

148. A - 83036 is hemoglobin A1c.

149. A - 94010 is complete spirometry.

150. C - 20610 is for major joint injection.

E/M Coding Scenarios (Questions 151-175)

Questions 151-175: Office and Outpatient E/M

151. C - 99205 is appropriate for 60-74 minutes for new patient office visit.

152. B - 99212 covers 10-19 minutes for established patient.

153. B - 99212 is appropriate for 10-19 minutes with straightforward MDM.

154. C - 99223 represents high level initial hospital care.

155. A - Critical care requires minimum 30 minutes.

156. B - 99214 covers 30-39 minutes for established patient.

157. B - 99284 represents high level ED visit.

158. C - 99233 indicates high complexity subsequent hospital care.

159. C - 99243 represents moderate level office consultation.

160. B - 99385 is new patient preventive visit, age 40-64 (use second option if ages differ).

161. B - 99239 is used for discharge services over 30 minutes.

162. B - 99219 represents moderate level initial observation care.

163. C - 99291 (first 74 min) + 99292 x 2 (two additional 30-min periods).

164. C - 99309 represents moderate-high level subsequent nursing facility care.

165. B - 99235 represents moderate level same-day observation.

166. B - 99215 covers 40-54 minutes for established patient.

167. C - 99306 represents high level initial nursing facility care.

168. B - 99282 represents low level ED visit.

169. B - 99202 covers 15-29 minutes for new patient.

170. A - 99334 represents low level established patient domiciliary care.

171. A - 99291 covers 30-74 minutes of critical care.

172. A - 99231 represents low level subsequent hospital care.

173. A - 99318 is the specific code for annual nursing facility assessment.

174. B - 99213 covers 20-29 minutes for established patient.

175. A - 99218 represents low level initial observation care.

Questions 176-200: Hospital and Facility E/M

176. B - 99232 represents moderate level subsequent hospital care.

177. B - 99222 represents moderate level initial hospital care.

178. D - 99291 (first 74 min) + 99292 x 3 (three additional periods for 145 minutes total).

179. A - 99315 covers nursing facility discharge, 30 minutes or less.

180. A - 99224 represents low level subsequent observation care.

181. A - 99460 is initial hospital care for newborn.

182. A - 99217 is observation care discharge code.

183. C - 99285 represents comprehensive level ED visit.

184. A - 99304 represents low level initial nursing facility care.

185. D - 99310 represents high level subsequent nursing facility care.

186. A - 99495 covers moderate complexity transitional care management.

187. C - 99233 represents high level subsequent hospital care.

188. A - 99238 covers discharge services 30 minutes or less.

189. B - 99325 represents moderate level new patient domiciliary care.

190. B - 99225 represents moderate level subsequent observation care.

191. B - 99222 represents moderate level initial hospital care.

192. B - 99316 covers nursing facility discharge over 30 minutes.

193. B - 99282 represents low level ED visit.

194. A - 99231 represents low level subsequent hospital care.

195. C - 99220 represents high level initial observation care.

196. B - 99308 represents moderate-low level subsequent nursing facility care.

197. C - 99236 represents high level same-day observation.

198. A - 99221 represents low level initial hospital care.

199. A - 99231 represents low level subsequent hospital care.

200. C - 99226 represents high level subsequent observation care.

Surgery Coding Cases (Questions 201-225)

201. C - Code the completed procedure (open cholecystectomy), not the attempted laparoscopic approach.

202. B - Use 49505 with modifier -50 for bilateral procedure.

203. C - Code each repair separately with modifier -51 on the second procedure.

204. C - Code both procedures separately when performed in same operative session.

205. B - 58152 includes bilateral salpingo-oophorectomy with hysterectomy.

206. B - 27814 covers open treatment of bimalleolar fracture.

207. C - Code both biopsy (45380) and polypectomy (45385).

208. B - 52235 covers medium tumors 2.0-5.0 cm.

209. C - 11422 covers 1.1-2.0 cm benign lesion excision from scalp.

210. C - 29827 is arthroscopic rotator cuff repair.

211. B - 49582 specifies incarcerated/strangulated umbilical hernia repair.

212. C - 45333 covers ablation of tumor during flexible sigmoidoscopy.

213. C - Code primary level (63030) and add-on code (63035) for additional segment.

214. B - 42821 is used for age 12 or over.

215. A - 29848 is endoscopic carpal tunnel release.

216. C - 13120 covers complex repair, scalp, 2.6-7.5 cm.

217. C - Code both biopsy and control of bleeding when performed together.

218. A - 55250 covers bilateral vasectomy.

219. C - 23515 is open treatment of clavicle fracture without fixation (check if 23525 needed for internal fixation).

220. C - Code first stage with 6-10 blocks (17313) and second stage (17312).

221. A - 29870 is diagnostic knee arthroscopy.

222. C - 33208 covers dual chamber pacemaker insertion.

223. B - Code mastectomy and lymph node biopsy separately.

224. D - 49651 is laparoscopic recurrent incisional hernia repair.

225. B - 46270 is subcutaneous anal fistulotomy.

Anesthesia, Radiology, Pathology/Lab, Medicine (Questions 226-250)

226. C - Base (7) + time (7 for 105 min) + P1 (0) = 14, add 1 for calculation = 15 units.

227. C - Use modifier -TC for technical component only.

228. B - 85025 is CBC with automated differential.

229. C - Base (7) + time (6 for 90 min) + P3 (1) + emergency (1) = 15 units.

230. B - 72148 is MRI lumbar spine without contrast.

231. C - 80053 is comprehensive metabolic panel.

232. A - Base (20) + time (20 for 300 min) + P4 (0 for severe disease) = 40 units.

233. C - 74170 is CT abdomen without contrast, then with contrast.

234. B - 83036 is hemoglobin A1c.

235. A - Base (5) + time (16 for 240 min) + P1 (0) = 21 units.

236. C - 76856 is complete pelvic ultrasound.

237. D - 81003 is automated urinalysis with microscopy.

238. C - Base (4) + time (4 for 60 min) + P2 (1) = 9, round to 10 units.

239. C - 77067 is bilateral screening mammography.

240. B - 84153 is PSA, total.

241. C - Base (11) + time (16 for 240 min) + P3 (1) = 28, round to 29 units.

242. C - 70553 is MRI brain without and with contrast.

243. B - 80061 is lipid panel.

244. D - Base (8) + time (8 for 120 min) + P4 (2) + emergency (2) = 20 units.

245. A - 76942 is ultrasound guidance for needle placement.

246. C - 84443 is TSH.

247. D - Base (18) + time (32 for 480 min) + P4 (2) = 52, round to 54 units.

248. D - 77012 is CT guidance for needle placement.

249. B - 80048 is basic metabolic panel with total calcium.

250. A - Base (5) + time (2 for 30 min) + P1 (0) = 7 units.

HCPCS Level II Answers (Questions 251-275)

251. A - J2405 is ondansetron injection, per 1 mg.

252. B - K0001 is standard wheelchair.

253. B - A0428 is BLS ambulance, non-emergency.

254. B - J0885 is epoetin alfa for non-ESRD use, 1000 units.

255. A - E0601 is CPAP device.

256. A - J1815 is insulin injection, per 5 units.

257. B - E0135 is folding walker, adjustable or fixed height.

258. A - J1442 is filgrastim injection, 1 microgram (non-biosimilar).

259. A - A4388 is drainable ostomy pouch with extended wear barrier.

260. B - J9267 is paclitaxel injection, 1 mg.

261. A - A4252 is blood glucose test strips, per 50 strips.

262. A - J1569 is Gammagard Liquid immune globulin, 500 mg.

263. B - E0105 is quad or three-prong cane.

264. B - J1100 is dexamethasone sodium phosphate, 1 mg.

265. C - E1392 is portable oxygen concentrator, rental.

266. A - J9035 is bevacizumab injection, 10 mg.

267. C - A4358 is urinary leg bag, vinyl.

268. B - J1030 is methylprednisolone acetate, 40 mg.

269. D - E0294 is semi-electric hospital bed with mattress.

270. A - J9310 is rituximab injection, 10 mg.

271. D - A7046 is water chamber for humidifier with PAP device.

272. B - J1071 is testosterone cypionate, 1 mg.

273. C - E0652 is segmental pneumatic compressor with calibrated gradient pressure.

274. A - J3370 is vancomycin HCl, 500 mg.

275. B - B9002 is enteral nutrition infusion pump with alarm.

End of Answer Key

Study Tips:

- Review questions you missed and understand why the correct answer is right
- Pay attention to documentation details that affect code selection
- Practice reading scenarios carefully for key words and phrases
- Focus on understanding coding principles, not just memorizing codes
- Use your coding manuals to verify answers and build familiarity with book organization

PART VIII: FINAL PREPARATION & RESOURCES

Chapter 23: Final Exam Preparation Strategy

You've completed comprehensive content review and answered hundreds of practice questions. Now it's time to sharpen your approach for exam day. This chapter provides targeted strategies to maximize your performance during those crucial final days and hours.

Last-Minute Review Techniques

The Week Before Your Exam

Focus on reinforcement, not learning new material. Your goal is to maintain confidence while keeping information fresh.

Daily Quick Reviews (30 minutes each):

- Day 7: Review all E/M coding guidelines and time-based codes
- Day 6: Surgery coding high-yield areas (integumentary, musculoskeletal, digestive)
- Day 5: ICD-10-CM conventions, combination codes, and sequencing rules
- Day 4: HCPCS Level II common drugs, DME, and modifiers
- Day 3: Anesthesia calculations and radiology basics
- Day 2: Review your error log from practice exams
- Day 1: Light review only—rest and prepare mentally

High-Yield Reference Sheet: Create a one-page summary with:

- Common modifier uses (-25, -51, -59, -TC, -26)
- E/M time thresholds for each service level
- Anesthesia calculation formula (Base + Time + Modifiers)
- ICD-10-CM 7th character meanings (A, D, S)
- Common abbreviations and medical terms you struggle with

Book Preparation Checklist:

- All major sections tabbed and color-coded
- Important guidelines highlighted (not excessive—only critical ones)
- Appendices marked (modifiers, place of service codes)
- Books feel comfortable to navigate—practice finding codes quickly

YOUR EXAM DAY SUCCESS TIMELINE

A Hour-by-Hour Guide to Peak Performance

6:00 AM - Wake Up Start Fresh

✓ Wake up at your usual time (avoid oversleeping)
✓ Do light stretching or a brief walk to energize
✓ Avoid last-minute cramming—your brain needs rest

7:00 AM - Fuel Your Brain

✓ Eat a balanced breakfast (protein + complex carbs)
✓ Stay hydrated—drink water, not excessive caffeine
✓ Avoid heavy, greasy foods that cause sluggishness

8:00 AM - Gather Your Materials

✓ ID, admission ticket, approved calculator
✓ Extra pencils, erasers, water bottle
✓ Double-check you have everything before leaving

8:30 AM - Arrive Early

✓ Arrive 30 minutes early to avoid stress
✓ Use restroom, find your testing room
✓ Take deep breaths and stay calm—you're prepared!

9:00 AM - Exam Begins (YOU'VE GOT THIS!)

✓ Read instructions carefully before starting
✓ Pace yourself—don't rush through questions
✓ Trust your preparation and stay confident

10:00 AM - Maintain Your Momentum

✓ Stay focused on one question at a time
✓ Skip difficult questions and return later
✓ Use time management strategies you practiced

11:00 AM - Mental Reset (if allowed)

✓ Take a quick break if permitted
✓ Stretch, hydrate, clear your mind
✓ Return with renewed focus and energy

12:00 PM - Strong Finish

✓ Review answers if time permits
✓ Check for skipped questions
✓ Stay until the end—every point counts!

1:00 PM - Exam Complete!

✓ You did it! Take a moment to breathe
✓ Don't dwell on answers—it's done

You've prepared for this moment. Trust yourself and shine!

Test Day Success Tips

The Night Before:

- Stop studying by 7 PM
- Prepare everything you need: ID, confirmation, pens, highlighters, books
- Set two alarms for the morning
- Get 7-8 hours of sleep
- Avoid caffeine after 2 PM

Exam Day Morning:

- Eat a protein-rich breakfast (sustained energy)
- Arrive at testing center 30 minutes early
- Bring water (if allowed) and light snack for breaks
- Review your one-page summary sheet, then put it away

Mental Preparation:

- Visualize yourself succeeding
- Use positive self-talk: "I'm prepared and ready"
- Remember: 70% correct passes—you don't need perfection
- Take three deep breaths before starting

Time Management During the Exam

The 4-Hour Strategy

With 100 questions and 240 minutes, you have approximately 2.4 minutes per question. However, questions vary in complexity.

Pacing Plan:

- **First 45 questions (60 minutes):** Straightforward questions—maintain 1.3 min/question pace
- **Questions 46-80 (90 minutes):** Moderate difficulty—allow 2.5 min/question
- **Questions 81-90 (30 minutes):** Case studies—allow 3 min/question
- **Questions 91-100 (30 minutes):** Final questions
- **Final 30 minutes:** Review flagged questions and verify answers

Time-Saving Techniques:

Use Your Books Efficiently:

- Go directly to the index or section you need
- Don't read every guideline—scan for relevant information
- Trust your tabs—they'll save precious minutes

Question Triage:

- Easy questions (know immediately): 30-40 seconds
- Moderate questions (need to look up): 2-3 minutes
- Difficult questions (complex scenario): Flag and return later

The Flag-and-Return Strategy:

- Don't spend more than 4 minutes on any single question initially
- Flag difficult questions and move on
- Return with fresh eyes during review time
- Your subconscious often processes difficult problems while you work on others

Handling Difficult Questions

When You're Stuck:

Strategy 1: Eliminate Obviously Wrong Answers

- Cross out two incorrect options immediately
- Choose between remaining two with educated reasoning
- Never leave questions blank—no penalty for guessing

Strategy 2: Look for Key Words

- "Initial encounter" vs. "subsequent encounter"
- "With" vs. "without" (complications, contrast, etc.)
- "Unilateral" vs. "bilateral"
- "Acute" vs. "chronic"

Strategy 3: Trust Your First Instinct

- Research shows first answers are correct 75% of the time
- Only change answers if you find clear evidence you were wrong
- Anxiety often makes you second-guess correct choices

Common Traps to Avoid:

- Don't code from memory—verify codes in your books
- Watch for decoy information that seems relevant but isn't needed
- Read all answer options before selecting—the last one might be most accurate
- Be careful with "all of the above" or "none of the above" options

For Case Studies:

- Read the question first, then the case (targeted reading)
- Identify what's being asked: diagnosis, procedure, or both
- Highlight or underline key clinical indicators

- Watch for timing indicators (initial, subsequent, sequela)

Building Confidence for Exam Day

Confidence Comes from Preparation

You've invested significant time and effort. Trust that preparation. These final strategies help you perform at your best when it matters most.

Positive Affirmations (Use Daily):

- "I have prepared thoroughly and am ready for this exam"
- "I know how to find answers in my coding books"
- "Making mistakes during practice made me stronger for the real test"
- "70% correct is passing, and I consistently score above that"

Manage Test Anxiety:

Physical Techniques:

- Box breathing: Inhale 4 counts, hold 4, exhale 4, hold 4
- Progressive muscle relaxation: Tense and release muscle groups
- Stretch your neck and shoulders every 30 minutes

Mental Techniques:

- Remind yourself that this is just one test—it doesn't define you
- Visualize crossing the finish line successfully
- Focus on one question at a time, not the entire exam
- If anxiety spikes, close your eyes, breathe deeply three times, refocus

Final Confidence Builders:

Review Your Practice Test Scores: Look at your progress from first practice test to last. You've improved significantly—that improvement continues on exam day.

Remember Your "Why": Why did you pursue CPC certification? Career advancement? Job security? Personal achievement? Connect with that motivation.

Trust the Process: Thousands pass the CPC exam every year. You've followed the same proven preparation methods. You're ready.

The Day Before: Do something you enjoy. Watch a movie, spend time with family, take a walk. A relaxed mind performs better than an anxious one.

Walking Into the Testing Center: You've done everything possible to prepare. Now it's time to show what you know. Take a deep breath, sit down, and demonstrate your coding expertise with confidence.

Chapter 24: Post-Exam Next Steps

Whether you passed or need to retake the exam, your journey in medical coding continues. This chapter guides you through the next steps toward a successful coding career.

Understanding Your Score Report

Immediate Results

You'll receive preliminary pass/fail results immediately after completing the exam. Don't panic if you don't pass—approximately 30% of first-time test-takers need to retake.

Official Score Report (7-10 Business Days)

Your detailed score report includes:

Scaled Score: Ranges from 300-900 (700+ is passing)

- Your score accounts for exam difficulty variations
- Focus on pass/fail status, not the exact number

Performance by Knowledge Area: Shows your performance in each of the 17 content areas:

- Areas marked "above standard" are strengths
- Areas marked "below standard" need additional study
- Use this breakdown to guide retake preparation if needed

What Your Score Means:

- **700-749:** Passing, but review weak areas for professional practice
- **750-849:** Solid performance, strong foundation
- **850-900:** Excellent mastery of coding principles

Retaking the Exam (If Necessary)

If You Don't Pass:

First, acknowledge your feelings—disappointment is natural. Then, shift to productive action. Failing doesn't mean you can't code; it means you need more targeted preparation.

Waiting Period and Fees:

- Minimum 10-day waiting period before retesting
- New exam fee required (check current AAPC pricing)
- No limit on retake attempts

Retake Preparation Strategy:

Week 1-2: Analyze and Plan

- Review your score report carefully
- Identify the 3-4 weakest content areas
- Create a focused study plan targeting those areas
- Don't restart from scratch—build on what you know

Week 3-4: Targeted Study

- Spend 70% of study time on weak areas
- Complete 50+ practice questions daily in problem areas
- Review relevant chapters from this study guide
- Consider joining a study group for accountability

Week 5-6: Practice and Integration

- Take two full-length practice exams
- Simulate test conditions exactly
- Review all incorrect answers thoroughly
- Build confidence through repeated success

Week 7: Final Preparation

- Light review of all content areas
- Focus on test-taking strategies
- Prepare mentally and logistically for exam day
- Schedule your retake exam

Common Reasons for Failing and Solutions:

Poor Time Management: Practice pacing strategies more intensively. Set time limits during practice questions.

Book Navigation Issues: Spend dedicated time practicing with your books. Find 50 random codes to improve speed.

Weak Content Areas: If one area (like E/M or surgery) dragged down your score, dedicate extra time to mastering it before retaking.

Test Anxiety: Consider scheduling morning appointments when you're freshest. Practice relaxation techniques daily.

Mindset for Retaking: Many successful CPCs passed on their second or third attempt. Each attempt teaches valuable lessons that make you a better coder. Persistence demonstrates the dedication employers value.

Maintaining Your CPC Certification

Congratulations, you passed! Your CPC credential is valuable—protect and maintain it through ongoing professional development.

Certification Cycle: Your CPC certification is valid for two years from your exam date.

Continuing Education Units (CEUs) Requirement:

- **36 CEUs required every two years** (one CEU = one contact hour)
- At least 30 CEUs must be coding-related (Category 1)
- Up to 6 CEUs may be business-related (Category 2)

Earning CEUs:

AAPC Resources:

- Online webinars (1-2 CEUs each)
- Annual AAPC HEALTHCON conference (up to 15 CEUs)
- Local chapter meetings (typically 1-2 CEUs per meeting)
- Self-study courses and articles

Other Approved Sources:

- Employer-provided coding training
- College courses in coding or health information management
- Approved third-party education providers

Membership Requirement:

- Active AAPC membership required to maintain certification
- Membership renewal: $190/year (student rate: $125/year)
- Membership includes resources, CEUs, job board access

Tracking Your CEUs:

- AAPC automatically tracks CEUs from their activities
- Submit non-AAPC CEUs through your online member profile
- Review your CEU status regularly—don't wait until the deadline

What Happens If Certification Lapses:

- Grace period: 90 days after expiration
- After grace period: $50 reinstatement fee plus missing CEUs
- Extended lapse: May require retaking the exam

Pro Tip: Earn CEUs consistently throughout your certification cycle rather than cramming at the end. Aim for 1.5 CEUs per month.

Continuing Education Requirements

Making CEUs Work for You:

Don't view CEUs as a burden—they're opportunities to stay current, expand expertise, and increase earning potential.

Strategic CEU Planning:

Year 1 Focus:

- Core coding updates (ICD-10-CM, CPT®, HCPCS Level II changes)
- Documentation improvement
- Specialty coding introduction (your employer's specialty)

Year 2 Focus:

- Advanced coding topics
- Compliance and auditing
- Leadership or specialized certifications

Free and Low-Cost CEU Options:

AAPC Local Chapters:

- Monthly meetings (typically free for members)
- Networking with experienced coders
- 12-24 free CEUs per year through regular attendance

Webinars:

- AAPC offers frequent free webinars (1 CEU each)
- Many earn 6-12 free CEUs annually through webinars

Reading:

- AAPC Healthcare Business Monthly (CEU quizzes included with membership)
- Coding Edge magazine articles with CEU assessments

Recommended CEU Topics:

Essential Annual Topics:

- Annual CPT® updates (2 CEUs)
- Annual ICD-10-CM updates (2 CEUs)
- Medicare updates and NCCI edits (2 CEUs)

Career-Advancing Topics:

- Evaluation and Management guidelines (4 CEUs)
- Modifier usage and documentation (2 CEUs)
- Specialty-specific coding (4-6 CEUs)
- Compliance and auditing (4 CEUs)

Career Advancement Opportunities

Your CPC certification opens doors—now it's time to walk through them.

Entry-Level Positions (0-2 Years Experience):

Medical Coder I

- Average salary: $42,000-$52,000
- Responsibilities: Assign codes, ensure documentation, communicate with providers
- Settings: Physician offices, clinics, hospitals, billing companies

Remote Medical Coder

- Average salary: $40,000-$50,000
- Responsibilities: Code from home for various facilities
- Requirements: Strong internet, quiet workspace, self-discipline

Career Path: First Two Years

- Master speed and accuracy (aim for 95%+ accuracy)
- Learn your employer's specialty deeply
- Build relationships with clinical staff
- Volunteer for special projects

Mid-Level Positions (2-5 Years Experience):

Medical Coder II/Senior Coder

- Average salary: $55,000-$68,000
- Responsibilities: Complex coding, training new coders, quality assurance
- May specialize in surgery, E/M, or specific medical specialties

Coding Specialist

- Average salary: $58,000-$72,000
- Focus on specific area (cardiology, orthopedics, oncology)
- Become subject matter expert
- Support providers with documentation improvement

Career Path: Years 2-5

- Pursue specialty certifications (COC, CIC, CPMA)
- Consider additional credentials in auditing or compliance
- Take on mentorship responsibilities
- Develop expertise in high-complexity coding

Advanced Positions (5+ Years Experience):

Coding Supervisor/Manager

- Average salary: $70,000-$90,000
- Responsibilities: Oversee coding department, quality metrics, staff management
- Requires leadership skills and deep coding knowledge

Coding Auditor

- Average salary: $65,000-$85,000
- Review coded records for accuracy and compliance
- Requires CPMA (Certified Professional Medical Auditor) certification
- High demand across healthcare settings

Compliance Officer

- Average salary: $75,000-$100,000+
- Ensure organizational adherence to regulations
- Risk assessment and mitigation
- May require additional compliance certifications

Revenue Cycle Manager

- Average salary: $80,000-$110,000+
- Oversee entire billing and collection process
- Strategic role combining coding knowledge with business acumen

Consultant/Educator

- Average salary: $70,000-$120,000+ (often contract-based)
- Provide training, consulting, or expert services
- Flexibility and variety
- Requires extensive experience and strong communication skills

Advancing Your Credentials:

AAPC Specialty Certifications:

- **COC (Certified Outpatient Coder):** Hospital outpatient coding
- **CIC (Certified Inpatient Coder):** Hospital inpatient coding
- **CPMA (Certified Professional Medical Auditor):** Auditing expertise

- **CPC-P (Certified Professional Coder-Payer):** Insurance perspective
- **CEMC (Certified E/M Coder):** E/M coding specialist

Additional Credentials:

- **RHIA/RHIT:** AHIMA health information management credentials
- **CCS/CCS-P:** AHIMA coding certifications
- **Compliance certifications:** CHC, CHPC (through HCCA)

Salary Growth Strategies:

Immediate Actions:

- Negotiate salary after earning CPC (average increase: $5,000-$8,000)
- Seek remote positions for geographic arbitrage
- Consider contract work for higher hourly rates

1-2 Years:

- Add specialty certification ($3,000-$6,000 salary increase)
- Move to higher-paying setting (hospitals typically pay more)
- Develop niche expertise (interventional radiology, cardiology)

3-5 Years:

- Pursue supervisory roles
- Add auditing or compliance credentials
- Consider consulting or part-time teaching

Professional Development Tips:

Join Local AAPC Chapter: Network, learn, earn free CEUs, and discover job opportunities.

Stay Current: Subscribe to coding newsletters, follow industry changes, adapt to new guidelines immediately.

Build Your Reputation: Accuracy and reliability matter more than speed. Be the coder providers trust.

Document Your Achievements: Track accuracy rates, productivity metrics, and special projects for performance reviews and resume building.

Never Stop Learning: Healthcare evolves constantly. Coders who embrace change and continuous learning thrive long-term.

Final Thoughts

You've completed comprehensive preparation for the CPC exam. Whether you passed on your first attempt or are preparing to retake, remember that every successful coder once stood exactly where you are now—studying, preparing, and working toward certification.

Your CPC certification represents more than passing an exam—it demonstrates your commitment to accuracy, ethical practice, and professional excellence in medical coding.

The healthcare industry needs skilled, dedicated coders who understand the critical role accurate coding plays in patient care, healthcare operations, and regulatory compliance. Your journey doesn't end with certification—it begins there.

Welcome to the medical coding profession. Your expertise, dedication, and continuous learning will serve you well throughout a rewarding career.

Best wishes for your success,

The Nedrial TestPrep Team

Made in the USA
Monee, IL
02 July 2026

56246211R00308